ALL THE BRAND-NAME FACTS
YOU NEED
RIGHT AT YOUR FINGERTIPS!

Calories count! With *The Brand-Name Calorie Counter* you can make your diet plans in advance and still include your favorite treats. The choice is yours because the information is here.

"PERENNIAL DIETERS! COMPULSIVE CALORIE COUNTERS! WEIGHT WATCHERS DROPOUTS! YOU ARE *MY* KIND OF PEOPLE AND THIS IS *OUR* LITERARY EVENT OF THE DECADE. . . . WITH THE DEDICATION OF A SCIENTIST, CORINNE NETZER HAS PENETRATED THE CALORIC MYSTERY OF THE SUPERMARKET."

—Gael Greene, *Life* magazine

"HELP HAS APPEARED IN A PAPERBACK BOOK THAT TAKES NOTE OF SUPERMARKET REALITIES. . . . NOW THOSE WHO ARE OVERWEIGHT CAN COUNT CALORIES IN ALMOST ALL PREPARED OR CONVENIENCE FOODS AND COMPARE VARIOUS BRANDS AS WELL."

—Morris Fishbein, M.D., *Medical World News*

Also by Corinne T. Netzer:

THE DIETER'S CALORIE COUNTER
THE BRAND-NAME CARBOHYDRATE GRAM COUNTER
THE CHOLESTEROL CONTENT OF FOOD
THE COMPLETE BOOK OF FOOD COUNTS
THE CORINNE T. NETZER 1991 CALORIE COUNTER
THE FAT CONTENT OF FOOD
THE CORINNE T. NETZER ENCYCLOPEDIA OF
    FOOD VALUES

THE
BRAND-
NAME
CALORIE
COUNTER

CORINNE T. NETZER

A DELL BOOK

Published by
Dell Publishing
a division of
Bantam Doubleday Dell Publishing Group, Inc.
666 Fifth Avenue
New York, New York 10103

ISBN: 0-440-21109-3

Printed in the United States of America

Published simultaneously in Canada

November 1991

10 9 8 7 6 5 4 3 2 1

RAD

INTRODUCTION

Eating is America's favorite pastime. If you stop and think about it, you'll probably realize that a good number of your waking hours are occupied with food. If you're not actually eating, then you're buying food, planning to buy it, preparing it, even fretting over its prices. It's almost impossible for any but the most iron-willed soul to escape the national food obsession.

It is, therefore, little wonder that every month an estimated ten million Americans embark on that battle of frustration known as a *diet*.

As a perennial dieter, I can tell you that there is definite hope, that you *will* lose weight if you stick to your diet. But that's the problem. Most people "fall off the wagon" after only two weeks of reducing. The sameness and boredom of crispy carrot sticks, broiled skinless chicken, and wedges of lettuce gets to them, and it's all over very quickly.

The purpose of *The Brand-Name Calorie Counter* is to help you stay on your diet by relieving the tedium. For instance, you might want to substitute a *Hormel* beef enchilada (140 calories) for that broiled chicken, or have a serving of *Green Giant* pasta primavera (110 calories) for lunch, or reward yourself with a *Sara Lee* chocolate mousse cake (180 calories). Dieting is not a pleasant experience, but I do believe the information contained herein can help to make it less painful by introducing variety— which is the spice not only of life but of dieting as well.

This fifth edition of *The Brand-Name Calorie Counter* is completely revised because the food industry is constantly growing and improving to meet the changing needs of the consumer. In addition, I have again included fast-food and chain restaurants so you may take your diet out to dinner. This section has been expanded, but if you don't find your favorites listed, it may be because the information wasn't available or because the product varies too much from one franchise location to another.

I've received letters from readers who tell me that they compile their weekly marketing list based on the information in *The Brand-Name Calorie Counter*. You may not opt to use the book in that way—but you might decide to make substitutions in whatever diet you're following, or you may try a new food or a different brand. You'll even find the data important in "maintaining" the new you after you've lost weight. Dieting is very personal, and how you choose to use this book is up to you, but with it you will have the information you need to plan your diet —and stay on it.

C.T.N.

CONTENTS

WHAT YOU SHOULD KNOW
ABOUT USING THIS BOOK

WHERE TO FIND WHAT

Most calorie counters list foods alphabetically. *The Brand-Name Calorie Counter* lists foods categorically. This means that all vegetables are grouped together; so are all frozen dinners, all nuts, all sauces, and so on. For example—and more important, for convenience when comparing similar foods—if you want to find the caloric content of various vegetables, you don't have to hopscotch from A (asparagus) to Z (zucchini); you simply turn to chapter 7, "Vegetables and Vegetable Products."

Occasionally, you may have trouble deciding what category a food belongs in; to locate such hard-to-categorize foods quickly, just flip to the index.

BE CAREFUL ABOUT MAKING COMPARISONS

It's only natural that you will want to use this counter to compare the caloric content of different foods and different brands. In some instances, you can make comparisons accurately by merely glancing at the listings. For example, all ice cream is listed in the same measure (one half cup); therefore, you can easily compare the caloric content of chocolate *Häagen-Dazs* with that of *Frusen Glädjé,* or *Breyers* or whatever.

To facilitate easy comparisons, categories have been listed in a uniform measure *whenever it was possible or feasible to do so.* However, it was neither feasible nor sensible to list certain foods in this manner. If all data on cookies, for example, were presented in a one-ounce measure, you would have to weigh an *Oreo* to learn its caloric content. For practicality's sake, cookies, snack cakes, bread, rolls, and various other foods are listed by the piece—in the size packaged by the manufacturer. This

WHAT YOU SHOULD KNOW   ix

means you can easily determine the calories in a single cookie, but you cannot compare different brands and varieties accurately. Why? Because, unless you weigh every cookie, you have no way of knowing if they are the same size.

To get the most from this book—and from your diet—you must recognize that similar foods are not necessarily packaged in the same or even similar sizes. Consider, for example, two varieties of *Pepperidge Farm* chocolate chunk pecan cookies, "Chesapeake" and "Special Collection." A Special Collection cookie contains 70 calories, while a Chesapeake has 120 calories. By the pound or ounce, the caloric content of the two may be identical, but by the piece a Chesapeake is nearly twice the size of the Special Collection. The point here is simple but important: if you're not certain that products are the same size, *don't make comparisons—they may not be accurate.*

You can, of course, compare any foods that are listed in the same standard measure. You can compare the calories in a half cup of cottage cheese with the calories in a half cup of fruit cocktail; or the calories in one ounce of Brie with the calories in one ounce of cream cheese. However, do not compare foods that are listed in *dissimilar units of measure.* Because even doctors and home economists sometimes confuse measures by capacity with measures by weight, it should be noted that you can't, for example, accurately compare four ounces of yogurt with a half cup of ice cream. Four ounces is a measure of how much something weighs. Half a cup is a measure of how much space something occupies. Think of it this way: Eight ounces of *Quaker* puffed rice cereal contains 864 calories and fills the capacity of about 16 eight-ounce measuring cups; an eight-ounce cup (or *eight fluid ounces)* of the same cereal contains 54 calories and weighs half an ounce. Clearly, eight ounces of puffed rice and an eight-ounce cupful of puffed rice are not the same! Just remember: The capacity of a standard eight-ounce measuring cup is eight *fluid* ounces, not eight *weight* ounces.

As noted before, you can compare foods listed in a similar measure—and you can, of course, convert a unit of measure to a smaller or larger amount. You may find the charts on the following page helpful in making conversions.

EQUIVALENTS BY CAPACITY
(all measures level)
1 quart = 4 cups
1 cup = 8 fluid ounces
    = ½ pint
    = 16 tablespoons
2 tablespoons = 1 fluid ounce
1 tablespoon = 3 teaspoons

EQUIVALENTS BY WEIGHT
1 pound = 16 ounces
3.57 ounces = 100 grams
1 ounce = 28.35 grams

You don't have to know that there are 28.35 grams in an ounce to use this book, but you may find the information handy when shopping or comparing package sizes. By federal law, the net weight (or volume) of a packaged food must be printed on the container. Most packages now list a food's net weight in metric measure as well as in ounces or pounds, and some labels give only the metric weight.

PAY ATTENTION TO PACKAGE SIZES
To get full value from *The Brand-Name Calorie Counter*, it's important to pay attention to package sizes. Specifically, whenever the caloric content of a food is listed by one ounce, you must check the label to learn how much the package weighs and then multiply its weight in ounces by the number of calories per ounce. Cheeses, for example, are listed in a one-ounce measure. To determine the caloric content of an eight-ounce package of *Kraft* American cheese, simply multiply eight by 110 and you will see that the entire package contains 880 calories.

Pay attention to weights, too, when a product is listed by the whole package. Many products (such as *Celentano* frozen lasagna) are available in various sizes. Also, one serving of a particular product, such as a frozen entree, may not be the same as one whole package. Sometimes entrees come packaged with two or more servings to a box or container.

PAY ATTENTION TO PACKAGE DIRECTIONS

Some products listed in *The Brand-Name Calorie Counter* require home preparation: condensed soups, entree mixes, sauce mixes, potato mixes, and many more. For convenience, the data on most of these products are given for the "finished" food when it is *prepared according to the basic package directions*. Should you make a change in a package recipe, you may also be changing the caloric content of a finished food. There is no reason why you shouldn't vary package directions—the point is, if you do so, be sure to determine how the change will affect the caloric content of the prepared food.

SOURCES AND ACCURACY OF DATA

The caloric values in this book are based on data obtained from producers and processors of brand-name foods. Every care has been exercised to evaluate the data as accurately and fully as possible; every effort has been made to present the material clearly and usefully.

Consumers should be aware, however, that a variety of factors can, to some extent, affect the accuracy of any and all analyses of food. For example, apples grown in different regions of the country may differ slightly in composition; therefore, the calories shown for any product that contains apples must be considered average or typical. Seasonal changes can also affect the composition of an apple; so, too, can the maturity of a crop when picked. For these and similar reasons, and because there is no practical way to analyze every sample of a processed food, it is an accepted practice within the food industry—and within the United States Department of Agriculture—to present nutritional data that is typical or "proximate."

As this edition of *The Brand-Name Calorie Counter* goes to press, the data have been checked to see that they are as up-to-date as possible. However, just as you strive to vary or improve your recipes, so do home economists in the food industry. As needed, corrections will be made in later editions of the book. Until then, you must be on the lookout for changes yourself. In particular, if you find that a favorite food is suddenly labeled "New" or "Improved," you may want to write the producer directly to ask if the food's caloric content has changed.

ABBREVIATIONS IN THIS BOOK

cont.	container
fl.	fluid
"	inch
lb.	pound
oz.	ounce
pkg.	package
pkt.	packet
tbsp.	tablespoon
tsp.	teaspoon
w/	with
w/out	without

Chapter 1

EGGS, PANCAKES, CEREALS, AND OTHER BREAKFAST FOODS

EGGS, SUBSTITUTE

	calories
(Featherweight), 2 eggs	120
(Fleischmann's Egg Beaters), 1/4 cup	25
w/cheese *(Fleischmann's Egg Beaters* Cheez), 1/2 cup .	130

BREAKFASTS, FROZEN, one package
See also "Breakfast Sandwiches," "French Toast, Frozen," "Pancakes, Frozen," and "Waffles, Frozen"

	calories
eggs, scrambled:	
w/bacon, and home fries *(Swanson Great Starts)*, 5.6 oz.	340
w/cheese, pancakes *(Swanson Great Starts)*, 3.4 oz. .	290
w/home fries *(Swanson Great Starts)*, 4.6 oz.	260
w/sausage, hash browns *(Swanson Great Starts)*, 6.5 oz.	430
reduced cholesterol eggs, w/mini oatbran muffins *(Swanson Great Starts)*, 4.75 oz.	250
French toast:	
w/links *(Weight Watchers)*, 4.5 oz.	270
w/sausage *(Swanson Great Starts)*, 5.5 oz.	380
cinnamon swirl, w/sausage *(Swanson Great Starts)*, 5.5 oz.	390
mini, w/sausage *(Swanson Great Starts)*, 2.5 oz. . . .	190

Breakfasts, Frozen, continued

oatmeal, w/lite links *(Swanson Great Starts)*, 4.6 oz. . .   310
omelet, w/cheese sauce, ham *(Swanson Great Starts)*, 7
   oz.   390
pancakes:
   w/bacon *(Swanson Great Starts)*, 4.5 oz.   400
   w/blueberry topping *(Weight Watchers)*, 4.75 oz. . . .   200
   w/links *(Weight Watchers)*, 4 oz.   220
   w/sausages *(Swanson Great Starts)*, 6 oz.   460
   silver dollar, w/sausage *(Swanson Great Starts)*, 3.75
     oz.   310
   w/strawberry topping *(Weight Watchers)*, 4.75 oz. . .   200
   whole wheat, w/lite links *(Swanson Great Starts)*, 5.5
     oz.   350
waffles:
   w/bacon *(Swanson Great Starts)*, 2.2 oz.   230
   Belgian, w/sausage *(Swanson Great Starts)*, 2.85 oz. .   280
   Belgian, and strawberries, w/sausage *(Swanson Great
     Starts)*, 3.5 oz.   210

BREAKFAST SANDWICHES, FROZEN & REFRIGERATED, one serving
See also "Sandwiches, Frozen"

                                                  calories

egg:
   w/beefsteak and cheese *(Swanson Great Starts
     Breakfast on a Muffin)*, 4.9 oz.   360
   w/Canadian bacon and cheese *(Swanson Great Starts
     Breakfast on a Biscuit)*, 5.2 oz.   420
   w/Canadian bacon and cheese *(Swanson Great Starts
     Breakfast on a Muffin)*, 4.1 oz.   290
   w/sausage and cheese *(Swanson Great Starts
     Breakfast on a Biscuit)*, 5.5 oz.   460
ham taco *(Owens Border Breakfasts)*, 2.17 oz.   90
ham and cheese *(Owens Border Breakfasts)*, 2 oz.   150
ham and cheese on bagel *(Swanson Great Starts)*, 3 oz.   240
sausage biscuit:
   (Owens Border Breakfasts), 2 oz.   210

(Swanson Great Starts Breakfast on a Biscuit), 4.7
  oz.   410
(Weight Watchers), 3 oz.   220
w/egg and cheese *(Owens Border Breakfasts),* 2.5 oz.   250
smoked *(Owens Border Breakfasts),* 2 oz.   200
sausage taco *(Owens Border Breakfasts),* 2.17 oz.   190

FRENCH TOAST, FROZEN, three ounces, except as noted
See also "Frozen Breakfasts"

	calories
(Aunt Jemima Original)	166
(Downyflake), 2 slices	270
w/cinnamon *(Weight Watchers)*	160
cinnamon swirl *(Aunt Jemima)*	171
raisin *(Aunt Jemima)*	172
sticks *(Farm Rich* Original)	300
sticks, apple cinnamon or blueberry *(Farm Rich)*	310

PANCAKES, FROZEN
*See also "Breakfasts, Frozen" and "Pancake &
Waffle Mix"*

	calories
(Aunt Jemima Original Microwave), 3.5 oz.	211
(Pillsbury Original Microwave), 3 pieces	240
batter *(Aunt Jemima* Original), 3.6 oz.	183
blueberry:	
(Aunt Jemima), 3.5 oz.	220
(Downyflake), 3 pieces	290
(Pillsbury Microwave), 3 pieces	250
batter *(Aunt Jemima),* 3.6 oz.	204
buttermilk:	
(Aunt Jemima Lite Microwave), 3.5 oz.	140
(Aunt Jemima Microwave), 3.5 oz.	210
(Pillsbury Microwave), 3 pieces	260
(Weight Watchers), 2.5 oz.	140

Pancakes, Frozen, buttermilk, continued
batter *(Aunt Jemima)*, 3.6 oz.................... 180
wheat, harvest *(Pillsbury* Microwave), 3 pieces 240

PANCAKE & WAFFLE MIX*, three 4″ pieces, except
as noted
See also "Pancakes, Frozen" and "Waffles, Frozen"

---

	calories
(Arrowhead Mills Griddle Lite), 1/2 cup	260
(Aunt Jemima Original)	116
(Aunt Jemima Original Complete)	253
(Bisquick Shake'N Pour)	260
(Bisquick Shake'N Pour Complete Waffle Mix), 2 pieces	280
(Estee), 3 pieces, 3″ each......................	100
(Featherweight)	140
(Hungry Jack Extra Lights)......................	210
(Hungry Jack Extra Lights Complete)	190
(Hungry Jack Panshakes)	250
(Martha White FlapStax), 1 piece	100
(Martha White Light Crust), 2 oz. dry	120
(Robin Hood/Gold Medal Pouch Mix), 1/8 pouch	100
apple cinnamon *(Bisquick Shake'N Pour)*	270
blueberry *(Bisquick Shake'N Pour)*	280
blueberry *(Hungry Jack)*	320
buckwheat *(Arrowhead Mills)*, 1/2 cup	270
buckwheat *(Aunt Jemima)*.......................	143
buttermilk:	
(Aunt Jemima)	122
(Aunt Jemima Complete)	231
(Aunt Jemima Lite Complete)	130
(Betty Crocker)	280
(Betty Crocker Complete), 1/2 cup dry ...	210
(Bisquick Shake'N Pour)	260
(Health Valley Biscuit & Pancake), 1 oz. .	100
(Hungry Jack)	240
(Hungry Jack Complete/Complete Packets) .	180
corn, blue *(Arrowhead Mills)*, 1/2 cup	330
multigrain *(Arrowhead Mills)*, 1/2 cup............	350
oat bran *(Arrowhead Mills)*, 1/2 cup	200

oat bran *(Bisquick Shake'N Pour)* 240
whole wheat *(Aunt Jemima)* 161

* Prepared according to package directions

WAFFLES, FROZEN, one piece, except as noted
See also "Pancake & Waffle Mix"

	calories
(Aunt Jemima Original)	173
(Downyflake), 2 pieces	120
(Eggo Homestyle)	120
(Eggo Nutri • Grain)	130
(Roman Meal), 2 pieces	280
all varieties *(Downyflake Jumbo)*, 2 pieces	170
apple & cinnamon *(Aunt Jemima)*	176
apple cinnamon *(Eggo)*	130
Belgian *(Weight Watchers)*, 1.5 oz.	120
blueberry:	
(Aunt Jemima)	175
(Downyflake), 2 pieces	180
(Eggo)	130
buttermilk *(Aunt Jemima)*	179
buttermilk *(Eggo)*	120
oat bran *(Eggo Common Sense)*	110
oat bran, fruit and nut *(Eggo Common Sense)*	120
raisin and bran *(Eggo Nutri • Grain)*	130
strawberry *(Eggo)*	130
whole-grain wheat *(Aunt Jemima)*	154

TOASTER MUFFINS & PASTRIES, one piece
See also "Muffins"

	calories
all varieties, except frosted *(Kellogg's Pop-Tarts)*	210
all varieties *(Toaster Strudel Breakfast Pastries)*	190
apple, Dutch, frosted *(Kellogg's Pop-Tarts)*	210
apple cinnamon *(Pepperidge Farm Croissant Toaster Tarts)*	170

Toaster Muffins & Pastries, continued

apple spice or banana nut *(Toaster Muffins)*   130
banana nut *(Thomas' Toast-R-Cakes)*   111
blueberry:
   (Thomas' Toast-R-Cakes)   108
   frosted *(Kellogg's Pop-Tarts)*   210
   wild Maine *(Toaster Muffins)*   120
bran *(Thomas' Toast-R-Cakes)*   103
brown sugar cinnamon, frosted *(Kellogg's Pop-Tarts)* . .   210
cheese *(Pepperidge Farm Croissant Toaster Tarts)*   190
cherry, frosted *(Kellogg's Pop-Tarts)*   200
chocolate fudge, frosted *(Kellogg's Pop-Tarts)*   200
chocolate vanilla creme, frosted *(Kellogg's Pop-Tarts)* .   200
corn *(Thomas' Toast-R-Cakes)*   120
corn, old fashioned, or raisin bran *(Toaster Muffins)* . .   120
grape, frosted *(Kellogg's Pop-Tarts)*   200
oat bran, w/raisins *(Awrey's Toastums)*   130
raspberry, frosted *(Kellogg's Pop-Tarts)*   200
strawberry *(Pepperidge Farm Croissant Toaster Tarts)* .   190
strawberry, frosted *(Kellogg's Pop-Tarts)*   200

CEREALS, READY-TO-EAT, one ounce, except as
noted
See also "Cereals, Cooking Type"

---

                                          calories

amaranth:
   flakes *(Health Valley)*   100
   w/bananas *(Health Valley)*   100
   w/raisins *(Health Valley Amaranth Crunch)*   110
bran *(see also "oat bran" and "rice bran," pages 9, 10):*
   (All-Bran)   70
   (Arrowhead Mills Bran Flakes)   100
   (Bran Buds)   70
   (Bran Chex)   90
   (Kellogg's 40%+ Bran Flakes)   90
   (Kellogg's Heartwise)   90
   (Nabisco 100% Bran)   70
   (Post Natural Bran Flakes)   90
   (Quaker Crunchy Bran)   89

apples and cinnamon or raisins *(Health Valley* 100%
  Natural)   70
apple spice or cinnamon *(Ralston Bran News)*   100
extra fiber *(All-Bran)*   50
w/fruit *(Fruitful Bran)*, 1.3 oz.   110
w/fruit and nuts *(Mueslix)*, 1.4 oz.   140
w/raisins *(Health Valley* Flakes)   100
w/raisins *(Kellogg's* Raisin Bran), 1.4 oz.   120
w/raisins *(Post* Natural Raisin Bran), 1.4 oz.   120
w/raisins *(Total Raisin Bran)*, 1.5 oz.   140
w/raisins and nuts *(Raisin Nut Bran)*   110
corn:
  (Arrowhead Mills Corn Flakes)   110
  (Arrowhead Mills Puffed Corn), .5 oz.   50
  (Corn Chex)   110
  (Corn Pops)   110
  (Country Corn Flakes)   110
  (Featherweight Corn Flakes), 1¼ cup   110
  (Health Valley Lites Puffed Corn), ½ cup   50
  (Honeycomb)   110
  (Kellogg's Corn Flakes)   100
  (Kellogg's Frosted Flakes)   110
  (Nutri • Grain)   100
  (Post Toasties)   110
  (Total Corn Flakes)   110
  blue *(Health Valley* Corn Flakes)   90
  chocolate flavor *(Cocoa Puffs)*   110
  w/fruit *(Health Valley Fruit Lites)*, .5 oz.   45
  w/nuts and honey *(Nut & Honey Crunch)*   110
granola, *see "mixed grain and natural style," below*
millet *(Arrowhead Mills* Puffed Millet), .5 oz.   50
mixed grain and natural style:
  (Almond Delight)   110
  (Apple Jacks)   110
  (Arrowhead Mills Arrowhead Crunch)   120
  (Arrowhead Mills Nature O's)   110
  (Cap'n Crunch)   113
  (Cap'n Crunch's Crunchberries)   113
  (Cap'n Crunch's Peanut Butter Crunch)   119
  (Cinnamon Toast Crunch)   120
  (Crispix)   110

Cereals, Ready-To-Eat, mixed grain and natural style, continued

(Crunchy Nut Oh!s)	127
(Double Chex)	100
(Familia Champion), 2 oz.	200
(Familia Crunchy)	116
(Familia No Added Sugar), 2 oz.	206
(Fiber One)	60
(Froot Loops)	110
(Golden Grahams)	110
(Grape-Nuts)	110
(Grape-Nuts Flakes)	100
(Health Valley Fiber 7 Flakes)	100
(Health Valley Healthy O's)	100
(Heartland)	130
(Honey Graham Chex)	110
(Honey Graham Oh!s)	122
(Just Right)	100
(Kaboom)	110
(King Vitaman)	110
(Kix)	110
(Nutri • Grain Nuggets)	100
(Product 19)	100
(Quaker 100% Natural)	127
(Special K)	110
(Sunflakes Multi-Grain)	100
(Trix)	110
w/almonds *(Honey Bunches of Oats)*	120
almond date or apple cinnamon *(Health Valley Healthy Crunch)*	100
w/almonds and raisins *(Nutri • Grain)*, 1.4 oz.	140
apple and cinnamon *(Quaker* 100% Natural)	126
w/apples and raisins *(Apple Raisin Crisp)*, 1.3 oz.	130
w/bananas, Hawaiian fruit *(Health Valley Sprouts 7)*	90
chocolate chip *(Cookie-Crisp)*	110
cinnamon and raisin *(Nature Valley* 100% Natural)	120
coconut *(Heartland)*	130
w/dates, raisins, walnuts, and oat clusters *(Fruit & Fibre)*, 1.25 oz.	120
w/fruit *(Health Valley Fruit & Fitness)*, 2 oz.	190
w/fruit and nuts *(Just Right)*, 1.3 oz.	140
w/fruit and nuts *(Mueslix Five Grain)*, 1.45 oz.	140

w/fruit and nuts *(Nature Valley* 100% Natural) . . .   130
w/fruit, tropical, and oat clusters *(Fruit & Fibre),*
  1.25 oz.   120
granola *(C.W. Post* Hearty)   130
granola, w/almonds *(Sun Country* 100% Natural) . .   130
granola, banana almond *(Sunbelt)*   130
granola, fruit and nut *(Sunbelt)*   120
granola, maple nut *(Arrowhead Mills),* 2 oz.   250
granola, w/raisins *(Sun Country)*   125
granola, w/raisins and dates *(Sun Country* 100%
  Natural)   123
honey roasted *(Honey Bunches of Oats)*   110
w/peaches, raisins, almonds, and oat clusters *(Fruit*
  & Fibre), 1.25 oz.   120
w/raisins *(Grape-Nuts)*   100
w/raisins *(Health Valley Sprouts 7)*   90
w/raisins *(Heartland)*   130
w/raisins and almonds *(Nutrific),* 1.5 oz.   140
raisin and date *(Quaker* 100% Natural)   123
raisin, dates, and almonds *(Ralston Muesli),* 1.45
  oz. = ½ cup   140
raisin, peaches, pecans *(Ralston Muesli),* 1.45 oz. . . .   150
raisin, walnuts, and cranberries *(Ralston Fruit*
  Muesli), 1.45 oz.   150
vanilla wafer *(Cookie-Crisp)*   110
oat:
  (Alpha-Bits)   110
  (Apple Cinnamon Cheerios)   110
  (Cheerios)   110
  (Cinnamon *Life)*   101
  (General Mills Oatmeal Crisp)   110
  (General Mills Toasted Oat)   130
  (Honey Nut Cheerios)   110
  (Life)   101
  (Oat Chex)   100
  (Post Oat Flakes)   110
  (Quaker Oat Squares)   105
  w/marshmallow *(Lucky Charms)*   110
  w/raisins *(General Mills* Oatmeal Raisin Crisp)   110
oat bran:
  (Arrowhead Mills Oat Bran Flakes)   110

Cereals, Ready-To-Eat, oat bran, continued

(Common Sense)	100
(Cracklin' Oat Bran)	110
(Health Valley Flakes)	100
(Health Valley Oat Bran O's)	90
almond crunch *(Health Valley Real)*	110
w/almonds and dates *(Health Valley Flakes)*	100
fruit, Hawaiian *(Health Valley Real)*	130
fruit and nut *(Health Valley Oat Bran O's)*	90
w/raisins *(Common Sense)*, 1.3 oz.	120
w/raisins *(General Mills Raisin Oat Bran)*, 1.5 oz.	150
w/raisins *(Health Valley Flakes)*	100
w/raisins *(Raisin Oat Bran Options)*, 1.45 oz.	130
w/raisins and nuts *(Health Valley Real)*	110

rice:

(Arrowhead Mills Puffed Rice), .5 oz.	50
(Featherweight Crisp Rice), 1 cup	110
(Health Valley Lites Puffed Rice), 1/2 cup	50
(Kellogg's Frosted Krispies)	110
(Kellogg's Rice Krispies)	110
(Quaker Puffed Rice), .5 oz.	54
(Rice Chex)	110
chocolate flavor *(Cocoa Krispies)*	110
w/fruit *(Health Valley Fruit Lites)*, .5 oz.	45
w/marshmallow bits *(Fruity Marshmallow Krispies)*, 1.3 oz.	140

rice bran *(Health Valley Rice Bran O's)*	110
rice bran, w/almonds and dates *(Health Valley)*	110

wheat:

(Arrowhead Mills Puffed Wheat), .5 oz.	50
(Arrowhead Mills Wheat Flakes)	110
(Clusters)	110
(Health Valley Lites Puffed Wheat), 1/2 cup	50
(Honey Smacks)	110
(Nutri • Grain)	100
(Quaker Puffed Wheat), .5 oz.	50
(Total)	100
(Wheat Chex)	100
(Wheaties)	100
brown sugar, nut, and honey filled *(Nut & Honey Crunch Biscuits)*	100

w/fruit *(Health Valley Fruit Lites)*, .5 oz. 45
fruit-filled, all varieties *(Kellogg's Squares)*,
   1 oz. = 1/2 cup 90
honey sweetened puffs *(Super Golden Crisp)* 110
w/raisins *(Crispy Wheats'n Raisins)* 100
w/raisins *(Nutri • Grain)*, 1.4 oz. 130
raspberry filled *(Fruit Wheats)* 90
wheat, shredded:
  (Frosted Mini-Wheats), 4 pieces 100
  (Nabisco), 1 piece 80
  (Nutri • Grain) 90
  (Quaker), 2 biscuits 132
  (S.W. Graham) 100
  bran *(Nabisco Shredded Wheat 'n Bran)* 90
  bite size *(Frosted Mini-Wheats)* 100
  cinnamon *(S.W. Graham)* 100
  mini *(Nabisco Spoon Size)* 90

CEREALS, COOKING-TYPE, dry, except as noted
*See also "Cereals, Ready-to-Eat" and "Cereal &
Grain Products"*

                                    calories
bran *(H–O Brand Super Bran)*, 1/3 cup 110
farina, *see "wheat," page 13*
grain, multi:
  four grain *(Arrowhead Mills)*, 1 oz. 94
  seven grain *(Arrowhead Mills)*, 1 oz. 100
oat bran:
  (Arrowhead Mills), 1 oz. 110
  (Quaker/Mother's), 1/3 cup or 2/3 cup cooked 92
  (3-Minute Brand Regular or Instant), 1 oz. 90
  (Wholesome 'N Hearty), 1 oz. 100
  apple and cinnamon *(Health Valley* Natural),
    1 oz. = 1/4 cup 100
  apple cinnamon *(Wholesome 'N Hearty* Instant),
    1 pkt. 130
  honey *(Wholesome 'N Hearty* Instant), 1 pkt. 110
  raisins and spice *(Health Valley* Natural), 1 oz. =
    1/4 cup 110

Cereals, Cooking-Type, continued

oatmeal and oats:

(Arrowhead Mills Instant), 1 oz.	100
(Arrowhead Mills Oat Flakes/Steel Cut Oats), 2 oz.	220
(H–O Brand Gourmet), 1/3 cup	100
(H–O Brand Instant), 1 pkt.	110
(H–O Brand Instant-box/Quick), 1/2 cup	130
(Instant Quaker), 1 pkt.	94
(Maypo 30 Second), 1 oz.	100
(Quaker Extra), 1 pkt.	95
(Quaker Quick/Old Fashioned), 1/3 cup or 2/3 cup cooked	99
(3-Minute Brand Quick or Old Fashioned), 1 oz.	100
(Total Instant), 1.2 oz.	110
(Total Quick), 1 oz.	90
apple and cinnamon *(H–O Brand* Instant), 1 pkt.	130
apple and cinnamon *(Instant Quaker),* 1 pkt.	118
apple and cinnamon *(Oatmeal Swirlers),* 1 pkt.	160
apple and cinnamon *(Total* Instant), 1.5 oz.	150
apple, date, and almond or apple spice *(Arrowhead Mills* Instant), 1 oz.	130
apples and spice *(Quaker Extra),* 1 pkt.	133
cherry *(Oatmeal Swirlers),* 1 pkt.	150
chocolate, milk *(Oatmeal Swirlers),* 1 pkt.	170
cinnamon raisin *(Total* Instant), 1.8 oz.	170
cinnamon, raisin, and almond *(Arrowhead Mills* Instant), 1 oz.	140
cinnamon and spice *(Instant Quaker),* 1 pkt.	164
cinnamon spice *(Oatmeal Swirlers),* 1 pkt.	160
w/fiber *(H–O Brand* Instant), 1 pkt.	110
w/fiber *(H–O Brand* Instant-box), 1/3 cup	100
w/fiber, apple and bran *(H–O Brand* Instant), 1 pkt.	130
w/fiber, raisin and bran *(H–O Brand* Instant), 1 pkt.	150
maple flavored *(Maypo* Vermont Style), 1 oz.	105
maple brown sugar *(H–O Brand* Instant), 1 pkt.	160
maple brown sugar *(Instant Quaker),* 1 pkt.	152
maple brown sugar *(Oatmeal Swirlers),* 1 pkt.	160
maple brown sugar *(Total* Instant), 1.6 oz.	160
w/oat bran *(3-Minute Brand* Quick), 1 oz.	100
peaches and cream *(Instant Quaker),* 1 pkt.	129
raisins *(3-Minute Brand),* 1 oz.	100

raisins and cinnamon *(Quaker Extra)*, 1 pkt. 129
raisins, dates, and walnut *(Instant Quaker)*, 1 pkt. . . . 141
raisins, w/oat bran *(3-Minute Brand)*, 1 oz. 100
raisins and spice *(H–O Brand* Instant)*, 1 pkt. 150
raisins and spice *(Instant Quaker)*, 1 pkt. 149
strawberry *(Oatmeal Swirlers)*, 1.6-oz. pkt. 150
strawberries and cream *(Instant Quaker)*, 1 pkt. . . . 129
sweet'n mellow *(H–O Brand* Instant, 1 pkt. 150
wheat:
  (Arrowhead Mills Bear Mush)*, 1 oz. 100
  (Cream of Wheat Instant/Quick)*, 1 oz. 100
  (Mix'n Eat Cream of Wheat Instant/Original)*, 1 pkt. 100
  (Wheat Hearts), 1 oz. or 3/4 cup cooked 110
  (Wheatena), 1 oz. 100
  all flavored varieties *(Mix'n Eat Cream of Wheat*
   Instant)*, 1 pkt. 130
  farina *(H–O Brand* Instant)*, 1 pkt. 110
  farina, cream *(H–O Brand)*, 3 tbsp. 120
  flakes *(Arrowhead Mills)*, 2 oz. 210
  whole *(Quaker/Mother's* Hot Natural)*, 1/3 cup or
   2/3 cup cooked 92
wheat and barley *(Maltex)*, 1 oz. 105

CEREAL & GRAIN PRODUCTS
See also "Cereals, Ready-to-Eat," "Cereals, Cooking-Type," and "Side Dishes, Mixes"

                                calories
amaranth seed *(Arrowhead Mills)*, 2 oz. 200
barley:
  flakes *(Arrowhead Mills)*, 2 oz. 200
  pearled *(Arrowhead Mills)*, 2 oz. 200
  pearled, medium or quick *(Quaker Scotch* Brand)*,
   1/4 cup 172
buckwheat groats *(Arrowhead Mills)*, 2 oz. 190
bulgur, *see "wheat," page 15*
corn, whole-grain, blue or yellow *(Arrowhead Mills)*,
  2 oz. 210
corn grits *(see also "hominy," page 14)*:
  (Albers Hominy Quick Grits)*, 1/4 cup 150

Cereal & Grain Products, corn grits, continued

white *(Arrowhead Mills)*, 2 oz.	200
white, enriched *(Quaker/Aunt Jemima* Regular/Quick)*, 3 tbsp.	101
white hominy product *(Quaker* Instant)*, 1 pkt.	79
yellow *(Arrowhead Mills)*, 2 oz.	200
yellow, enriched *(Quaker* Quick)*, 3 tbsp.	101
w/imitation bacon bits *(Quaker* Instant)*, 1 pkt.	101
w/real cheddar cheese flavor *(Quaker* Instant)*, 1 pkt.	104
w/imitation ham bits *(Quaker* Instant)*, 1 pkt.	99

cornmeal:

buttermilk, white, self-rising, mix *(Aunt Jemima)*, 3 tbsp.	101
white, bolted, mix *(Aunt Jemima)*, 1 oz.	99
white, self-rising *(Aunt Jemima)*, 1 oz.	98
white, self-rising, enriched, bolted *(Aunt Jemima)*, 1 oz.	99
white or yellow *(Albers)*, 1 oz.	100
white or yellow, enriched *(Quaker/Aunt Jemima)*, 1 oz. = 3 tbsp.	102
whole-grain, blue, yellow or hi-lysine *(Arrowhead Mills)*, 2 oz.	210
yellow, bolted *(Tone's)*, 1 tsp.	9
yellow, bolted, mix *(Aunt Jemima)*, 1 oz.	97
flax seed *(Arrowhead Mills)*, 1 oz.	140

hominy *(see also "corn grits," page 13)*:

golden *(Allens)*, 1/2 cup	80
golden *(Van Camp's)*, 1 cup	128
w/red and green peppers *(Van Camp's)*, 1 cup	129
Mexican *(Allens)*, 1/2 cup	80
white *(Allens)*, 1/2 cup	70
white *(Van Camp's)*, 1 cup	138
millet, hulled *(Arrowhead Mills)*, 1 oz.	90
oat flakes or groats *(Arrowhead Mills)*, 2 oz.	220
quinoa seed *(Arrowhead Mills)*, 2 oz.	200
rye, flakes *(Arrowhead Mills)*, 2 oz.	190
rye, whole-grain *(Arrowhead Mills)*, 2 oz.	190
teff seed *(Arrowhead Mills)*, 2 oz.	200
wheat bran *(Arrowhead Mills)*, 2 oz.	50

wheat bran, toasted *(Kretschmer)*, 1 oz.   57
wheat, bulgur *(Arrowhead Mills)*, 2 oz.   200
wheat, cracked *(Arrowhead Mills)*, 2 oz.   180
wheat germ:
   (Kretschmer), 1 oz. = ¼ cup   103
   honey crunch *(Kretschmer)*, 1 oz. = ¼ cup   105
   raw *(Arrowhead Mills)*, 2 oz.   210

Chapter 2

BREADSTUFFS, CRACKERS, AND FLOUR PRODUCTS

> **BREAD,** one slice, except as noted
> *See also "Bread Dough, Ready-To-Bake" and "Sweet Breads, Mixes"*

	calories
apple walnut *(Arnold)*	64
(Arnold Bran'nola Original)	85
barbecue *(Colombo Brand BBQ Loaf)*, 2 oz.	139
bran, whole *(Brownberry Natural)*	58
bran and oat *(Oatmeal Goodness Light)*	40
brown, canned *(S&W New England)*, 2 slices	76
brown, plain, canned *(B&M)*, 1.6 oz.	92
(Brownberry Bran'nola)	85
(Brownberry Health Nut)	71
cinnamon oatmeal *(Oatmeal Goodness)*	90
cinnamon raisin:	
(Arnold)	67
(Weight Watchers)	60
cinnamon or cinnamon raisin swirl *(Pepperidge Farm)*	90
corn and molasses *(Pepperidge Farm)*	70
date nut roll *(Dromedary)*, 1/2" slice	80
French:	
(DiCarlo Parisian)	70
extra sour *(Colombo Brand)*, 2 oz.	150
extra sour, sliced *(Colombo Brand)*, 2 oz.	153
sweet *(Colombo Brand French Stick)*, 2 oz.	154
twin *(Pepperidge Farm)*, 1 oz.	80
garlic *(Colombo Brand)*, 2 oz.	185

grain:
    mixed *(Roman Meal* Round Top) 67
    mixed *(Roman Meal* Thin Sliced Sandwich) 55
    multi *(Roman Meal* Sun Grain) 68
    multi *(Weight Watchers)* 40
    nutty *(Arnold Bran'nola)* 85
    nutty *(Brownberry Bran'nola* Nutty Grains) 85
    seven *(Pepperidge Farm* Hearty Slice) 90
(Hollywood Dark or Light) 70
honey bran *(Pepperidge Farm)* 90
Italian:
    (Arnold Francisco International), 1-oz. slice 72
    (Brownberry Light) 44
    (Wonder Family) 70
    brown and serve *(Pepperidge Farm* Deli Classics),
      1 oz.. 80
    light *(Arnold* Bakery) 45
    thick sliced *(Arnold* Francisco International) 66
(Monk's Hi-Fibre), 1 slice, approx. 1 oz. 70
oat:
    (Arnold Bran'nola Country) 90
    (Brownberry Bran'nola Country). 90
    crunchy *(Pepperidge Farm,* 1½ lb.) 95
oat bran:
    (Awrey's) 50
    (Roman Meal Split-Top) 68
    honey *(Roman Meal)* 71
    honey nut *(Roman Meal)*. 72
oatmeal:
    (Pepperidge Farm) 70
    (Pepperidge Farm, 1½ lb.) 90
    (Pepperidge Farm Light Style) 45
    (Pepperidge Farm Very Thin) 40
    and bran *(Oatmeal Goodness)* 90
    light *(Arnold* Bakery) 44
    sunflower seed *(Oatmeal Goodness)* 90
orange raisin *(Brownberry)* 67
pita:
    oat bran *(Sahara),* ½ piece 66
    wheat, whole *(Sahara),* 1 piece, approx. 2 oz. 150
    white *(Sahara),* ½ piece or 1 mini piece 79

Bread, continued

pumpernickel:
(Arnold)	70
(Pepperidge Farm Family)	80
small *(Pepperidge Farm* Party), 4 slices	60

raisin:
bran *(Brownberry)*	61
cinnamon *(Brownberry)*	66
w/cinnamon *(Monk's)*	70
walnut *(Brownberry)*	68

rice bran:
(Roman Meal)	70
golden *(Monk's)*	70
honey nut *(Roman Meal)*	71

rye:
(Beefsteak Hearty/Mild/Soft)	70
(Braun's Old Allegheny)	70
(Pepperidge Farm Family)	80
(Weight Watchers)	40
(Wonder)	70
caraway *(Brownberry* Natural)	73
Dijon *(Pepperidge Farm)*	50
dill *(Arnold)*	71
Jewish, seeded *(Levy's)*	76
Jewish, seedless *(Levy's)*	75
onion *(Beefsteak)*	70
seedless *(Brownberry* Natural Thin Sliced)	45
seedless *(Pepperidge Farm* Family)	75
small *(Pepperidge Farm* Party), 4 slices	60
wheatberry *(Beefsteak)*	70

sourdough *(DiCarlo)*	70
sourdough French *(Boudin),* 2 slices or 2 oz.	130
sunflower and bran *(Monk's)*	70
Vienna *(Pepperidge Farm* Deli Classics)	70
Vienna *(Pepperidge Farm* Light Style)	45

wheat:
(Arnold Brick Oven)	57
(Beefsteak Hearty/Soft)	70
(Brownberry Hearth), 1 oz.	70
(Brownberry Natural)	80
(Country Grain)	70

(Fresh & Natural)	70
(Home Pride Butter Top/7 Grain/Stoneground)	70
(Pepperidge Farm, 1½ lb.)	90
(Pepperidge Farm Family, 2 lb.)	70
(Pepperidge Farm Light Style)	45
(Pepperidge Farm Very Thin)	35
(Weight Watchers)	40
apple honey *(Brownberry)*	69
cracked *(Pepperidge Farm)*	70
cracked *(Wonder)*	70
dark *(Arnold Bran'nola)*	83
hearty *(Arnold Bran'nola)*	88
hearty *(Brownberry Bran'nola)*	88
honey wheatberry *(Arnold)*	77
light golden *(Arnold* Bakery)	44
multigrain *(Beefsteak)*	70
oatmeal *(Oatmeal Goodness)*	90
oatmeal *(Oatmeal Goodness* Light)	40
sesame *(Pepperidge Farm)*	95
soft *(Brownberry)*	74
sprouted *(Pepperidge Farm)*	70
whole *(Arnold* Stoneground 100%)	48
whole *(Daily),* 2 oz., approx. 1 slice	140
whole *(Monk's* 100% Stone Ground)	70
whole *(Pepperidge Farm* Thin Sliced)	60
whole *(Wonder* 100%/Soft 100%)	70
whole *(Wonder* High Fiber/Light)	40
whole *(Wonder* Family)	70
white:	
(Arnold Brick Oven)	61
(Arnold Country White)	98
(Arnold Light Premium)	42
(Beefsteak Robust)	70
(Brownberry Light Premium)	42
(Brownberry Natural)	59
(Home Pride Butter Top)	70
(Monk's)	60
(Pepperidge Farm Large Family, 2 lb.)	70
(Pepperidge Farm Thin Sliced, 1 lb.)	80
(Pepperidge Farm Thin Sliced, 8 oz.)	70
(Pepperidge Farm Very Thin)	40

Bread, white, continued
(Weight Watchers)	40
(Wonder)	70
(Wonder High Fiber/Light)	40
(Wonder Thin Sliced)	50
w/buttermilk *(Wonder)*	70
country *(Pepperidge Farm)*	95
extra fiber *(Arnold* Brick Oven)	55
sandwich *(Pepperidge Farm)*	65
toasting *(Pepperidge Farm)*	90

BREAD DOUGH, READY TO BAKE*
See also "Bread" and "Sweet Breads, Mixes"

	calories
brown and serve:	
(du Jour Austrian/du Jour French), 1 slice	70
French *(Pepperidge Farm)*, 2 slices	180
Italian *(Pepperidge Farm)*, 2 slices	150
frozen, honey walnut or white *(Bridgford)*, 1 oz.	76
frozen, white *(Rich's)*, 2 slices	120
refrigerated:	
cornbread twists *(Pillsbury)*, 1 twist	70
French, crusty *(Pillsbury)*, 1" slice	60
wheat or white *(Pipin' Hot)*, 1" slice	70

* *Prepared according to package directions*

SWEET BREADS, MIXES*
See also "Bread," "Muffins, Mixes," and "Rolls, Frozen, Mixes or Refrigerated"

	calories
banana *(Pillsbury)*, 1/12 loaf	170
blueberry nut *(Pillsbury)*, 1/12 loaf	150
cherry nut *(Pillsbury)*, 1/12 loaf	180
cornbread:	
(Aunt Jemima Easy), 1 serving	196
(Dromedary), 2" × 2" square	130

(Martha White Cotton Pickin'), ¼ pan   170
(Pillsbury/Ballard), ⅛ recipe   140
   white or yellow *(Robin Hood/Gold Medal* Pouch
      Mix), ⅙ mix   150
cranberry or date *(Pillsbury),* 1/12 loaf   160
date nut *(Dromedary),* 1/12 loaf   183
gingerbread *(Betty Crocker* Classic), 1/9 mix   220
gingerbread *(Pillsbury),* 3″ square   190
nut *(Pillsbury),* 1/12 loaf   170

* *Prepared according to package directions*

BAGELS, FROZEN, one piece

	calories
all varieties *(Lender's* Bagelettes), .9 oz.	70
plain:	
(Lender's Big'n Crusty), 3⅛ oz.	240
(Sara Lee), 2.5 oz.	190
(Sara Lee), 3.1 oz.	230
plain or egg *(Lender's),* 2 oz.	150
blueberry *(Lender's),* 2.5 oz.	190
cinnamon'n raisin *(Lender's* Big'n Crusty), 3⅛ oz. . . .	250
cinnamon raisin *(Sara Lee),* 2.5 oz.	200
cinnamon and raisin *(Sara Lee),* 3.1 oz.	240
egg:	
(Lender's Big'n Crusty), 3⅛ oz.	250
(Sara Lee), 2.5 oz.	200
(Sara Lee), 3.1 oz.	250
garlic *(Lender's),* 2 oz.	160
garlic *(Lender's* Big'n Crusty), 3⅛ oz.	250
oat bran:	
(Lender's), 2.5 oz.	170
(Sara Lee), 2.5 oz.	180
(Sara Lee), 3.1 oz.	220
onion:	
(Lender's), 2 oz.	160
(Lender's Big'n Crusty), 3⅛ oz.	230
(Sara Lee), 2.5 oz.	190
(Sara Lee), 3.1 oz.	230

Bagels, Frozen, continued

poppy seed or sesame seed *(Lender's)*, 2 oz.	160
poppy seed or sesame seed *(Sara Lee)*, 2.5 oz.	190
poppy seed *(Sara Lee)*, 3.1 oz.	230
pumpernickel *(Lender's)*, 2 oz.	160
raisin'n honey *(Lender's)*, 2.5 oz.	200
rye *(Lender's)*, 2 oz.	150
sesame seed *(Sara Lee)*, 3.1 oz.	240
soft *(Lender's)*, 2.5 oz.	210
wheat'n raisin *(Lender's)*, 2.5 oz.	190

BISCUITS, one piece, except as noted
See also "Rolls"

---

	calories
packaged:	
(Wonder)	80
buttermilk *(Weight Watchers)*, 2 pieces	100
country *(Awrey's 3")*, 2 oz.	160
round or square *(Awrey's 2")*, 1 oz.	80
sliced or unsliced *(Awrey's)*, 2 oz.	160
square *(Awrey's 3")*, 2 oz.	160
frozen *(Bridgford)*, 2 oz.	180
mix:	
(Arrowhead Mills), 2 oz.	100
(Bisquick), 1/2 cup	240
(Martha White BixMix), 1 piece*	100
(Robin Hood/Gold Medal Pouch Mix), 1/8 mix*	90
buttermilk *(Health Valley Biscuit & Pancake)*, 1 oz.	100
refrigerated:	
(Ballard Ovenready)	50
(Big Country Butter Tastin')	100
(Pillsbury Big Premium Heat 'n Eat)	140
(Pillsbury Country)	50
(Roman Meal)	90
baking powder *(1869 Brand)*	100
butter or buttermilk *(Pillsbury)*	50
buttermilk *(Ballard Ovenready)*	50
buttermilk *(Big Country)*	100
buttermilk *(1869 Brand)*	100

buttermilk *(Hungry Jack* Extra Rich)	50
buttermilk *(Pillsbury* Heat 'n Eat)	85
buttermilk *(Pillsbury* Tender Layer)	50
buttermilk, flaky *(Hungry Jack)*	90
buttermilk, fluffy *(Hungry Jack)*	90
(1869 Brand Butter Tastin')	100
flaky *(Hungry Jack)*	80
flaky *(Hungry Jack Butter Tastin')*	90
flaky, honey *(Hungry Jack)*	90
fluffy *(Pillsbury* Good 'n Buttery)	90
oat bran, honey nut *(Roman Meal)*	131
Southern style *(Big Country)*	100
white *(Roman Meal* Premium)	127

* *Prepared according to package directions.*

MUFFINS, one piece, except as noted
See also "Muffins, Frozen & Refrigerated," "Muffins, Mixes," and "Toaster Muffins & Pastries"

---

	calories
apple:	
(Awrey's), 2.5 oz.	220
(Awrey's), 1.5 oz.	130
cinnamon, mini *(Hostess),* 5 pieces or 1 pkg.	160
streusel *(Awrey's* Grande), 4.2 oz.	340
banana nut *(Awrey's* Grande), 4.2 oz.	370
banana walnut, mini *(Hostess),* 5 pieces or 1 pkg.	160
blueberry:	
(Awrey's), 2.5 oz.	210
(Awrey's), 1.5 oz.	130
(Awrey's Grande), 4.2 oz.	360
mini *(Hostess),* 5 pieces or 1 pkg.	150
cranberry *(Awrey's),* 1.5 oz.	120
corn *(Awrey's),* 2.5 oz.	220
corn *(Awrey's),* 1.5 oz.	130
English:	
(Hi Fiber)	110
(Pepperidge Farm)	140
(Roman Meal Original)	146

Muffins, English, continued

(Thomas')	130
(Wonder)	130
cinnamon apple (Pepperidge Farm)	140
cinnamon chip (Pepperidge Farm)	160
cinnamon raisin (Hi Fiber)	110
cinnamon raisin (Pepperidge Farm)	150
cinnamon and raisin oatmeal (Oatmeal Goodness)	140
honey and oatmeal (Oatmeal Goodness)	140
multi-grain (Hi Fiber)	120
oat bran (Thomas')	116
raisin (Thomas')	153
rye (Thomas')	120
sourdough (Pepperidge Farm)	135
wheat, honey (Thomas')	129

oat bran:

(Awrey's), 2.75 oz.	180
(Hostess)	170
all varieties (Health Valley Oat Bran Fancy Fruit Muffins)	180
pineapple raisin oat bran (Awrey's), 2.75 oz.	180
raisin (Wonder Raisin Rounds)	140

raisin bran:

(Awrey's), 2.5 oz.	190
(Awrey's), 1.5 oz.	110
(Awrey's Grande), 4.2 oz.	320
rice bran, raisin (Health Valley Rice Bran Fancy Fruit Muffins)	215
sourdough (Wonder)	130

MUFFINS, FROZEN & REFRIGERATED, one piece
See also "Muffins" and "Muffins, Mixes"

---

	calories
frozen:	
apple oat bran (Sara Lee)	190
apple spice (Sara Lee)	220
blueberry (Pepperidge Farm Old Fashioned)	170
blueberry (Sara Lee)	200
blueberry (Sara Lee Free & Light)	120

cheese streusel *(Sara Lee)* 220
chocolate chunk *(Sara Lee)* 220
cinnamon swirl *(Pepperidge Farm Old Fashioned)* .. 190
corn *(Pepperidge Farm Old Fashioned)* 180
corn, golden *(Sara Lee)* 250
oat bran *(Sara Lee)* 220
oat bran, w/apple *(Pepperidge Farm Old Fashioned)* 190
raisin bran *(Pepperidge Farm Old Fashioned)* 170
raisin bran *(Sara Lee)* 220
refrigerated, English *(Roman Meal)*, 1/2 piece 71
refrigerated, English, honey nut and oat bran *(Roman
    Meal)*, 1/2 piece 81

MUFFINS, MIXES*
*See also "Muffins," "Muffins, Frozen & Refrigerated,"
and "Sweet Breads, Mixes"*

	calories
all varieties, except bran *(Martha White)*, 1/6 pkg.	140
apple cinnamon *(Betty Crocker)*, 1/12 pkg.	120

apple streusel, Dutch *(Betty Crocker Bake Shop)*,
    1/12 pkg. 200
applesauce *(Robin Hood/Gold Medal Pouch Mix)*,
    1/6 pkg. 160
banana *(Robin Hood/Gold Medal Pouch Mix)*, 1/6 pkg. 150
banana nut *(Betty Crocker)*, 1/12 pkg. 120
blueberry:
    (Duncan Hines Bakery Style), 1 piece 190
    (Robin Hood/Gold Medal Pouch Mix), 1/6 pkg. 170
    streusel *(Betty Crocker Bake Shop)*, 1/12 pkg. 210
    wild *(Betty Crocker)*, 1/12 pkg. 120
    wild *(Duncan Hines)*, 1 piece 110
bran:
    (Martha White), 1/6 pkg. 150
    and honey *(Duncan Hines)*, 1 piece 120
    and honey *(Duncan Hines Bakery Style)*, 1 piece ... 200
caramel *(Robin Hood/Gold Medal Pouch Mix)*, 1/6 pkg. 150
carrot nut *(Betty Crocker)*, 1/12 pkg. 150
chocolate chip *(Betty Crocker)*, 1/12 pkg. 150
cinnamon streusel *(Betty Crocker)*, 1/10 pkg. 200

Muffins, Mixes*, continued

cinnamon swirl *(Duncan Hines* Bakery Style), 1 piece	200
corn:	
(Dromedary), 1 piece	120
(Flako), 1 serving	116
(Robin Hood/Gold Medal), 1/6 pkg.	130
blue *(Arrowhead Mills)*, 1 piece	110
cranberry orange nut *(Duncan Hines* Bakery Style),	
1 piece	200
honey bran *(Robin Hood/Gold Medal* Pouch Mix),	
1/6 pkg.	170
oat *(Robin Hood/Gold Medal* Pouch Mix), 1/6 pkg. . . .	150
oat bran:	
(Betty Crocker), 1/8 pkg.	190
all varieties *(Hain)*, 1 piece	140
apple spice *(Arrowhead Mills)*, 1 piece . . . . . : . .	120
oatmeal raisin *(Betty Crocker)*, 1/12 pkg.	140
pecan crunch *(Duncan Hines* Bakery Style), 1 piece . .	220
strawberry crown *(Betty Crocker)*, 1/10 pkg.	150
wheat bran *(Arrowhead Mills)*, 2 pieces	270

* Prepared according to package directions

ROLLS, one piece, except as noted
See also "Rolls, Frozen, Mixes, & Refrigerated" and "Snack Cakes & Pastries"

	calories
assorted *(Brownberry* Hearth)	124
brown and serve:	
(Pepperidge Farm Hearth)	50
buttermilk *(Wonder)*	80
club *(Pepperidge Farm)*	100
French *(Pepperidge Farm*, 3/pkg.), 1/2 piece	120
French *(Pepperidge Farm*, 2/pkg.), 1/2 piece	180
French, petite *(du Jour)*	230
gem style *(Wonder)*	80
Italian, crusty *(du Jour)*	80
cinnamon, homestyle *(Awrey's)*	240
cinnamon swirl *(Awrey's* Grande)	340

crescent, butter *(Pepperidge Farm* Deli Classics) 110
croissant:
    (Pepperidge Farm Sandwich Quartet) 170
    butter *(Awrey's),* 3 oz. 300
    butter *(Awrey's),* 2 oz. 200
    butter *(Awrey's),* 1 oz. 100
    butter, petite *(Pepperidge Farm* All Butter) 120
    margarine *(Awrey's),* 2.5 oz. 250
    margarine *(Awrey's),* 1.25 oz. 120
    wheat *(Awrey's),* 2.5 oz. 240
dinner:
    (Arnold 24 Dinner Party) 51
    (Pepperidge Farm Old Fashioned) 50
    (Roman Meal) 69
    (Wonder) 80
    black forest *(Awrey's)* 50
    country style *(Pepperidge Farm* Classic) 50
    cracked wheat *(Awrey's)* 50
    crusty *(Awrey's)* 70
    plain *(Awrey's)* 60
    poppy seed *(Awrey's)* 59
    wheat *(Home Pride)* 70
    white *(Home Pride)* 80
    sesame seed *(Awrey's)* 60
egg *(Levy's* Old Country Deli), 1 oz. 146
egg, sandwich *(Arnold* Dutch) 123
finger, w/poppy seeds *(Pepperidge Farm)* 50
49er, sour *(Colombo* Brand), 1.2 oz. 90
49er, sweet *(Colombo* Brand), 1.2 oz. 96
frankfurter, *see "hot dog," page 28*
French style:
    (Francisco International) 108
    (Pepperidge Farm Deli Classics, 9/pkg) 100
    (Pepperidge Farm Deli Classics, 4/pkg), ½ piece . . . 120
hamburger:
    (Arnold) 115
    (Pepperidge Farm) 130
    (Roman Meal Original) 113
    (Wonder) 120
    (Wonder Light) 80
hoagie *(Wonder)* 400

Rolls, continued

hoagie, soft *(Pepperidge Farm* Deli Classics)   210
hot dog:
   (Arnold)   100
   (Arnold New England Style)   108
   (Country Grain)   100
   (Pepperidge Farm)   140
   (Roman Meal Original)   104
   (Wonder/Wonder Light)   80
   Dijon *(Pepperidge Farm)*   160
   oat bran *(Awrey's)*   110
kaiser *(Arnold* Francisco)   184
kaiser *(Brownberry* Hearth)   152
Luigi *(Colombo* Brand–Twin Pack), 2 oz.   146
onion *(Levy's* Old Country Deli), 1 oz.   153
pan *(Wonder)*   80
Parker House *(Pepperidge Farm)*   60
party *(Pepperidge Farm)*   30
sandwich:
   oat bran *(Awrey's)*   120
   onion, w/poppy seeds *(Pepperidge Farm)*   150
   potato *(Pepperidge Farm)*   160
   salad *(Pepperidge Farm* Deli Classics)   110
   sesame seed *(Pepperidge Farm)*   140
soft *(Pepperidge Farm* Family)   100
sourdough, French style *(Pepperidge Farm* Deli
   Classics)   100
steak, sour *(Colombo* Brand), 2.6 oz.   200
steak, sweet *(Colombo* Brand), 2.6 oz.   206
twist, golden *(Pepperidge Farm* Deli Classics)   110

ROLLS, FROZEN, MIXES, OR REFRIGERATED
See also "Rolls"

	calories
apple, sweet, frozen *(Weight Watchers)*, 1/2 pkg.	190
butterflake, refrigerated *(Pillsbury)*, 1 piece	140
cinnamon:	
(Pepperidge Farm, 2/pkg.), 1 piece	280
all butter, frozen *(Sara Lee)*, 1 piece	230

all butter, icing packet *(Sara Lee)*, 1 pkt.   50
bun, frozen *(Rich's Ever Fresh)*, 1 piece   293
iced, refrigerated *(Hungry Jack)*, 2 pieces   290
iced, refrigerated *(Pillsbury)*, 1 piece   110
crescent, refrigerated *(Pillsbury)*, 1 piece   100
croissants, butter, frozen, 1 piece:
  (Sara Lee), 1.5 oz.   170
  petite *(Pepperidge Farm)*, 1 piece   140
  petite *(Sara Lee)*, 1 oz.   120
honeybun, mini, frozen *(Rich's Ever Fresh)*, 1 piece . . .   133
hot, mix* *(Dromedary)*, 2 pieces   239
hot, mix* *(Pillsbury)*, 2 pieces   270
Parkerhouse, frozen *(Bridgford)*, 1-oz. piece   85

* *Prepared according to package directions*

BREADSTICKS, one piece, except as noted	
	calories
plain *(Stella D'oro)*	41
plain, dietetic *(Stella D'oro)*	46
onion *(Stella D'oro)*	40
pizza *(Fattorie & Pandea)*, 3 pieces	59
pizza *(Stella D'oro)*	43
sesame:	
(Fattorie & Pandea), 3 pieces	65
(Stella D'oro)	51
dietetic *(Stella D'oro)*	49
soft, refrigerated *(Pillsbury)*	100
soft, refrigerated *(Roman Meal)*	117
wheat *(Stella D'oro)*	42
wheat, whole *(Fattorie & Pandea)*, 3 pieces	57
refrigerated *(Roman Meal)*	117

CROUTONS
See also "Crumbs & Meal" and "Stuffing & Stuffing Mixes"

	calories
all varieties, except cheddar and Romano *(Pepperidge Farm)*, ½ oz.	70
Caesar salad *(Brownberry)*, 1 oz.	62
cheddar cheese *(Brownberry)*, 1 oz.	63
cheddar and Romano *(Pepperidge Farm)*, ½ oz.	60
garlic'n cheese *(Flavor Tree* Salad Nuggets), ¼ cup	167
onion *(Flavor Tree* Salad Nuggets), ¼ cup	163
onion and garlic *(Brownberry)*, 1 oz.	60
seasoned *(Brownberry)*, 1 oz.	59
sesame *(Flavor Tree* Salad Nuggets), ¼ cup	160
toasted *(Brownberry)*, 1 oz.	56

STUFFING & STUFFING MIXES
See also "Croutons" and "Crumbs & Meal"

	calories
dry, 1 oz.:	
apple and raisin *(Pepperidge Farm* Distinctive)	110
chicken, classic *(Pepperidge Farm* Distinctive)	110
corn *(Brownberry)*	103
corn bread, cube, or herb *(Pepperidge Farm)*	110
country style *(Pepperidge Farm)*	100
herb *(Brownberry)*	100
herb, country garden *(Pepperidge Farm* Distinctive)	120
vegetable, harvest, and almond *(Pepperidge Farm* Distinctive)	110
wild rice and mushroom *(Pepperidge Farm* Distinctive)	130
frozen, ½ cup:	
chicken *(Green Giant Stuffing Originals)*	170
cornbread *(Green Giant Stuffing Originals)*	170
mushroom *(Green Giant Stuffing Originals)*	150
wild rice *(Green Giant Stuffing Originals)*	160
mix, dry:	
(Croutettes), .7 oz.	70

Cajun style *(Golden Dipt)*, ¼ cup   40
cheddar and French *(Golden Dipt)*, ¼ cup   80
chicken or herb *(Betty Crocker)*, ⅙ pkg.   110
herb, garden *(Golden Dipt)*, ¼ cup   40
mix*, ½ cup:
  beef *(Stove Top)*   180
  broccoli and cheese *(Stove Top* Microwave)   170
  chicken flavor *(Betty Crocker)*   180
  chicken flavor *(Stove Top)*   180
  chicken flavor *(Stove Top* Flexible Serving)   170
  chicken flavor *(Stove Top* Microwave)   160
  cornbread *(Stove Top)*   170
  cornbread *(Stove Top* Flexible Serving)   180
  cornbread, homestyle *(Stove Top* Microwave)   160
  herb, homestyle *(Stove Top* Flexible Serving)   170
  herb, savory *(Stove Top)*   170
  herb, traditional *(Betty Crocker)*   190
  long grain and wild rice *(Stove Top)*   180
  mushroom and onion *(Stove Top)*   180
  mushroom and onion *(Stove Top* Microwave)   170
  pork *(Stove Top)*   170
  pork *(Stove Top* Flexible Serving)   170
  w/rice *(Stove Top)*   180
  San Francisco style *(Stove Top Americana)*   170
  turkey *(Stove Top)*   170

* *Prepared according to package directions*

CRUMBS & MEAL
See also "Croutons" and "Stuffing & Stuffing Mixes"

                                     calories
breadcrumbs:
  plain *(Devonsheer)*, 1 oz.   108
  plain or Italian, dry, grated *(Tone's)*, 1 tsp.   8
  Italian style *(Devonsheer)*, 1 oz.   104
  Italian style, whole wheat *(Jaclyn's)*, ½ oz.   28
corn flake crumbs *(Kellogg's)*, 1 oz.   100
cracker crumbs and meal:
  (Golden Dipt), 1 oz.   100

Crumbs & Meal, cracker crumbs and meal, continued

matzo *(Manischewitz Farfel)*, 1 cup   180
matzo meal *(Manischewitz Daily)*, 1 cup   514

SHELLS & WRAPPERS, one piece, except as noted
See also "Pastry and Pie Crusts"

---

	calories
egg roll wrapper *(Nasoya)*	23
frankfurter wrap *(Weiner Wrap)*	60
taco salad shell *(Azteca)*	200

taco shell:
    (Gebhardt)   30
    (Lawry's)   50
    (Lawry's Super)   86
    (Old El Paso)   55
    (Old El Paso Super Size)   100
    (Ortega)   50
    (Tio Sancho)   64
    (Tio Sancho Super)   94
    corn *(Azteca)*   60
    miniature *(Old El Paso)*, 3 pieces   70

tortilla:
    corn *(Azteca)*   45
    corn *(Old El Paso)*   60
    flour *(Azteca)*, 9" diam.   130
    flour *(Azteca)*, 7" diam.   80
    flour *(Old El Paso)*   150

tostaco shell *(Old El Paso)*   100

tostada shell:
    (Lawry's)   73
    (Old El Paso), 2 pieces   110
    (Ortega)   50
    (Tio Sancho)   67

wonton skin *(Nasoya)*   23

SEASONED BATTER & COATING MIXES
See also "Condiments & Seasonings"

	calories
beer batter *(Golden Dipt)*, 1 oz.	100
breading *(Golden Dipt)*, 1 oz.	90
chicken:	
(Featherweight), 1/4 pkg.	18
(Golden Dipt), 1 oz.	90
(Shake'n Bake), 1/4 pouch	80
(Shake'n Bake Oven Fry Extra Crispy), 1/4 pouch	110
barbecue *(Shake'n Bake)*, 1/4 pouch	90
batter, Cajun *(Tone's)*, 1 tsp.	12
homestyle *(Shake'n Bake Oven Fry)*, 1/4 pouch	80
corn dog batter *(Golden Dipt Corny Dog)*, 1 oz.	100
country, mild *(Shake'n Bake)*, 1/4 pouch	80
fish:	
(Featherweight), 1/4 pkg.	18
(Shake'n Bake), 1/4 pouch	70
batter, Cajun *(Tone's)*, 1 tsp.	12
batter, fish & chips *(Golden Dipt)*, 1 1/4 oz.	120
blackened redfish *(Golden Dipt)*, 1/4 tsp.	2
broiled *(Golden Dipt)*, 1/4 tsp.	2
fish fry *(Golden Dipt)*, 2/3 oz.	60
fish fry, Cajun style *(Golden Dipt)*, 2/3 oz.	60
seafood *(Golden Dipt)*, 2/3 oz.	60
seafood *(Tone's)*, 1 tsp.	10
seafood, all purpose *(Golden Dipt)*, 1/4 tsp.	2
seafood, Chesapeake *(Tone's)*, 1 tsp.	8
seafood, lemon pepper *(Golden Dipt)*, 1/4 tsp.	8
shrimp and crab, Cajun style *(Golden Dipt)*, 1/4 tsp.	2
herb, Italian *(Shake'n Bake)*, 1/4 pouch	80
onion ring batter *(Golden Dipt)*, 1 oz.	100
pork:	
(Shake'n Bake Original Recipe), 1/8 pouch	40
barbecue *(Shake'n Bake* Original Recipe), 1/8 pouch	40
extra crispy *(Shake'n Bake Oven Fry)*, 1/4 pouch	120
tempura batter *(Golden Dipt)*, 1 oz.	100

FLOUR, one cup, except as noted
See also "Cereal & Grain Products" and "Baking Powder, Baking Soda, & Starch"

---

	calories
all varieties, except self-rising *(Pillsbury's Best)*	400
all-purpose:	
(Ballard)	400
(Ceresota/Heckers), 4 oz.	390
(Red Band)	390
(White Deer)	400
regular or unbleached *(Gold Medal)*	400
regular or unbleached *(Robin Hood)*	400
amaranth *(Arrowhead Mills)*, 2 oz.	200
barley *(Arrowhead Mills)*, 2 oz.	200
bread *(Gold Medal Better For Bread)*	400
buckwheat, whole-grain *(Arrowhead Mills)*, 2 oz.	190
chickpea *(Arrowhead Mills)*, 2 oz.	200
corn:	
(Quaker Masa Harina De Maiz), 1.3 oz. or ⅓ cup .	137
(Quaker Masa Trigo), 1.3 oz. or ⅓ cup	149
white *(Tone's* Masa Harina), 1 tsp.	8
millet, whole-grain *(Arrowhead Mills)*, 2 oz.	185
oat, whole-grain *(Arrowhead Mills)*, 2 oz.	200
oat blend *(Gold Medal)*	390
rice *(Featherweight)*	500
rice, brown *(Arrowhead Mills)*, 2 oz.	200
rye, stone ground *(Robin Hood)*	360
rye, whole-grain *(Arrowhead Mills)*, 2 oz.	190
rye and wheat *(Pillsbury's Best* Bohemian Style)	400
self-rising:	
(Ballard/Pillsbury's Best)	380
(Gold Medal)	380
(Red Band)	380
(Robin Hood)	380
enriched *(Aunt Jemima)*, 1 oz., approx. ¼ cup	109
soy *(Arrowhead Mills)*, 2 oz.	250
teff, whole-grain *(Arrowhead Mills)*, 2 oz.	200
wheat gluten, vital *(Arrowhead Mills)*, 1 oz.	100
white:	
(Drifted Snow)	400

(Softasilk), 1 oz. or ¼ cup	100
(Wondra)	400
whole wheat:	
(Ceresota/Heckers), 4 oz.	400
(Gold Medal)	350
blend *(Gold Medal)*	380
pastry *(Arrowhead Mills)*, 2 oz.	180
stone ground *(Arrowhead Mills)*, 2 oz.	200
unbleached *(Arrowhead Mills)*, 2 oz.	200

YEAST, BAKER'S

	calories
(Fleischmann's Active Dry/RapidRise), .25 oz.	20
(Red Star Active Dry), .25 oz.	20
fresh or household *(Fleischmann's)*, .6 oz.	15

BAKING POWDER, BAKING SODA, & STARCH,
one teaspoon, except as noted

	calories
baking powder:	
(Davis)	8
(Featherweight Low Salt)	8
(Tone's)	5
baking soda *(Tone's)*	0
cornstarch *(Argo/Kingsford)*, 1 tbsp.	30
cornstarch *(Tone's)*	10
potato starch *(Featherweight)*, 1 cup	620

CRACKERS
See also "Rice & Grain Cakes"

	calories
bacon flavor *(Keebler* Toasteds), 4 pieces	60
bacon flavor thins *(Nabisco)*, 7 pieces	70
w/bacon and cheese *(Handi-Snacks)*, 1 pkg.	130
bran *(FiberRich)*, 1 piece	18

Crackers, continued
butter flavor:
(Escort), 3 pieces	70
(Keebler Club Low Salt), 4 pieces	60
(Keebler Toasteds Buttercrisp), 4 pieces	60
(Keebler Town House Regular/Low Salt), 4 pieces . .	70
(Pepperidge Farm Flutters), .75 oz.	100
(Ritz Regular/Low Salt), 4 pieces	70
(Ritz Bits Regular/Low Salt), 22 pieces	70
dairy *(Nabisco American Classic),* 4 pieces	70
thins *(Pepperidge Farm* Distinctive), 4 pieces	70

cheese or cheese flavor:
(Cheese Nips), 13 pieces	70
(Combos), 1.8 oz.	240
(Hain), 1 oz.	130
(Pepperidge Farm Snack Sticks), 8 pieces	130
(Ritz Bits), 22 pieces	70
(Rokeach), 25 pieces or 1 oz.	140
(Tid Bits), 16 pieces	70
cheddar *(Better Cheddars),* 10 pieces	70
cheddar *(Guppies),* .25 oz.	40
cheddar *(Keebler Town House Jrs.),* 8 pieces	80
cheddar, smoked *(Pepperidge Farm* Goldfish), 1 oz. .	130
cheddar or Parmesan *(Pepperidge Farm* Goldfish),	
1 oz.	120
Swiss *(Nabisco Swiss Cheese),* 7 pieces	70
thins *(Pepperidge Farm* Goldfish Thins), 4 pieces . . .	50

cheese sandwich:
cheddar *(Keebler Town House* & Cheddar), 1 piece .	70
and peanut butter *(Keebler),* 2 pieces	70
wheat and American cheese *(Keebler),* 1 piece	70
and cheese *(Handi-Snacks),* 1 pkg.	130
chicken flavored *(Chicken in a Biskit),* 7 pieces	80

chowder, *see "soup and oyster," page 40*
(Crisp & Light Crackerbread Regular/Salt Free), 1 slice	17

crispbread *(see also specific grains):*
(Dar-Vida), 1 piece	20
(Kavli Norwegian), 1 thick piece	35
(Kavli Norwegian), 2 thin pieces	40
(Wasa Breakfast), 1 piece	50
(Wasa Extra Crisp), 1 piece	25

(Wasa Fiber Plus), 1 piece	35
dark, regular or w/caraway *(Finn Crisp),* 2 pieces	38
garlic flavor *(Weight Watchers),* 2 pieces	30
high fiber *(Ryvita* Crisp Bread), 1 piece	23
high fiber *(Ryvita* Snackbread), 1 piece	14
croissant *(Carr's),* 1 piece	25
(Estee Unsalted), 4 pieces	60
(FFV Schooners), 33 pieces, approx. .5 oz.	60
(Featherweight Low Salt), 2 pieces	30
garlic *(Manischewitz Garlic Tams),* 10 pieces	153
graham, see *"Cookies, graham cracker," page 245*	
grain, mixed *(Harvest Crisps* 5 Grain), 6 pieces	60
grain, multi *(Pepperidge Farm* Wholesome), 4 pieces	70
(Hain Rich Regular/No Salt Added), 1 oz.	130
herb, garden *(Pepperidge Farm Flutters),* .75 oz.	100
high fiber, see *specific listings*	
(Manischewitz Tam-Tams), 10 pieces	147
(Manischewitz Tam-Tams No Salt), 10 pieces	138
matzo, 1 board, except as noted:	
(Manischewitz Daily Unsalted)	110
(Manischewitz Passover)	129
American *(Manischewitz)*	115
dietetic, thin *(Manischewitz)*	91
egg *(Manischewitz* Passover)	132
egg *(Manischewitz* Passover Crackers), 10 pieces	108
egg n' onion *(Manischewitz)*	112
miniature *(Manischewitz),* 10 pieces	90
tea, thin *(Manischewitz* Daily)	103
thin *(Manischewitz)*	100
whole wheat, w/bran *(Manischewitz)*	110
melba toast, .5 oz., except as noted:	
(Devonsheer Regular/Unsalted), 1 piece	16
(Devonsheer Rounds)	53
(Devonsheer Unsalted Rounds)	52
bacon *(Old London* Rounds)	53
garlic *(Devonsheer* Rounds)	56
garlic *(Old London* Rounds)	56
honey bran *(Devonsheer),* 1 piece	16
honey bran *(Devonsheer* Rounds)	52
oat *(Harvest Crisps),* 6 pieces or .5 oz.	60
onion *(Devonsheer* Rounds)	51

Crackers, melba toast, continued

onion *(Old London* Rounds)	52
pumpernickel *(Old London)*	54
rye *(Devonsheer* Regular/Unsalted), 1 piece	16
rye *(Devonsheer* Rounds)	53
rye *(Old London/Old London* Rounds)	52
sesame *(Devonsheer)*, 1 piece	16
sesame *(Devonsheer* Rounds)	57
sesame *(Old London* Regular/Unsalted)	55
sesame *(Old London* Rounds)	56
vegetable *(Devonsheer)*, 1 piece	16
wheat *(Estee* 6 calorie), 1 piece	6
wheat *(Estee* Snax), 1 oz.	100
wheat *(Old London)*	51
wheat, whole *(Devonsheer* Regular/Unsalted), 1 piece	16
white *(Old London* Regular/Unsalted)	51
white *(Old London* Rounds)	48
whole-grain *(Old London)*	52
whole-grain *(Old London* Rounds)	54
whole-grain *(Old London* Unsalted)	53
oat *(Oat Thins)*, 8 pieces or .5 oz.	70
oat bran *(Oat Bran Krisp)*	60
onion:	
(Hain Regular/No Salt Added), 1 oz.	130
(Keebler Toasteds), 4 pieces	60
(Manischewitz Onion Tams), 10 pieces	150
oyster, *see "soup and oyster," page 40*	
peanut butter:	
(Combos), 1.8 oz.	240
(Handi-Snacks), 1 pkg.	190
cheese *(Little Debbie)*, 1.4 oz.	190
toasty *(Little Debbie)*, 1.4 oz.	200
sandwich *(Ritz Bits)*, 6 pieces or .5 oz.	80
toast and *(Keebler)*, 2 pieces	70
(Pepperidge Farm Original Goldfish), 1 oz.	130
pizza *(Pepperidge Farm* Goldfish), 1 oz.	130
poppy, toasted *(Nabisco American Classic)*, 4 pieces	70
pretzel *(Pepperidge Farm* Goldfish), 1 oz.	110
pretzel *(Pepperidge Farm* Snack Sticks), 8 pieces	120
pumpernickel *(Pepperidge Farm* Snack Sticks), 8 pieces	140
rice, harvest *(Weight Watchers* Crispbread), 2 pieces	30

rice, toasted *(Pepperidge Farm* Wholesome), 4 pieces . . 60
rice bran *(Health Valley)*, 7 pieces 130
rye:
    (Hain Regular/No Salt Added), 1 oz. 120
    (Keebler Toasteds), 4 pieces 60
    (Rykrisp), .5 oz. 40
    dark *(Ryvita* Crisp Bread), 1 piece 26
    golden *(Wasa* Crispbread), 1 piece 35
    hearty *(Wasa* Crispbread), 1 piece 45
    light *(Finn Crisp* Hi-Fiber), 1 piece 35
    light *(Ryvita* Crisp Bread), 1 piece 26
    light *(Wasa* Crispbread Lite), 1 piece 25
    original *(Finn Crisp* Hi-Fiber), 1 piece 40
    seasoned *(Rykrisp/Rykrisp* Twindividuals), .5 oz. . . . 45
    sesame *(Rykrisp)*, .5 oz. 50
    sesame, toasted *(Ryvita* Crisp Bread), 1 piece 31
saltine:
    all varieties *(Premium)*, 5 pieces 60
    all varieties *(Zesta)*, 5 pieces 60
    (Premium Bits), 16 pieces 70
    (Rokeach), 10 pieces 120
sandwich, *see specific listings*
sesame:
    (Dar-Vida Crispbread), 1 piece 22
    (FFV Crisp), 1 piece 60
    (Hain Regular/No Salt Added), 1 oz. 140
    (Keebler Toasteds), 4 pieces 60
    (Pepperidge Farm Distinctive), 4 pieces 80
    (Pepperidge Farm Snack Sticks), 8 pieces 140
    bread wafer *(Meal Mates)*, 3 pieces 70
    golden *(Nabisco American Classic)*, 4 pieces 70
    golden *(Pepperidge Farm Flutters)*, .75 oz. 110
    savory *(Wasa* Crispbread), 1 piece 30
    wafer *(FFV* Crisp), 4 pieces 60
sesame and cheese *(Twigs* Snack Sticks), 5 pieces 70
sesame wheat *(Wasa* Crispbread), 1 piece 50
snack *(Rokeach)*, 9 pieces 130
soda or water:
    (Carr's Table Water, Bite Size), 2 pieces 25
    (Crown Pilot), .5-oz. piece 70
    (FFV Ocean Crisps), 1 piece 60

Crackers, soda or water, continued
    (North Castles English), 1 piece 10
    (Pepperidge Farm Distinctive English Water Biscuit),
        4 pieces 70
    (Royal Lunch), .5-oz. piece 60
    (Sailor Boy Pilot), 1 piece 100
soup and oyster:
    (Dandy), 20 pieces or .5 oz. 60
    (OTC), 1 piece 25
    (Oysterettes), 18 pieces or .5 oz. 60
sour cream and chive *(Hain* Regular/No Salt Added),
    1 oz. 130
sourdough *(Hain* Regular/Low Salt), 1 oz. 130
toast *(Uneeda* Biscuits Unsalted Tops), 3 pieces 60
vegetable:
    (Hain Regular/No Salt Added), 1 oz. 130
    (Vegetable Thins), 7 pieces 70
    garden *(Pepperidge Farm* Wholesome), 5 pieces 60
water, *see "soda or water," page 39*
(Waverly Regular/Low Salt), 4 pieces 70
wheat:
    (FFV Crispy Wafer), 6 pieces 70
    (FFV Stoned Wheat Wafer), 4 pieces 60
    (Health Valley Stoned Wheat Regular/No Salt
        Added), 13 pieces 120
    (Manischewitz Wheat Tams), 10 pieces 150
    (Red Oval Farms Stoned Wheat Thins), 1 piece 30
    (Ryvita Original Snackbread), 1 piece 20
    (Sociables), 6 pieces 70
    (Triscuit Regular/Low Salt), 3 pieces 60
    (Triscuit Bits), 8 pieces 60
    (Wheat Thins Regular/Low Salt), 8 pieces 70
    (Wheatsworth Stone Ground), 4 pieces 70
    cracked *(Nabisco American Classic),* 4 pieces 70
    cracked *(Pepperidge Farm* Distinctive), 3 pieces 100
    hearty *(Pepperidge Farm* Distinctive), 4 pieces 100
    herb *(Health Valley* Stoned Wheat Regular/No Salt
        Added), 13 pieces 120
    nutty *(Wheat Thins),* 7 pieces 70
    sesame *(Health Valley* Stoned Wheat Regular/No
        Salt Added), 13 pieces 130

toasted *(Pepperidge Farm Flutters)*, .75 oz.	110
toasted, w/onion *(Pepperidge Farm* Distinctive), 4 pieces.	80
vegetable, seven grain *(Health Valley* Stoned Wheat Regular/No Salt Added), 13 pieces	120
whole *(Carr's)*, 2 pieces	70
whole *(Keebler Wheatables)*, 12 pieces	70
whole *(Manischewitz)*, 10 pieces	90
whole-grain *(Keebler Harvest Wheats)*, 4 pieces	60
whole-grain *(Wasa* Crispbread), 1 piece	30
wheat 'n bran *(Triscuit)*, 3 pieces	60
zwieback toast *(Nabisco)*, 2 pieces	60

RICE & GRAIN CAKES, one piece, except as noted
See also "Crackers"

---

	calories
corn or rye cake *(Quaker* Grain Cakes)	35
rice cake:	
(Hain Regular/Unsalted)	40
(Hain Regular/Unsalted Mini), .5 oz.	50
(Quaker Regular/Unsalted)	35
all varieties *(Lundberg* Sodium Free/Very Low Sodium)	60
apple cinnamon *(Hain* Mini), .5 oz.	50
barbecue *(Hain* Mini), .5 oz.	70
barley and oats *(Mother's)*	34
brown rice *(Konriko* Original Unsalted)	30
buckwheat *(Mother's* Unsalted)	35
cheese *(Hain* Mini), .5 oz.	60
corn *(Quaker/Mother's)*	35
five grain *(Hain)*	40
honey nut *(Hain* Mini), .5 oz.	60
multigrain *(Quaker/Mother's)*	34
multigrain *(Quaker/Mother's* Unsalted)	35
rye *(Quaker)*	34
sesame *(Hain* Regular/Unsalted)	40
sesame *(Quaker/Mother's* Regular/Unsalted)	35
teriyaki *(Hain* Mini), .5 oz.	50
wheat cake *(Quaker* Grain Cakes)	34

Chapter 3

CREAM, MILK, AND MILK BEVERAGES

MILK, eight fluid ounces, except as noted
See also "Cream" and "Flavored Milk Beverages"

	calories
buttermilk, cultured:	
(Crowley/Crowley Unsalted)	110
lowfat 2% *(Knudsen)*	120
lowfat 1.5% *(Borden* Golden Churn)	120
lowfat 1.5% *(Friendship* Unsalted)	120
lowfat, 2% fat:	
(Borden Hi-Protein)	140
(Crowley/Crowley Tone Acidophilus)	120
(Knudsen/Knudsen Sweet Acidophilus)	140
(Viva)	120
lowfat, 1% fat:	
(Borden)	100
(Crowley/Crowley Lactaid)	100
(Knudsen Nice n' Light, High Nutrient)	130
calcium added *(Darigold)*	100
protein fortified *(Crowley)*	120
skim:	
(Borden)	90
(Borden Skim-Line)	100
(Crowley)	90
(Knudsen)	80
(Weight Watchers)	90
whole:	
(Borden/Borden Hi-Calcium)	150
(Crowley)	150

(Knudsen)	160
condensed, sweetened, canned, 1/3 cup:	
(Borden)	320
(Carnation)	320
(Diehl Jerzee)	320
(Eagle)	320
dry, nonfat, instant:	
(Carnation), 5 level tbsp.	80
(Sanalac Dairy Fresh), .8 oz.	80
(Weight Watchers Dairy Creamer), 1 pkt.	10
evaporated, canned, 1/2 cup:	
(Carnation)	170
(Diehl)	170
(Pet)	170
imitation, filled *(Diehl)*	150
lowfat *(Carnation)*	110
skim *(Carnation)*	100
skim *(Diehl)*	100
skim *(Pet Light)*	100

CREAM
See also "Milk" and "Creamers, Nondairy"

	calories
half and half *(Crowley)*, 1 fl. oz.	35
sour, *see "Sour Cream," below*	

SOUR CREAM
See also "Cream"

	calories
(Bison), 1 oz.	50
(Crowley), 1 oz.	50
(Friendship), 1 oz. or 2 tbsp.	55
half and half *(Sealtest Light)*, 1 tbsp.	25
light *(Crowley)*, 1 oz.	30
light *(Weight Watchers)*, 1 oz. or 2 tbsp.	35

CREAMERS, NONDAIRY, one teaspoon, except as noted
See also "Cream"

	calories
(Crowley), ½ oz.	16
(Diehl)	10
(N-Rich)	10
liquid *(Coffee-mate),* 1 tbsp.	16
liquid, frozen *(Rich's Coffee Rich/Farm Rich/*	
Poly Rich), ½ oz.	20
powdered:	
(Coffee-mate)	10
(Coffee-mate Lite)	8
(Cremora)	10

FLAVORED MILK BEVERAGES, eight fluid ounces, except as noted
See also "Cocoa & Flavored Mixes, Dry"

	calories
all flavors *(Sego),* 10 fl. oz.	225
chocolate flavor:	
(Frostee)	200
mix* *(Nestlé Quik)*	230
mix* *(Nestlé Quik* Sugar Free)	140
regular or malt, mix* *(Pillsbury* Instant Breakfast)	290
chocolate milk, dairy pack:	
(Hershey's)	210
(Meadow Gold)	210
lowfat 2% *(Borden* Dutch Brand)	180
lowfat 2% *(Hershey's)*	190
lowfat 1% *(Knudsen)*	190
cocoa mix**:	
(Hills Bros), 6 fl. oz.	110
(Hills Bros Sugar Free), 6 fl. oz.	60
eggnog, canned *(Borden),* 4 fl. oz.	160
eggnog, dairy pack *(Crowley),* 6 fl. oz.	270
milkshake, frozen:	
chocolate *(MicroMagic),* 7 fl. oz.	200

chocolate or strawberry *(MicroMagic)*, 11.5 fl. oz. . .   340
vanilla *(MicroMagic)*, 11.5 fl. oz.   380
strawberry flavor:
    (Frostee)   180
    mix* *(Nestlé Quik)*   220
    mix* *(Pillsbury* Instant Breakfast)   290
vanilla flavor, mix* *(Pillsbury* Instant Breakfast)   300

* Prepared according to package directions, with whole milk
** Prepared according to package directions

Chapter 4

YOGURT

YOGURT & YOGURT DRINKS
See also "Frozen Yogurt"

	calories
plain:	
(Bison Lowfat), 1 cup	150
(Bison Nonfat), 1 cup	120
(Columbo Nonfat Lite), 8 oz.	110
(Colombo Whole Milk), 8 oz.	160
(Crowley), 1 cup	160
(Crowley Lowfat), 1 cup	140
(Crowley Nonfat), 1 cup	120
(Dannon Lowfat), 8 oz.	140
(Dannon Nonfat), 8 oz.	110
(Friendship Lowfat 1.5%), 1 cup	150
(Weight Watchers Nonfat), 1 cup	90
(Yoplait), 6 oz.	130
(Yoplait Nonfat), 8 oz.	120
all flavors:	
(Bison Lowfat), 1 cup	210
(Dannon Fresh Flavors), 8 oz.	200
(Dannon Fruit on the Bottom), 8 oz.	240
(Dannon Fruit on the Bottom), 4.4 oz.	130
(Friendship Lowfat), 1 cup	210
(New Country Regular/Lowfat/Supreme), 6 oz.	150
(Ripple 70), 6 oz.	70
(Weight Watchers Ultimate 90), 1 cup	90
(Yoplait Custard Style), 4 oz.	130
(Yoplait Fat Free), 6 oz.	150

all fruit flavors:

    (Colombo Nonfat Fruit on the Bottom), 8 oz. 190

    (Colombo Nonfat Lite Minipack), 4.4 oz. 100

    (Colombo Whole Milk Fruit on the Bottom), 8 oz. . 230

    (Crowley Nonfat), 1 cup 100

    (Crowley Sundae Style), 1 cup 250

    (Crowley Swiss Style), 1 cup 240

    (Yoplait), 6 oz. 190

    (Yoplait Light), 6 oz. 90

    except cherry and mixed berries *(Yoplait Custard*
        Style), 6 oz. 190

berries, mixed:

    (Dannon Extra Smooth), 4.4 oz. 130

    (Yoplait Breakfast Yogurt), 6 oz. 210

    (Yoplait Custard Style), 6 oz. 180

berries or fruit, orchard, w/wheat, nuts, and raisins
    (Dannon Hearty Nuts & Raisins), 8 oz. 260

cherry *(Yoplait Custard Style),* 6 oz. 180

cherry, w/almonds *(Yoplait Breakfast Yogurt),* 6 oz. . . 200

cherry-vanilla *(Lite-Line* Swiss Style 1%), 1 cup 240

fruit, tropical *(Yoplait Breakfast Yogurt),* 6 oz. 210

peach *(Lite-Line* Swiss Style 1%), 1 cup 230

raspberry *(Meadow Gold* Lowfat 1.5%), 1 cup 250

strawberry:

    (Crowley Nonfat), 1 cup 190

    (Dannon Extra Smooth), 4.4 oz. 130

    (Lite-Line Lowfat 1%), 1 cup 240

strawberry-almond *(Yoplait Breakfast Yogurt),* 6 oz. . . 200

strawberry-banana *(Yoplait Breakfast Yogurt),* 6 oz. . . . 220

vanilla:

    (Colombo French), 8 oz. 215

    (Crowley Lowfat), 1 cup 200

    (Dannon Fresh Flavors), 4.4 oz. 110

    (Yoplait/Yoplait Custard Style), 6 oz. 180

    (Yoplait Nonfat), 8 oz. 180

    w/wheat, nuts, and raisins *(Dannon* Hearty Nuts &
        Raisins), 8 oz. 270

yogurt drink, all flavors *(Dan'up),* 8 oz. 190

FROZEN YOGURT, 1/2 cup, except as noted
See also "Yogurt & Yogurt Drinks"

---

	calories
plain *(Crowley* Peaks of Perfection), 3.5 fl. oz.	90
all flavors:	
(Crowley), 3 fl. oz.	80
(Dreyer's Inspirations), 3 oz.	80
except cherry or chocolate *(Sealtest Free)*	100
soft-serve *(Crowley* Peaks of Perfection), 3.5 fl. oz. . .	100
soft-serve *(Dannon* Nonfat)	90
all flavors, except chocolate, soft-serve *(Dannon)*	100
caramel chunk *(Colombo* Gourmet), 3 fl. oz.	120
cherry, black *(Breyers)*	120
cherry, black, or chocolate *(Sealtest Free)*	110
chocolate:	
(Bison), 3.5 fl. oz.	94
(Breyers)	120
soft-serve *(Dannon)*	120
chocolate chunk, Bavarian *(Colombo* Gourmet),	
3 fl. oz.	120
chocolate or vanilla *(Häagen-Dazs),* 3 fl. oz.	130
mocha Swiss almond *(Colombo* Gourmet), 3 fl. oz. . . .	120
Heath Bar crunch *(Colombo* Gourmet), 3 fl. oz.	130
peach *(Breyers)*	110
peach or strawberry *(Häagen-Dazs),* 3 fl. oz.	120
peanut butter crunch *(Colombo* Gourmet), 3 fl. oz. . . .	140
raspberry, red *(Breyers)*	120
raspberry, wild, cheesecake *(Colombo* Gourmet),	
3 fl. oz.	100
strawberry or strawberry-banana *(Breyers)*	110
strawberry passion *(Colombo* Gourmet), 3 fl. oz.	100
vanilla *(Breyers)*	120
vanilla almond crunch *(Häagen-Dazs),* 3 fl. oz.	150
vanilla dream *(Colombo* Gourmet), 3 fl. oz.	90

Chapter 5

CHEESE AND
CHEESE PRODUCTS

CHEESE*, one ounce, except as noted
See also "Cheese, Substitute & Imitation," "Cheese Food," "Cheese Product," and "Cheese Spreads"

---

	calories
American, processed:	
(Borden)	110
(Dorman's/Dorman's Loaf Low Sodium)	110
(Hoffman's)	110
(Kraft Deluxe)	110
(Land O'Lakes)	110
hot pepper *(Sargento)*	110
sharp *(Old English)*	110
asiago, wheel *(Frigo)*	110
babybel *(Laughing Cow)*	91
babybel, mini *(Laughing Cow)*, ¾ oz.	74
(Bel Paese Domestic Traditional)	101
(Bel Paese Imported)	90
(Bel Paese Lite)	76
(Bel Paese Medallion Process)	71
blue:	
(Dorman's Danablu 50%)	100
(Dorman's Danablu 60%)	108
(Frigo)	100
(Kraft)	100
(Sargento)	100
blue castello or saga *(Dorman's* 70%)	134
bonbel *(Laughing Cow)*	100
bonbel, mini *(Laughing Cow)*, ¾ oz.	74

Cheese*, continued

bonbino *(Laughing Cow)*	103
brick:	
(Dorman's)	110
(Kraft)	110
(Land O'Lakes)	110
Brie *(Dorman's)*	81
Brie *(Sargento)*	100
burger cheese *(Sargento)*	110
Cajun *(Sargento)*	110
caljack *(Churney)*	100
Camembert:	
(Dorman's 45%)	82
(Dorman's 50%)	89
(Sargento)	90
caraway *(Kraft)*	100
cheddar:	
(Alpine Lace Cheddar Flavored)	100
(Darigold)	110
(Dorman's)	110
(Dorman's Chedda-Delite)	90
(Featherweight Low Sodium)	110
(Frigo)	110
(Kraft)	110
(Land O'Lakes)	110
(Laughing Cow)	110
(Sargento/Sargento New York)	110
all varieties *(Weight Watchers* Natural)	80
mild, reduced fat *(Kraft* Light Naturals)	80
reduced fat *(Dorman's* Low Sodium)	80
sharp or extra sharp *(Axelrod)*	110
sharp, reduced fat *(Kraft* Light Naturals)	90
sharp, slicing *(Boar's Head)*	110
smokey or super sharp, processed *(Hoffman's)*	110
Vermont *(Churny)*	110
cheddar jack *(Dorman's* Chedda-Jack)	90
colby:	
(Alpine Lace Colby-Lo)	80
(Dorman's)	110
(Kraft)	110
(Land O'Lakes)	110

(Sargento)	110
(Weight Watchers Natural)	80
reduced fat *(Kraft* Light Naturals)	80
colby jack *(Sargento)*	110
cottage, *see "Cottage Cheese," page 59*	
cream cheese:	
(Crowley)	110
(Darigold)	99
(Dorman's 65%)	90
(Dorman's 70%)	102
(Philadelphia Brand)	100
w/chives or pimento *(Philadelphia Brand)*	90
cream cheese, soft:	
(Friendship)	103
(Philadelphia Brand)	100
all flavors, except w/chives and onion or w/honey *(Philadelphia Brand)*	90
w/chives and onion or w/honey *(Philadelphia Brand)*	100
cream cheese, whipped:	
(Philadelphia Brand)	100
all flavors *(Philadelphia Brand)*	90
danbo *(Dorman's 20%)*	62
danbo *(Dorman's 45%)*	98
(Dorman's Crema Dania 70%)	134
Edam:	
(Dorman's)	100
(Dorman's 45%)	91
(Kaukauna)	100
(Kraft)	90
(Land O'Lakes)	100
(Laughing Cow)	100
(May-Bud)	100
(Sargento)	100
farmer:	
(Friendship Regular/No Salt Added), 1/2 cup	160
(Kaukauna)	100
(May-Bud)	90
(Sargento)	100
feta:	
(Churny Natural)	75

Cheese*, feta, continued
  (Dorman's 45%)   91
  (Sargento)   80
fontina *(Sargento)*   110
gjetost *(Sargento)*   130
Gouda:
  (Dorman's)   100
  (Kraft)   110
  (Land O'Lakes)   100
  (Laughing Cow)   110
  (May-Bud)   100
  (Sargento)   100
  all varieties *(Kaukauna)*   100
  mini *(Laughing Cow)*, ¾ oz.   80
grated *(Polly-O)*   130
havarti:
  (Casino)   120
  (Dorman's 45%)   91
  (Dorman's 60%)   118
  (Sargento)   120
hot pepper *(Hickory Farms)*   106
Italian style, grated *(Sargento)*   110
Jarlsberg *(Norseland Jarlsberg)*   97
(Laughing Cow Reduced mini), ¾ oz.   45
Limburger *(Sargento)*   90
Limburger, natural *(Mohawk Valley* Little Gem)   90
mascarpone *(Galbani* Imported)   128
Monterey Jack:
  (Alpine Lace Monti-Jack-Lo)   80
  (Darigold)   110
  (Dorman's)   100
  (Kaukauna)   110
  (Land O'Lakes)   110
  (May-Bud)   110
  (Sargento)   110
  (Weight Watchers Natural)   80
  all varieties *(Axelrod)*   100
  all varieties *(Kraft)*   110
  w/peppers, mild *(Casino)*   110
  reduced fat *(Dorman's* Low Sodium)   80
  reduced fat *(Kraft* Light Naturals)   80

mozzarella:

(Dorman's)	90
(Polly-O Lite)	70
(Weight Watchers Natural)	70
fresh *(Polly-O Fior di Latte)*	80
low moisture *(Casino)*	90
shredded *(Weight Watchers)*	70
whole milk *(Crowley)*	90
whole milk *(Polly-O)*	90
whole milk *(Sargento)*	90
whole milk, low moisture *(Frigo)*	90
part skim *(Crowley)*	70
part skim *(Polly-O)*	80
part skim, low moisture *(Alpine Lace)*	70
part skim, low moisture *(Frigo)*	80
part skim, low moisture *(Kraft)*	80
part skim, low moisture *(Land O'Lakes)*	80
part skim, low moisture *(Sargento)*	80
part skim, reduced fat *(Frigo)*	60
part skim, w/jalapeño pepper *(Kraft)*	80
part skim or reduced fat *(Dorman's* Low Sodium)	80

Muenster:

(Alpine Lace)	100
(Dorman's Regular/Low Sodium)	110
(Dorman's 50%)	100
(Kaukauna)	110
(Land O'Lakes)	100
red rind *(Sargento)*	100
reduced fat *(Dorman's* Low Sodium)	80

Neufchâtel:

garlic and herbs or garden vegetable *(Kaukauna)*	80
light *(Philadelphia Brand)*	80

Parmesan:

(Kraft)	110
fresh *(Sargento)*	110
grated *(Frigo)*	130
grated *(Kraft)*	130
grated *(Polly-O)*	130
grated *(Sargento)*	130
Reggiano *(Galbani* Imported)	105
wheel or fresh grated *(Frigo)*	110

Cheese*, continued

Parmesan and Romano, grated *(Frigo)*	130
Parmesan and Romano, grated *(Sargento)*	110
pimiento, processed *(Kraft* Deluxe)	100
pasta, Italian, grated *(Frigo* Parmazest)	120
pizza, shredded *(Frigo)*	90
pizza, shredded, low fat *(Frigo)*	65
pot cheese *(Sargento)*	25
Primavera *(Bel Paese* Lite)	68
provolone:	
(Alpine Lace Provo-Lo)	70
(Dorman's Regular/Low Sodium)	90
(Kraft)	100
(Land O'Lakes)	100
(Sargento)	100
regular or smoked *(Frigo)*	100
Queso blanco *(Sargento)*	100
Queso de papa *(Sargento)*	110
ricotta:	
(Polly-O Lite), 2 oz.	80
(Sargento)	40
(Sargento Lite)	23
whole milk *(Crowley)*, 2 oz.	100
whole milk *(Frigo)*	50
whole milk *(Polly-O)*, 2 oz.	100
low fat *(Frigo)*	20
part skim *(Crowley)*, 2 oz.	80
part skim *(Frigo)*	45
part skim *(Polly-O)*, 2 oz.	90
part skim *(Sargento)*	30
Romano:	
(Kraft Natural)	110
(Sargento)	110
grated *(Frigo)*	130
grated *(Kraft)*	130
grated *(Polly-O)*	130
wedge *(Frigo)*	110
Slim Jack *(Dorman's)*	90
smoked *(Sargento* Smokestick)	100
string:	
(Frigo)	80

(Polly-O), 1-oz. stick	90
low moisture *(Kraft)*	80
regular or smoked *(Sargento)*	80
Swiss:	
(Alpine Lace Swiss-Lo)	100
(Boar's Head Domestic)	110
(Boar's Head No Salt Added)	100
(Casino)	110
(Dorman's Regular/No Salt Added)	100
(Dorman's Reduced Fat)	90
(Kraft Light Naturals)	90
(Kraft 75% Very Low Sodium)	110
(Land O'Lakes)	110
(Sargento/Sargento Finland)	110
(Weight Watchers Natural)	90
processed *(Borden)*	100
processed *(Kraft* Deluxe)	90
regular or aged *(Kraft)*	110
smoked *(Dorman's)*	100
taco:	
(Sargento)	110
shredded *(Frigo)*	110
shredded *(Kraft)*	110
taleggio *(Tal-Fino* Brand Imported)	89
Tilsiter *(Sargento)*	100
Tybo *(Dorman's* 45%)	98
Tybo, red wax *(Sargento)*	100

* Note: Unless otherwise noted, the figure listed for any cheese above applies to all of the forms in which it may be packaged—slices, loaves, wedges, and the like. Be careful not to confuse "real" cheese with a "cheese spread" or "cheese food" that bears the same or a similar name. Generally, it isn't hard to differentiate between cheese and cheese spreads, but cheese foods sometimes pose a problem (especially when they're packaged in slices). Check the label if you're confused about a product; if it is a cheese food, the label will say so.

CHEESE, SUBSTITUTE & IMITATION, one ounce
See also "Cheese Food" and "Cheese Product"

	calories
all varieties:	
(Churny Delicia)	80
except creamed cheese *(Weight Watchers)*	50
imitation *(Frigo)*	90
American *(Golden Image)*	90
cheddar:	
imitation *(Sargento)*	90
mild, imitation *(Golden Image)*	110
shredded *(Fisher Ched-O-Mate)*	90
cheese food:	
(Cheeztwin)	90
(Fisher Sandwich-Mate)	90
(Lite-Line Low Cholesterol)	90
colby *(Dorman's* LoChol)	90
colby, imitation *(Golden Image)*	110
cream cheese, imitation, all flavors *(Tofutti Better than Cream Cheese)*	80
creamed cheese *(Weight Watchers)*	35
mozzarella, imitation *(Sargento)*	80
mozzarella, shredded *(Fisher Pizza-Mate)*	90
Muenster or Swiss *(Dorman's* LoChol)	100
(Nucoa Heart Beat)	50

CHEESE FOOD, one ounce
See also "Cheese Product"

	calories
all varieties:	
(Cracker Barrel)	90
(Kaukauna Lite)	70
(Velveeta)	100
cold pack *(Kaukauna* Cup)	100
cold pack *(Wispride)*	100
except salami *(Land O'Lakes)*	90
except sharp *(Kraft* Singles)	90

American:
(Borden Slices) 100
(Borden Singles) 90
(Darigold) 80
colored (Hoffman's) 100
grated (Kraft) 130
sharp (Borden Singles) 90
w/bacon (Hoffman's Chees'N Bacon) 90
w/bacon (Kraft/Kraft Cheez'N Bacon) 90
w/caraway (Hoffman's Swisson Rye) 90
w/garlic (Kraft) 90
w/jalapeño pepper (Hoffman's) 90
w/jalapeño pepper (Kraft) 90
(Nippy) 90
w/onion (Hoffman's Chees'N Onion) 100
salami (Hoffman's Chees'N Salami) 90
salami (Land O'Lakes) 100
sharp (Kraft Singles) 100
smoked (Smokelle) 90

CHEESE-NUT BALL OR LOG, one ounce

	calories
ball or log, all varieties (Cracker Barrel)	90
ball or log, all varieties (Kaukauna)	100
log, cheddar, sharp or port wine (Sargento)	100
log, Swiss almond (Sargento)	90

CHEESE PRODUCT, processed, one ounce
*See also "Cheese, Substitute & Imitation" and
"Cheese Food"*

	calories
all varieties (Light N' Lively Singles)	70
all varieties (Lite-Line)	50
American flavor:	
(Alpine Lace)	90
(Borden Light)	70
(Harvest Moon)	70

Cheese Product, American flavor, continued

(Lite-Line Reduced Sodium/Sodium Lite)	70
cream cheese, light *(Philadelphia Brand)*	60
pizza topping *(Lunch Wagon)*	80
sandwich slices *(Lunch Wagon)*	90

> **CHEESE SPREADS,** one ounce, except as noted
> *See also "Dips"*

---

calories

all varieties:

(Cheez Whiz)	80
(Squeeze-A-Snak)	80
(Weight Watchers Cup), 1 oz. or 2 tbsp.	70

American, processed:

(Kraft)	80
sharp or pimiento *(Sargento* Cracker Snacks)	110
w/bacon *(Kraft)*	80
blue *(Roka)*	70
brick *(Sargento* Cracker Snacks)	100
cream, *see "Cheese, cream cheese" page 51*	
w/garlic *(Kraft)*	80
w/jalapeño pepper *(Kraft)*	70
w/jalapeño pepper, loaf *(Kraft)*	80
(Land O'Lakes Golden Velvet)	80
(Laughing Cow Cheezbits), 1/6 oz.	13
Limburger *(Mohawk Valley)*	70
Mexican or pimiento *(Velveeta)*	80
(Micro Melt)	80
Neufchâtel, *see "Cheese, Neufchâtel" page 53*	
olives and pimiento *(Kraft)*	60
pimiento or pineapple *(Kraft)*	70
sharp *(Old English)*	80
Swiss *(Sargento* Cracker Snacks)	100
(Velveeta)	80
(Velveeta Slices)	90

COTTAGE CHEESE, 1/2 cup, except as noted

	calories
creamed:	
(Bison 4% fat)	120
(Borden 4% fat Regular/Unsalted)	120
(Breakstone's), 4 oz.	110
(Crowley 4% fat)	120
(Friendship California Style 4%)	120
chive *(Bison)*	120
garden salad *(Bison)*	110
w/peaches or pineapple *(Crowley* 4% fat)	140
w/pineapple *(Bison)*	140
w/pineapple *(Friendship* 4%)	140
dry curd, unsalted *(Borden)*	80
lowfat:	
2% *(Breakstone's)*, 4 oz.	100
2% *(Weight Watchers)*	100
1½% *(Lite-Line)*	90
1% *(Bison)*	90
1% *(Crowley* Regular/No Salt Added)	90
1% *(Friendship* Regular/No Salt Added)	90
1% *(Weight Watchers)*	90
calcium fortified, 1% *(Crowley)*	90
lactose reduced, 1% *(Friendship)*	90
w/pineapple, 1% *(Crowley)*	110
w/pineapple, 1% *(Friendship)*	110
nonfat *(Knudsen)*, 4 oz.	70
pot style, large curd, lowfat 2% *(Friendship)*	100

CHEESE DISHES, FROZEN
See also "Dinners, Frozen" and "Entrees, Frozen"

	calories
blintzes:	
(King Kold), 2.5-oz. piece	113
(King Kold No Salt Added), 2.5-oz. piece	96
nuggets, mozzarella, breaded *(Banquet Cheese Hot Bites)*, 2.63 oz.	240

Cheese Dishes, Frozen, continued

sticks, breaded:

cheddar *(Farm Rich)*, 3 oz.	300
hot pepper *(Farm Rich)*, 3 oz.	260
mozzarella *(Farm Rich)*, 3 oz.	240
provolone *(Farm Rich)*, 3 oz.	270

Chapter 6

FRUIT AND
FRUIT PRODUCTS

FRUIT, CANNED OR IN JARS, 1/2 cup, except as noted
See also "Fruit, Dried" and "Fruit, Frozen"

---

	calories
apple:	
baked, whole *(Lucky Leaf/Musselman's)*, 1 apple . .	110
baked style *(White House)*, 3.5 oz.	118
chipped or diced *(Lucky Leaf/Musselman's)*, 4 oz. .	50
chipped, in water *(White House)*, 4 oz.	50
dessert, sliced *(Lucky Leaf/Musselman's)*, 4 oz.	70
rings, spiced *(White House)*, 3.5 oz.	180
rings, spiced, red/green *(Lucky Leaf/Musselman's)*, 4 oz.	100
sliced, sweetened *(White House)*, 4 oz.	54
sliced, in water *(White House)*, 4 oz.	40
sliced, unpeeled *(Lucky Leaf/Musselman's)*, 4 oz. . .	90
applesauce:	
(Del Monte)	90
(Del Monte Lite)	50
(Featherweight)	50
(Hunt's Snack Pack), 4.25 oz.	80
(Lucky Leaf/Musselman's Regular or Chunky), 4 oz.	80
(Lucky Leaf/Musselman's Unsweetened), 4 oz.	50
(Mott's), 6 oz.	150
(Mott's Chunky), 6 oz.	86
(Mott's Natural), 6 oz.	80

Fruit, Canned or in Jars, applesauce, continued

(S&W)	90
(S&W Nutradiet/S&W Unsweetened)	55
(Stokely)	90
(Stokely Unsweetened)	45
(Tree Top Original)	80
(White House Regular or Chunky), 4 oz.	80
(White House Unsweetened), 4 oz.	50
in apple juice (White House), 4 oz.	50
cinnamon (Mott's), 6 oz.	152

apricot:

whole, peeled (Del Monte)	100
halves, unpeeled (Del Monte)	100
halves, unpeeled (Del Monte Lite)	60
in water, unpeeled, halves (S&W/Nutradiet)	35
in water, peeled, whole (S&W/Nutradiet)	28
in juice (Featherweight)	50
in juice, unpeeled (Libby Lite)	60
in heavy syrup, halves (S&W)	110
in heavy syrup, whole, peeled (S&W)	100
blackberry, in water (Allens)	25
blueberry, in water (Lucky Leaf/Musselman's), 4 oz.	40
blueberry, in heavy syrup (S&W)	111

cherry:

sour, red, pitted (White House), 3.5 oz.	43
sour, red, pitted, in water (Stokely)	45
tart, red, pitted (Lucky Leaf/Musselman's), 4 oz.	50
sweet, dark (Del Monte)	90
sweet, light, w/pits (Del Monte)	100
sweet, packaged (Mott's Cherry Fruit Pak), 3.75 oz.	72
cherry, black, fruit concentrate (Hain), 1 oz. or 2 tbsp.	67
citrus salad (Florigold), 8 oz.	120
crabapple, spiced (Lucky Leaf/Musselman's), 4 oz.	110
cranberry fruit concentrate (Hain), 1 oz. or 2 tbsp.	45

cranberry sauce:

whole or jellied (Ocean Spray), 2 oz.	90
whole or jellied (S&W Old Fashioned)	90
cranberry sauce, w/apple, orange, raspberry or strawberry (Ocean Spray Cran-Fruit), 2 oz.	100
figs, in heavy syrup, whole (Del Monte)	100
figs, kadota, in heavy syrup, whole (S&W Fancy)	100

fruit, mixed:
    (Del Monte Fruit Cup), 5 oz.   100
    chunky *(Del Monte)*   80
    chunky *(Del Monte Lite)*   50
    chunky *(S&W/Nutradiet)*   40
    in juice, chunky *(Libby Lite)*   50
    in sweetened clarified juice *(S&W)*   90
fruit cocktail:
    (Del Monte)   80
    (Del Monte Lite)   50
    (S&W/Nutradiet Regular/Unsweetened)   40
    in juice *(Featherweight)*   50
    in juice *(Libby Lite)*   50
    in sweetened clarified juice *(S&W)*   90
    in heavy syrup *(S&W)*   90
fruit compote *(Rokeach)*, 4 oz.   120
fruit for salad or fruit salad, tropical *(Del Monte)*   90
grapefruit sections:
    (S&W/Nutradiet/S&W Unsweetened)   40
    in juice *(Featherweight)*   40
    in light syrup *(S&W)*   80
    in light syrup *(Stokely)*   90
grapes, in heavy syrup *(S&W* Premium Thompson) . .   100
orange, Mandarin, *see "tangerine," page 64*
peach:
    (Mott's Peach Fruit Pak), 3.75 oz.   75
    freestone, halves or slices *(Del Monte)*   90
    freestone, halves or slices *(Del Monte Lite)*   60
    freestone, halves or slices *(S&W/Nutradiet)*   30
    yellow cling *(Del Monte* Fruit Cup), 5 oz.   110
    yellow cling, halves or slices *(Del Monte)*   80
    yellow cling, halves or slices *(Del Monte Lite)*   50
    yellow cling, halves or slices *(S&W/Nutradiet)*   30
    yellow cling, spiced, w/pits *(Del Monte)*, 3½ oz. . . .   80
    in juice, yellow cling, halves or slices *(Featherweight)*   50
    in juice, yellow cling, halves or slices *(Libby Lite)* . .   50
    in juice, yellow cling, sliced, sweetened *(S&W)*   90
    in heavy syrup, halves or slices *(S&W)*   100
    in heavy syrup, whole, spiced *(S&W)*   90
pear:
    Bartlett, halves or slices *(Del Monte)*   80

Fruit, Canned or in Jars, pear, continued

Bartlett, halves or slices *(Del Monte Lite)*	50
Bartlett, peeled *(S&W/Nutradiet)*	35
peeled halves or quarters *(S&W/Nutradiet)*	35
in juice, halves *(Featherweight)*	60
in juice, halves or slices *(Libby Lite)*	60
in juice, slices, sweetened *(S&W* Natural Style)	80
in heavy syrup, halves *(S&W)*	100

pineapple:

(Mott's Pineapple Fruit Pak), 3.75 oz.	86
in juice, all cuts *(Dole)*	70
in juice, spears *(Del Monte),* 2 spears	50
in juice, slices *(S&W* 100% Hawaiian)	70
in juice, slices, chunks, tidbits, or crushed *(Del Monte)*	70
in juice, crushed *(Empress)*	70
in syrup, all cuts *(Del Monte)*	90
in syrup, all cuts *(Dole)*	95
in heavy syrup, slices *(S&W* 100% Hawaiian), 2 slices	90
unsweetened, sliced *(S&W/Nutradiet)*	60

plum:

whole or halves, unpeeled *(S&W/Nutradiet)*	52
purple, in juice, whole *(Featherweight)*	80
purple, in light syrup *(Stokely)*	100
purple, in heavy syrup *(Stokely)*	130
purple, in extra heavy syrup, whole or halves, unpeeled *(S&W* Fancy)	135

tangerine:

(Del Monte Mandarin Orange), 5½ oz.	100
(S&W Natural Style)	60
in water *(Featherweight* Mandarin Orange)	35
in light syrup *(Dole)*	76
in light syrup *(Empress),* 5½ oz.	100
in heavy syrup *(S&W)*	76
unsweetened *(S&W/Nutradiet)*	28

FRUIT, DRIED (UNCOOKED)
See also "Fruit Snacks"

calories

apple:
chips *(Weight Watchers)*, .75-oz. pkg.	70
chunks *(Sun • Maid/Sunsweet)*, 2 oz.	150
slices *(Del Monte)*, 2 oz.	140
apricot *(Del Monte)*, 2 oz.	140
apricot *(Sun • Maid/Sunsweet)*, 2 oz.	140
banana chips, freeze-dried *(Mountain House)*, ½ cup .	248
currant, zante *(Del Monte)*, ½ cup	200

date, pitted:
(Bordo), 2 oz.	204
(Dole), ½ cup	280
(Dromedary), 1 oz. or 5 dates	100
chopped *(Dromedary)*, ¼ cup	130
diced *(Bordo)*, 2 oz..	203
figs, Calimyrna *(Blue Ribbon/Sun • Maid)*, ½ cup . . .	250
figs, Mission *(Blue Ribbon/Sun • Maid)*, ½ cup	210

fruit, mixed:
(Del Monte), 2 oz..	130
(Sun • Maid/Sunsweet) 2 oz.	150
bits *(Sun • Maid/Sunsweet)*, 2 oz..	150

raisins, seedless:
(Sun • Maid), ½ cup	290
Golden *(Del Monte)*, 3 oz..	260

FRUIT, FROZEN
See also "Fruit Bars, Frozen"

calories

apple, escalloped *(Stouffer's)*, 4 oz..	130
apple, glazed, in raspberry sauce *(The Budget Gourmet Side Dish)*, 5 oz.	110
apple fritter *(Mrs. Paul's)*, 2 pieces	240
apple sticks, breaded, fried *(Farm Rich)*, 4 oz.	260
cherry *(Lucky Leaf)*, 4 oz.	130
fruit, mixed, in syrup *(Birds Eye* Quick Thaw Pouch), 5 oz..	120

Fruit, Frozen, continued

raspberry, red, in lite syrup *(Birds Eye* Quick Thaw
      Pouch), 5 oz.   100
strawberry:
   in lite syrup, whole *(Birds Eye),* 4 oz.   80
   in lite syrup, halves *(Birds Eye* Quick Thaw Pouch),
      5 oz.   90
   in syrup, halves *(Birds Eye* Quick Thaw Pouch),
      5 oz.   120

FRUIT BARS, FROZEN, one serving
*See also "Frozen Yogurt" and "Ice Cream & Frozen
Confections"*

---

	calories
all flavors *(Dole Fresh Lites)*	25
all flavors *(Dole SunTops)*	40
all flavors *(Minute Maid Fruit Juicee),* 2.25 fl. oz.	60
berry, wild *(Sunkist* Fruit & Juice Bar)	103
coconut *(Sunkist),* 4 fl. oz.	170
lemonade *(Sunkist),* 4 fl. oz.	90
orange *(Sunkist* Juice Bar), 4 fl. oz.	100
piña colada *(Dole Fruit'n Juice)*	90
pineapple *(Dole Fruit'n Juice)*	70
raspberry or strawberry *(Dole Fruit'n Juice)*	70
wildberry *(Sunkist),* 4 fl. oz.	140
and cream:	
blueberry *(Dole* Fruit & Cream)	90
chocolate/banana *(Dole* Fruit & Cream)	175
chocolate/strawberry *(Dole* Fruit & Cream)	140
peach, raspberry or strawberry *(Dole* Fruit & Cream)	90
strawberry *(Sunkist),* 4 fl. oz.	90
and yogurt, cherry *(Dole* Fruit & Yogurt)	80
and yogurt, raspberry or strawberry *(Dole* Fruit &
Yogurt)	70

FRUIT JUICES, six fluid ounces, except as noted
See also "Fruit & Fruit-Flavored Drinks"

	calories
all flavors, except peach, nectar *(Libby's)*	110
apple:	
(Indian Summer)	90
(Kraft Pure 100%)	80
(Minute Maid), 8.45 fl. oz.	128
(Minute Maid Juices to Go), 9.6 fl. oz.	145
(Minute Maid On The Go), 10 fl. oz.	152
(Mott's)	88
(Mott's Natural Style)	76
(Ocean Spray)	90
(Red Cheek Natural/100% Pure)	97
(S&W 100% Pure Unsweetened)	85
(Tree Top)	90
(TreeSweet)	90
(Veryfine 100%), 8 fl. oz.	107
(White House)	87
blend *(Libby's Juicy Juice)*	90
sparkling *(Welch's)*	100
chilled or frozen* *(Minute Maid)*	91
chilled or frozen* *(Sunkist),* 8 fl. oz.	79
chilled or frozen* *(Tree Top)*	90
apple cider:	
(Indian Summer)	80
(Lucky Leaf/Musselman's)	90
cinnamon *(Indian Summer)*	90
sparkling *(Lucky Leaf)*	80
canned or frozen* *(Tree Top)*	90
apple-cherry:	
(Musselman's Breakfast Cocktail)	100
(Red Cheek)	113
cider *(Indian Summer)*	100
apple-citrus, canned or frozen* *(Tree Top)*	90
apple-cranberry:	
(Apple & Eve)	80
(Lucky Leaf)	130
(Mott's)	83
canned or frozen* *(Tree Top)*	100

Fruit Juices, apple-cranberry, continued

cider *(Indian Summer)*	100
apple-grape:	
(Libby's Juicy Juice)	90
(Mott's)	86
(Red Cheek)	109
canned or frozen* *(Tree Top)*	100
apple-pear, canned or frozen* *(Tree Top)*	90
apple-raspberry:	
(Mott's)	83
(Red Cheek)	113
canned or frozen* *(Tree Top)*	80
apricot nectar *(Del Monte)*	100
apricot nectar *(S&W)*	100
apricot-pineapple nectar *(S&W/Nutradiet)*, 4 fl. oz.	35
berry *(Libby's Juicy Juice)*	90
boysenberry *(Smucker's* Naturally 100%), 8 fl. oz.	120
cherry:	
black *(Smucker's* Naturally 100%), 8 fl. oz.	130
blend *(Dole Pure & Light* Mountain Cherry)	87
blend *(Libby's Juicy Juice)*	90
cranberry *(Lucky Leaf)*	110
cranberry *(Smucker's* Naturally 100%), 8 fl. oz.	130
fruit juice, tropical *(Libby's Juicy Juice)*	100
grape:	
(Kraft Pure 100% Unsweetened)	104
(Lucky Leaf)	130
(Minute Maid), 8.45 fl. oz.	150
(Sippin' Pak), 8.45 fl. oz.	130
(Veryfine 100%), 8 fl. oz.	153
(Welch's USDA)	120
blend *(Libby's Juicy Juice)*	100
Concord *(S&W* Unsweetened)	100
purple *(Welch's)*	120
red *(Welch's)*, 8.45 fl. oz.	170
red or white *(Welch's)*	120
sparkling, red *(Welch's)*	128
sparkling, white *(Welch's)*	120
white *(Welch's)*, 8.45 fl. oz.	160
chilled or frozen* *(Minute Maid)*	100
frozen* *(Sunkist)*	69

frozen* purple or white *(Welch's)* 100
grapefruit:
    (Del Monte) 70
    (Kraft Pure 100%) 70
    (Minute Maid) 78
    (Minute Maid On The Go), 10 fl. oz. 130
    (Mott's), 9.5-fl.-oz. can 118
    (Ocean Spray) 70
    (S&W) 80
    (Stokely) 76
    (Sunkist Fresh Squeezed), 8 fl. oz. 96
    (Tree Top) 80
    (Veryfine 100%), 8 fl. oz. 101
    pink *(Ocean Spray Pink Premium)* 60
    regular or pink *(TreeSweet)* 72
    chilled or frozen*, pink *(Minute Maid)* 78
    frozen* *(Minute Maid)* 83
    frozen* *(Sunkist)* 56
    frozen* *(TreeSweet)* 78
guava, bottled or frozen* *(Welch's Orchard* Tropicals) . 100
lemon:
    (ReaLemon), 1 fl. oz. 6
    (Lucky Leaf) 30
    (Minute Maid 100% Pure), 1 tbsp. 4
    chilled *(ReaLemon* 100%), 1 fl. oz. 6
    frozen* *(Sunkist)*, 1 fl. oz. 7
lime *(ReaLime)*, 1 fl. oz. 6
lime, bottled *(Rose's)*, 1 fl. oz. 48
orange:
    (Del Monte Unsweetened) 80
    (Minute Maid), 8.45 fl. oz. 129
    (Ocean Spray) 90
    (S&W) 83
    (Sippin' Pak), 8.45 fl. oz. 110
    (Stokely Unsweetened) 89
    (Sunkist) 84
    (Tree Top) 90
    (TreeSweet) 78
    (Veryfine 100%), 8 fl. oz. 121
    blend *(Minute Maid* Juices to Go), 9.6 fl. oz. 149
    blend *(Minute Maid On The Go)*, 10 fl. oz. 155

Fruit Juices, orange, continued

blend *(Veryfine* 100%), 8 fl. oz.	120
chilled *(Citrus Hill* Plus Calcium/Select)	90
chilled *(Crowley),* 8 fl. oz.	110
chilled *(Kraft* Pure 100% Unsweetened)	80
chilled *(Sunkist)*	84
chilled *(Sunkist* Fresh Squeezed)	77
chilled or frozen* *(Minute Maid)*	91
frozen* *(Sunkist),* 8 fl. oz.	112
frozen* *(TreeSweet)*	84
w/calcium, chilled or frozen* *(Minute Maid)*	93
reduced acid, chilled or frozen* *(Minute Maid)*	89
orange-banana *(Smucker's* Naturally 100%), 8 fl. oz. .	120
orange-grapefruit, chilled *(Kraft* Pure 100%)	80
orange-pineapple, chilled *(Kraft* Pure 100%)	80
peach *(Smucker's* Naturally 100%), 8 fl. oz.	120
peach, orchard blend *(Dole* Pure & Light)	90
peach nectar *(Libby's)*	100
pineapple:	
(Del Monte Unsweetened)	100
(Dole)	103
(Minute Maid), 8.45 fl. oz.	139
(Minute Maid On The Go), 10 fl. oz.	165
(Mott's), 9.5-fl.-oz. can	169
(S&W Unsweetened)	100
(Veryfine 100%), 8 fl. oz.	125
chilled or frozen* *(Dole)*	100
chilled or frozen* *(Minute Maid)*	99
pineapple-grapefruit *(Dole)*	90
pineapple-pink grapefruit *(Dole)*	101
pineapple-orange *(Dole)*	100
pineapple-orange, chilled or frozen* *(Minute Maid)* . . .	98
pineapple-orange-banana *(Dole)*	90
prune:	
(Del Monte Unsweetened)	120
(Lucky Leaf)	150
(Mott's/Mott's Country Style)	130
(S&W Unsweetened)	120
(Sunsweet)	130
raspberry, red *(Smucker's* Naturally 100%), 8 fl. oz. . .	120
raspberry blend *(Dole* Pure & Light Country)	87

raspberry-cranberry *(Apple & Eve)*   90
tangerine, chilled *(Dole Pure & Light* Mandarin)   97
tangerine, chilled or frozen* *(Minute Maid)*   91

* Diluted according to package directions

FRUIT SNACKS
See also "Fruit, Dried"

---

                                                            calories
all varieties:
  (Fruit Corners/Fruit Roll-Ups Peel-Outs), 1 roll   50
  (Fruit Wrinkles), 1 pouch   100
  (Squeezit), 6.75 oz.   110
  (Weight Watchers), 1 pouch   50
all varieties, except yogurt-coated *(Sunkist Fun Fruits)*,
  1 pouch   100
apple roll *(Flavor Tree)*, 1 piece   75
apricot roll *(Flavor Tree)*, 1 piece   76
cherry roll *(Flavor Tree)*, 1 piece   75
fruit punch roll *(Flavor Tree)*, 1 piece   74
grape roll *(Flavor Tree)*, 1 piece   76
raspberry roll *(Flavor Tree)*, 1 piece   75
strawberry roll *(Flavor Tree)*, 1 piece   74
strawberry, yogurt coated *(Sunkist Fun Fruits* Creme
  Supremes), 1 pouch   114

FRUIT & FRUIT FLAVORED DRINKS, six fluid
ounces, except as noted
See also "Fruit Juices" and "Soft Drinks & Mixers"

---

                                                            calories
all flavors, mix*:
  (Crystal Light Sugar Free), 8 fl. oz.   4
  (Kool-Aid), 8 fl. oz.   100
  (Kool-Aid Presweetened), 8 fl. oz.   80
  (Kool-Aid Sugar Free), 8 fl. oz.   4
apple drink *(Hi-C* Candy Apple Cooler)   94
apple juice cocktail *(Welch's Orchard)*, 10 fl. oz.   170

citrus fruit juice drink:
  (Five Alive), 8.45 fl. oz. 123
  (Hi-C Citrus Cooler) 95
  chilled or frozen* *(Five Alive)* 87
  berry, chilled or frozen* *(Five Alive)* 88
  tropical, chilled or frozen* *(Five Alive)* 85
citrus punch, chilled or frozen* *(Minute Maid)* 93
cranberry juice cocktail:
  (Ocean Spray) 110
  (Ocean Spray Low Calorie) 40
  (Veryfine), 8 fl. oz. 160
  chilled or frozen* *(Sunkist)* 110
  frozen* *(Welch's)* 100
  frozen* *(Welch's* No Sugar Added) 40
cranberry juice drink blend *(Ocean Spray Cran-Tastic)* 110
cranberry-apple juice cocktail, frozen* *(Welch's)* 120
cranberry-apple juice drink:
  (Ocean Spray CranApple) 130
  (Ocean Spray CranApple Low Calorie) 40
cranberry-apricot juice drink *(Ocean Spray Cranicot)* . . 110
cranberry-blueberry juice cocktail, frozen* *(Welch's)* . . 110
cranberry-grape juice cocktail, frozen* *(Welch's)* 110
cranberry-grape juice drink *(Ocean Spray Cran-Grape)* 130
cranberry-raspberry drink *(Ocean Spray Cran-*
    Raspberry) 110
cranberry-raspberry drink *(Ocean Spray Cran-*
    Raspberry Low Calorie) . . . . '. 40
cranberry-raspberry juice cocktail, frozen* *(Welch's)* . . 110
fruit drink:
  (Hi-C Double Fruit Cooler) 93
  (Hi-C Double Fruit Cooler), 8.45 fl. oz. 131
  (Hi-C Ecto Cooler) 95
  (Hi-C Ecto Cooler), 8.45 fl. oz. 134
  (Hi-C Hula Cooler) 97
fruit juice cocktail *(Welch's Orchard* Harvest Blend
    Cocktails-In-A-Box), 8.45 fl. oz. 150
fruit juice cocktail, bottled or frozen* *(Welch's Orchard*
    Harvest Blend) 110
fruit juice drink *(Tang* Fruit Box), 8.45 fl. oz. 140
fruit punch:
  (Minute Maid), 8.45 fl. oz. 128

Fruit & Fruit Flavored Drinks, fruit punch, continued

  (Minute Maid Juices to Go), 11.5 fl. oz. 174
  (Minute Maid On The Go), 10 fl. oz. 152
  (Veryfine 100% Juice Punch), 8 fl. oz. 122
  blend *(Libby's Juicy Juice)* 100
  blend *(Libby's Juicy Juice),* 8.45 oz. 140
  Concord *(Minute Maid),* 8.45 fl. oz. 131
  Concord *(Minute Maid* Juices to Go), 11.5 fl. oz. . . 178
  Concord *(Minute Maid On The Go),* 10 fl. oz. 155
  tropical *(Minute Maid),* 8.45 fl. oz. 130
  tropical *(Minute Maid* Juices to Go), 11.5 fl. oz. . . . 176
  chilled or frozen* *(Minute Maid)* 91
fruit punch cocktail:
  (Welch's Orchard Fruit Harvest Punch), 10 fl. oz. . . 180
  (Welch's Orchard Fruit Harvest Punch Cocktails-In-
    A-Box), 8.45 fl. oz. 150
  island fruit *(Hawaiian Punch)* 90
fruit punch drink:
  (Bama), 8.45 fl. oz. 130
  (Hi-C), 8.45 fl. oz. 135
  (Hi-C) 96
  (Hi-C Hula Punch), 8.45 fl. oz. 122
  (Hi-C Hula Punch) 87
  (Mott's), 10-fl.-oz. bottle 170
  (Mott's), 9.5-fl.-oz. can 161
  (Wylers) 84
  mountain berry *(Kool-Aid Koolers),* 8.45 fl. oz. 140
  rainbow *(Kool-Aid Koolers),* 8.45 fl. oz. 130
  red *(Hawaiian Punch* Fruit Juicy) 90
  red *(Hawaiian Punch* Fruit Juicy Lite) 60
  tropical *(Kool-Aid Koolers),* 8.45 fl. oz. 130
  tropical *(Wyler's)* 157
  tropical or wild fruit *(Hawaiian Punch)* 90
  chilled *(Crowley),* 8 fl. oz. 130
  chilled *(Minute Maid* Light'N Juicy) 14
  tropical, mix* *(Wyler's* Crystals), 8 fl. oz. 85
grape drink:
  (Bama), 8.45 fl. oz. 120
  (Crowley), 8 fl. oz. 130
  (Minute Maid Light'N Juicy) 13
  (Veryfine), 8 fl. oz. 130

grape juice cocktail:
  (Welch's Orchard) 110
  (Welch's Orchard Cocktails-In-A-Box), 8.45 fl. oz. ... 150
  frozen* *(Welch's* No Sugar Added) 40
grape juice drink:
  (Hi-C) 96
  (Hi-C), 8.45 fl. oz. 136
  (Kool-Aid Koolers), 8.45 fl. oz. 140
  (Tang Fruit Box), 8.45 fl. oz. 130
  frozen* *(Sunkist)* 69
grape-apple drink *(Mott's),* 10-fl.-oz. bottle 167
grape-apple drink *(Mott's),* 9.5-fl.-oz. can 158
grapeade, chilled or frozen* *(Minute Maid)* 94
grapefruit juice cocktail, pink:
  (Minute Maid Juices to Go), 11.5 fl. oz. 163
  (Minute Maid Juices to Go), 9.6 fl. oz. 136
  (Ocean Spray) 80
  (TreeSweet Lite) 40
  (Veryfine), 8 fl. oz. 120
  chilled or frozen* *(Minute Maid)* 85
grapefruit juice drink *(Citrus Hill* Plus Calcium) 70
guava fruit drink *(Ocean Spray Mauna La'i)* 100
guava-passion fruit drink *(Ocean Spray Mauna La'i)* .. 100
guava-strawberry tropical refresher *(Veryfine),* 8 fl. oz. 120
lemon drink, chilled *(Crowley),* 8 fl. oz. 130
lemon-lime drink *(Veryfine),* 8 fl. oz. 120
lemonade:
  (Hi-C), 8.45 fl. oz. 109
  (Minute Maid Light'N Juicy) 8
  (Shasta), 12 fl. oz. 146
  (Sunkist), 8 fl. oz. 141
  (Veryfine), 8 fl. oz. 120
  (Wyler's) 64
  chilled, regular, pink, or country *(Minute Maid)* ... 81
  frozen* *(Sunkist),* 8 fl. oz. 92
  frozen*, regular, pink, or country *(Minute Maid)* .. 77
lemonade flavor drink mix*:
  (Wyler's Crystals, 4 servings/pkg.), 8 fl. oz. 92
  regular, pink, or punch *(Country Time),* 8 fl. oz. ... 80
  regular or pink *(Country Time* Sugar Free), 8 fl. oz. 4
limeade, frozen* *(Minute Maid)* 71

Fruit & Fruit Flavored Drinks, continued

orange drink:
(Bama), 8.45 fl. oz.	120
(Crowley), 8 fl. oz.	130
(Hawaiian Punch)	100
(Hi-C)	95
(Hi-C), 8.45 fl. oz.	134
(Veryfine), 8 fl. oz.	130

orange flavor drink, breakfast:
chilled or frozen* *(Bright & Early)*	90
mix*, crystals *(Tang)*	90
mix*, crystals *(Tang Sugar Free)*	6

orange juice cocktail *(Welch's Orchard)*, 10 fl. oz.	150

orange juice drink:
(Citrus Hill Lite Premium)	60
(Kool-Aid Koolers), 8.45 fl. oz.	110
(Minute Maid Light'N Juicy)	16
(Tang Fruit Box), 8.45 fl. oz.	130
tropical *(Tang Fruit Box)*, 8.45 fl. oz.	150

orange-apricot, orange-grapefruit, or orange-pineapple juice cocktail *(Musselman's Breakfast)*	90
papaya punch *(Veryfine)*, 8 fl. oz.	120
passion fruit juice cocktail *(Welch's Orchard Tropicals Cocktails-In-A-Box)*, 8.45 fl. oz.	140
passion fruit juice cocktail, bottled or frozen* *(Welch's Orchard Tropicals)*	100
passion fruit-orange refresher *(Veryfine)*, 8 fl. oz.	110
peach drink *(Hi-C)*	101
pineapple-banana juice cocktail *(Welch's Orchard Tropicals Cocktails-In-A-Box)*, 8.45 fl. oz.	140
pineapple-banana juice cocktail, bottled or frozen* *(Welch's Orchard Tropicals)*	100
pineapple-grapefruit juice cocktail *(Ocean Spray)*	110
pineapple-grapefruit juice drink *(Del Monte)*	90
pineapple-orange drink *(Veryfine)*, 8 fl. oz.	130
pineapple-orange juice drink *(Del Monte)*	90
raspberry juice cocktail *(Welch's Orchard)*, 10 fl. oz.	160
strawberry, wild, flavor drink, mix* *(Wyler's Crystals)*, 8 fl. oz.	85
strawberry juice drink *(Tang Fruit Box)*, 8.45 fl. oz.	120

* Prepared or diluted according to package directions

Chapter 7

VEGETABLES AND VEGETABLE PRODUCTS

> **VEGETABLES, CANNED OR IN JARS,** 1/2 cup,
> except as noted
> *See also "Vegetables, Dried & Mixes" and
> "Vegetables, Frozen"*

	calories
artichoke hearts, marinated *(S&W)*, 3.5 oz.	225
asparagus:	
(Green Giant Green/50% Less Salt)	20
(Stokely Regular/No Salt or Sugar Added)	20
all varieties *(Del Monte)*	20
green *(S&W* Fancy)	18
green, colossal *(S&W* Fancy)	20
points, all green *(S&W/Nutradiet)*	17
white *(Green Giant)*	16
bamboo shoots *(La Choy)*, 1.5 oz.	8
bean salad:	
four bean *(Joan of Arc/Read)*	100
green bean, German-style *(Joan of Arc/Read)*	90
three bean *(Green Giant)*	70
three bean *(Joan of Arc/Read)*	90
bean sprouts *(La Choy)*, 2 oz.	6
beans, black *(Progresso)*, 8 oz.	205
beans, burrito *(Del Monte* Burrito Filling)	110
beans, chili:	
(Hunt's), 4 oz.	102
(S&W)	130
Caliente style *(Green Giant/Joan of Arc)*	100
in chili gravy *(Dennison's)*, 7.5 oz.	180

Vegetables, Canned or in Jars, beans, chili, continued

hot *(Allens)*	90
Mexican style *(Allens)*	135
Mexican style *(Van Camp's)*, 1 cup	210
in sauce *(Hormel)*, 5 oz.	130
spiced *(Gebhardt)*, 4 oz.	113
beans, garbanzo, *see "chickpeas," page 81*	
beans, great northern:	
(Allens)	105
(Green Giant)	80
(Joan of Arc)	80
w/pork *(Allens)*	100
w/pork *(Luck's)*, 7.25 oz.	220
beans, green:	
(Green Giant 50% Less Salt)	18
(Stokely Regular/No Salt or Sugar)	20
whole *(S&W Vertical Pack)*	20
whole, cut or French style *(Del Monte)*	20
whole, stringless *(S&W)*	20
cut *(Featherweight)*	25
cut *(Green Giant Pantry Express)*	12
cut *(S&W Premium Golden/S&W Nutradiet)*	20
cut *(Del Monte No Salt Added)*	20
cut or French style *(Allens)*	20
cut or French style *(S&W Premium Blue Lake)*	20
cut, French, or kitchen sliced *(Green Giant)*	16
almondine *(Green Giant)*	45
dilled *(S&W)*	60
Italian *(Allens)*	18
Italian, cut *(Del Monte)*	25
seasoned, French style *(Del Monte)*	20
w/shelled beans and pork *(Luck's)*, 8 oz.	200
shelly beans *(Allens)*	35
w/potatoes and mushrooms, in sauce *(Green Giant Pantry Express)*	50
beans, kidney:	
(Hunt's), 4 oz.	120
(S&W/Nutradiet)	90
red *(Progresso)*, 8 oz.	190
red, dark *(S&W Premium/Lite 50% Less Salt)*	120
red, dark *(Van Camp's)*, 1 cup	182

red, dark or light *(Green Giant)* 90
red, dark or light *(Joan of Arc)* 90
red, dark or light *(Stokely)* 110
red, dark or light *(Allens)* 105
red, light *(Van Camp's)*, 1 cup 184
red, baked *(B&M)*, 8 oz. 290
red, New Orleans style *(Van Camp's)*, 1 cup 178
white *(Progresso* Cannellini), 8 oz. 180
beans, lima:
   (Featherweight) 80
   (Joan of Arc) 80
   (S&W) 100
   (Stokely Regular/No Salt or Sugar Added) 80
   butterbeans *(Green Giant)* 80
   butterbeans *(Van Camp's)*, 1 cup 162
   butterbeans, large *(Allens)* 110
   Fordhook *(Stokely)* 80
   green *(Del Monte)* 70
   green, all sizes, or green and white *(Allens)* 90
   green, small *(S&W* Fancy) 80
   green, small, w/pork *(Luck's)*, 7.5 oz. 220
   w/ham *(Dennison's)*, 7.5 oz. 250
   w/pork *(Luck's)*, 7.5 oz. 230
beans, mung, sprouted *(La Choy)*, 2 oz. 8
beans, navy *(Allens)* 160
beans, October, w/pork *(Luck's)*, 7.25 oz. 230
beans, pinto:
   (Allens) 105
   (Gebhardt), 4 oz. 197
   (Green Giant/Joan of Arc) 90
   (Old El Paso) 100
   (Progresso), 8 oz. 165
   baked style, w/pork *(Luck's,* 15 oz.), 7.5 oz. 220
   Picante style *(Green Giant/Joan of Arc)* 100
beans, red:
   (Allens) 115
   (Green Giant/Joan of Arc) 90
   (Van Camp's), 1 cup 194
   small *(Hunt's)*, 4 oz. 91
beans, refried:
   (Bearitos Organic), 1 oz. 30

Vegetables, Canned or in Jars, beans, refried, continued

(Bearitos Organic No Salt), 1 oz.	29
(Gebhardt), 4 oz.	130
(Rosarita), 4 oz.	130
plain or spicy *(Del Monte)*	130
plain or w/green chilies *(Old El Paso),* ¼ cup	50
jalapeño *(Gebhardt),* 4 oz.	110
w/sausage *(Old El Paso),* ¼ cup	180
spicy *(Bearitos* Organic), 1 oz.	31
vegetarian *(Old El Paso),* ¼ cup	45
beans, shellie *(Stokely)*	35
beans, wax:	
(Allens)	15
(Stokely Regular/No Salt or Sugar Added)	20
golden, cut or French style *(Del Monte)*	20
beans, yellow eye, baked style *(B&M),* 8 oz.	362
beets:	
(Stokely No Salt or Sugar Added)	40
whole, sliced or cut *(Stokely)*	40
whole, small, diced or julienne *(S&W)*	40
whole, tiny, or sliced *(Del Monte)*	35
sliced *(Featherweight)*	45
sliced *(S&W/Nutradiet)*	35
sliced, small, tender *(S&W* Premium)	40
diced *(Stokely)*	35
Harvard *(Stokely)*	70
pickled *(Stokely)*	100
pickled *(Stokely* Jars)	90
pickled, whole, extra small *(S&W)*	70
pickled, crinkle sliced, w/liquid *(Del Monte)*	80
pickled, w/red wine vinegar *(S&W* Regular or Party)	70
blackeye peas:	
(Green Giant)	90
fresh, w/or w/out snaps *(Allens)*	100
mature *(Joan of Arc)*	90
mature, plain or w/pork *(Allens)*	105
mature, w/pork *(Luck's),* 7.5 oz.	200
cannellini beans, *see "beans, kidney, white," page 79*	
carrots:	
(Stokely Regular/No Salt or Sugar Added)	35
all styles *(Allens)*	30

whole, sliced, or diced *(Del Monte)*   30
whole, tiny, diced, or julienne *(S&W* Fancy)   30
sliced *(Featherweight)*   30
sliced *(S&W/Nutradiet)*   30
chickpeas or garbanzos:
   (Allens)   110
   (Green Giant)   90
   (Old El Paso)   190
   (S&W/Nutradiet)   100
   large *(S&W* Lite 50% Less Salt)   110
collards, chopped *(Allens)*   20
collards, chopped, w/pork *(Luck's)*, 7.5 oz.   90
corn:
   (Del Monte Regular/No Salt Added Vacuum Pack) .   90
   (Green Giant 50% Less Salt, No Sugar Added)   50
   (Green Giant Delicorn)   80
   in brine *(Green Giant)*   70
   kernel *(Featherweight)*   80
   kernel *(Green Giant/Green Giant Niblets* Vacuum
     Pack)   80
   kernel *(S&W/Nutradiet)*   80
   golden, kernel *(Del Monte* No Salt Added)   80
   golden, kernel *(Green Giant* 50% Less Salt)   70
   golden, kernel *(Green Giant* No Salt or Sugar)   80
   golden, kernel *(Stokely* No Salt or Sugar Added) . . .   80
   golden, kernel *(Green Giant Pantry Express)*   80
   golden, kernel *(Green Giant* Vacuum Pack)   70
   golden, kernel *(Stokely* Vacuum-Pack)   90
   golden or white, kernel *(Del Monte)*   70
   golden or white, kernel *(Stokely)*   90
   sweet select *(Green Giant)*   60
   white *(Green Giant* Vacuum Pack)   80
   young tender, kernel *(S&W* Premium)   90
   cream-style *(Green Giant)*   100
   cream-style *(S&W/Nutradiet)*   100
   cream-style *(S&W* Premium Homestyle No Starch) .   120
   cream-style *(S&W* Premium Homestyle Starch
     Added)   105
   cream-style, golden *(Del Monte* Regular/No Salt) . .   80
   cream-style, golden or white *(Stokely)*   100
   cream-style, white *(Del Monte)*   90

Vegetables, Canned or in Jars, corn, continued

w/green beans, carrots and pasta, in tomato sauce *(Green Giant Pantry Express)*	80
w/peppers *(Green Giant Mexicorn)*	80
garden salad *(Joan of Arc/Read)*	70
garden salad, marinated *(S&W)*	60
kale, chopped *(Allens)*	25

mushrooms:

(B in B), ¼ cup	12
whole, pieces, and stems *(Green Giant)*, ¼ cup	12
pieces and stems *(Allens)*	20
pieces and stems *(Empress)*, 2 oz.	14
in butter sauce *(Green Giant)*	30
w/garlic *(B in B)*, ¼ cup	12
mustard greens, chopped *(Allens)*	20
onions, whole, small *(S&W)*	35
onions, sweet *(Heinz)*, 1 oz.	40
peas, cream, fresh *(Allens)*	90
peas, crowder, fresh *(Allens)*	80

peas, field, fresh:

w/ or w/out snaps *(Allens)*	100
tiny, w/snaps *(Allens)*	70

peas, green or sweet:

(Del Monte Regular/No Salt Added)	60
(Green Giant 50% Less Salt)	50
(Stokely No Salt or Sugar Added)	50
dry early June *(Allens)*	80
early or sweet *(Stokely)*	60
early June *(S&W Petit Pois)*	70
early June, sweet, or sweet mini *(Green Giant)*	50
mini sweet, in brine *(Green Giant)*	60
seasoned *(Del Monte)*	60
small *(Del Monte)*	50
sweet *(Featherweight)*	70
sweet *(S&W Perfection)*	70
sweet, w/pearl onions *(Green Giant)*	50
sweet, w/tiny pearl onions *(S&W)*	60
peas, purple hull, fresh *(Allens)*	100
pepper rings, hot *(Vlasic)*, 1 oz.	4
peppers, cherry, mild *(Vlasic)*, 1 oz.	8

peppers, chili, green, hot:
    whole or diced *(Del Monte)* 20
    whole *(Old El Paso)*, 1 chili 8
    whole, diced, sliced, or strips *(Ortega)*, 1 oz. 10
    chopped *(Old El Paso)*, 2 tbsp. 8
peppers, hot, whole or diced *(Ortega)*, 1 oz. 8
peppers, jalapeño:
    whole *(Old El Paso)*, 2 peppers 14
    whole or diced *(Ortega)*, 1 oz. 10
    whole or sliced *(Del Monte)* 30
    hot *(Vlasic)*, 1 oz. 10
    marinated *(La Victoria)*, 1 tbsp. 4
    nacho *(La Victoria)*, 1 tbsp. 2
peppers, pepperoncini, salad *(Vlasic)*, 1 oz. 4
peppers, sweet *(Heinz* Sweet Pepper Mementos), 1 oz. . 6
potato salad, German *(Joan of Arc/Read)* 120
potato salad, homestyle *(Joan of Arc/Read)* 340
potatoes:
    (Stokely) 50
    whole or sliced *(Del Monte)* 45
    whole, new, extra small *(S&W)* 45
    sliced, diced, or double diced, white *(Allens)* 45
    sliced or diced *(Taylor's Brand)*, 1 cup 90
    au gratin *(Green Giant Pantry Express)* 120
    scalloped, and ham *(Hormel Micro Cup)*, 7.5 oz. ... 260
pumpkin:
    (Del Monte) 35
    (Libby's) 42
    (Stokely) 40
sauerkraut:
    (Claussen) 17
    (Del Monte) 25
    (Snow Floss) 28
    (Stokely Bavarian) 30
    shredded *(Allens)* 21
    shredded and chopped *(Stokely)* 20
spinach:
    (Allens Low Sodium) 28
    (S&W Premium Northwest) 25
    (Stokely) 30
    leaf *(Featherweight)* 35

Vegetables, Canned or in Jars, spinach, continued

leaf, whole or chopped *(Del Monte* Regular/No Salt)	25
sliced or chopped, curly *(Allens)*	28
succotash *(S&W* Country Style)	80
succotash *(Stokely)*	90

sweet potato:

whole *(Taylor's Brand* Vacuum Pack), 1 cup	210
in water, cut *(Allens)*	70
in light syrup *(Joan of Arc/Princella/Royal Prince)* .	110
in syrup, whole or cut *(Allens)*	90
in syrup, whole and cut *(Taylor's Brand),* 1 cup . . .	240
in syrup, cut *(Kohl's)*	110
in heavy syrup *(Joan of Arc/Princella/Royal Prince)*	130
in extra heavy syrup *(S&W* Southern)	139
in pineapple orange sauce *(Joan of Arc/Princella/* *Royal Prince)*	210
candied *(Joan of Arc/Princella/Royal Prince)*	240
candied *(S&W)*	180
mashed *(Joan of Arc/Princella/Royal Prince)*	90

tomato:

(Featherweight)	20
whole *(Hunt's* Regular/No Salt Added), 4 oz.	20
whole *(S&W/Nutradiet)*	25
whole *(Stokely)*	25
whole, peeled, regular or Italian style pear *(Contadina)*	25
whole, peeled *(Del Monte)*	25
whole, peeled, regular or Italian style pear *(S&W)* . .	25
crushed *(Hunt's),* 4 oz.	25
crushed, in puree *(Contadina)*	30
cut, peeled *(S&W* Ready-Cut)	25
diced, in rich puree *(S&W)*	35
wedges *(Del Monte)*	30
aspic, supreme *(S&W)*	60
w/green chilies *(Old El Paso),* ¼ cup	14
w/jalapeños (Ortega), 1 oz.	8
paste, see *"Tomato Paste & Puree,"* page 100	
pickled, kosher *(Claussen),* 1 oz.	5
pickled, kosher *(Claussen),* 1 average piece	9
puree, see *"Tomato Paste & Puree,"* page 100	
stewed *(Del Monte* Regular/No Salt Added)	35

stewed *(Hunt's* Regular/No Salt Added), 4 oz.	35
stewed *(Stokely)*	35
stewed, all varieties, except Mexican *(S&W)*	35
stewed, all varieties *(Contadina)*	35
stewed, Mexican style *(S&W)*	40
turnip greens:	
chopped *(Allens)*	21
chopped, w/diced turnips *(Allens)*	19
w/diced turnips *(Stokely)*	20
turnips *(Stokely)*	20
turnips, diced *(Allens)*	16
vegetables, mixed:	
(Del Monte)	40
(Featherweight)	40
(Green Giant Garden Medley)	40
(Green Giant Pantry Express)	35
(S&W Old Fashioned Harvest)	35
(Stokely Regular/No Salt or Sugar Added)	40
Chinese *(La Choy)*	12
chop suey *(La Choy)*	9
water chestnut, Chinese *(La Choy)*, 1.28 oz.	18
zucchini, in tomato sauce *(Del Monte)*	30

VEGETABLES, DRIED & MIXES*
*See also "Vegetables, Canned or in Jars,"
"Vegetables, Frozen," and "Side Dishes, Mixes"*

	calories
beans, black, mix *(Fantastic Foods)*, 1/2 cup**	157
beans, green, freeze-dried *(Mountain House)*, 1/2 cup . .	35
beans, kidney, red, raw *(Arrowhead Mills)*, 2 oz. dry . .	190
beans, pinto, raw *(Arrowhead Mills)*, 2 oz. dry	200
beans, refried, mix, instant *(Fantastic Foods)*, 1/2 cup . .	207
celery flakes *(Tone's)*, 1 tsp. dry	9
chickpeas *(Arrowhead Mills)*, 2 oz. dry	200
corn, dried *(John Cope's)*, 1 oz. dry or 4 oz. prepared .	101
lentils, green *(Arrowhead Mills)*, 2 oz. dry	190
lentils, red *(Arrowhead Mills)*, 2 oz. dry	195
onion, minced, w/green onion *(Lawry's)*, 1 tsp. dry . . .	7
peas, green, freeze-dried *(Mountain House)*, 1/2 cup . . .	70

Vegetables, Dried & Mixes*, continued

peas, split, green *(Arrowhead Mills)*, 2 oz. dry	200
potato mix, 1/2 cup, except as noted:	
(Betty Crocker Potato Buds)	130
au gratin *(Betty Crocker)*	150
au gratin *(Fantastic Foods)*	196
au gratin *(Idahoan)*	130
au gratin, tangy *(French's)*	130
bacon and cheddar *(Betty Crocker* Twice Baked) . . .	210
butter, herbed *(Betty Crocker* Twice Baked)	220
cheddar, mild, w/onion *(Betty Crocker* Twice Baked)	190
cheddar, smokey *(Betty Crocker)*	140
cheddar, spicy *(Idahoan)*	140
cheddar and bacon *(Betty Crocker)*	140
cheddar and bacon casserole *(French's)*	130
country style *(Fantastic Foods)*	85
hash brown *(Idahoan* Quick One-Pan)	140
hash brown, w/onions *(Betty Crocker)*	160
herb and butter *(Idahoan)*	150
julienne *(Betty Crocker)*	130
mashed *(Country Store* Flakes), 1/3 cup flakes	70
mashed *(French's Idaho)*	130
mashed *(French's Idaho* Spuds)	140
mashed *(Hungry Jack* Flakes)	140
mashed *(Idahoan)*	140
mashed *(Idahoan Instamash)*	80
scalloped *(Idahoan)*	140
scalloped, regular or cheesy *(Betty Crocker)*	140
scalloped, cheese, real *(French's)*	140
scalloped, creamy Italian *(French's)*	120
scalloped, crispy top, w/savory onion mix *(French's)*	140
scalloped, 'n ham *(Betty Crocker)*	160
sour cream and chives *(Betty Crocker)*	140
sour cream and chives *(Betty Crocker* Twice Baked)	200
sour cream and chives *(French's)*	150
sour cream and chives *(Idahoan)*	130
Stroganoff, creamy *(French's)*	130
western *(Idahoan)*	120
potato pancake *(French's Idaho)*, 3 cakes, 3" each	90
salad, mix:	
Caesar *(Suddenly Salad)*, 1/2 cup	170

ranch and bacon *(Suddenly Salad)*, 1/2 cup   210
soybean *(Arrowhead Mills)*, 2 oz. dry   230
soybean flakes *(Arrowhead Mills)*, 2 oz. dry   250
vegetable flakes, dehydrated *(French's)*, 1 tbsp. dry . . .   12

* *Prepared according to package directions, except as noted*
** *Prepared without added ingredients*

VEGETABLES, FROZEN
See also "Entrees, Frozen" and "Vegetable Dishes, Frozen"

---

	calories
artichoke hearts *(Birds Eye* Deluxe), 3 oz.	30
artichoke hearts *(Seabrook)*, 3 oz.	25
asparagus:	
spears *(Southern)*, 3.5 oz.	27
spears or cuts *(Birds Eye)*, 3.3 oz.	25
spears or cuts *(Seabrook)*, 3.3 oz.	25
cuts *(Green Giant Harvest Fresh)*, 1/2 cup	25
beans, green:	
(Green Giant), 1/2 cup	14
whole *(Birds Eye* Deluxe), 3 oz.	25
whole *(Birds Eye* Farm Fresh), 4 oz.	30
whole *(Southern)*, 3.5 oz.	33
whole, cut, or French style *(Seabrook)*, 3 oz.	25
cut *(Birds Eye* Portion Pack), 3 oz.	25
cut *(Green Giant Harvest Fresh)*, 1/2 cup	16
cut *(Stokely Singles)*, 3 oz.	30
cut or French style *(Birds Eye)*, 3 oz.	25
French style *(Southern)*, 3.5 oz.	34
Italian *(Birds Eye)*, 3 oz.	30
Italian *(Seabrook)*, 3 oz.	30
petite *(Birds Eye* Deluxe), 2.6 oz.	20
in butter sauce *(Green Giant* One Serving), 5.5 oz. . .	60
in butter sauce, cut *(Green Giant)*, 1/2 cup	30
beans, green, Bavarian style w/spaetzle, in sauce *(Birds Eye* International), 3.3 oz.	100
beans, green, French, w/toasted almonds *(Birds Eye* Combinations), 3 oz.	50

Vegetables, Frozen, continued

beans, green, and mushroom, creamy *(Green Giant*
    Garden Gourmet), 1 pkg.   220
beans, lima:
    (Green Giant), 1/2 cup   100
    (Green Giant Harvest Fresh), 1/2 cup   80
    (Health Valley), 1/2 cup   94
    baby *(Birds Eye),* 3.3 oz.   130
    baby *(Seabrook),* 3.3 oz.   130
    baby *(Southern),* 3.5 oz.   135
    baby, butter *(Seabrook),* 3.3 oz.   140
    Fordhook *(Birds Eye),* 3.3 oz.   100
    Fordhook *(Seabrook),* 3.3 oz.   100
    Fordhook *(Southern),* 3.5 oz.   105
    speckled *(Seabrook),* 3.3 oz.   120
    speckled *(Southern),* 3.5 oz.   135
    tiny *(Seabrook),* 3.3 oz.   110
    in butter sauce *(Green Giant),* 1/2 cup   100
    in butter sauce, baby *(Stokely Singles),* 4 oz.   140
beans, pinto *(Seabrook),* 3.2 oz.   160
beans, wax, cut *(Seabrook),* 3 oz.   25
blackeye peas *(Seabrook),* 3.3 oz.   130
blackeye peas *(Southern),* 3.5 oz.   136
broccoli:
    (Health Valley), 1/2 cup   26
    spears *(Green Giant Harvest Fresh),* 1/2 cup   20
    spears *(Southern),* 3.5 oz.   30
    spears, baby *(Birds Eye* Deluxe), 3.3 oz.   30
    spears, baby *(Seabrook),* 3.3 oz.   30
    spears, whole *(Birds Eye* Farm Fresh), 4 oz.   30
    spears, cuts, or chopped *(Birds Eye),* 3.3 oz.   25
    spears, cuts, or chopped *(Seabrook),* 3.3 oz.   25
    florets *(Birds Eye* Deluxe), 3.3 oz.   25
    cuts *(Birds Eye* Portion Pack), 3 oz.   20
    cuts *(Green Giant Harvest Fresh),* 1/2 cup   16
    cuts *(Green Giant* Polybag), 1/2 cup   12
    cuts *(Stokely Singles),* 3 oz.   25
    chopped *(Southern),* 3.5 oz.   28
    in butter sauce *(Green Giant* One Serving), 4.5 oz. . .   45
    in butter sauce, spears *(Birds Eye* Butter Sauce
      Combinations), 3.3 oz.   45

in butter sauce, spears *(Green Giant)*, 1/2 cup   40
in cheese sauce *(Birds Eye* Cheese Sauce
  Combinations), 5 oz.   130
in cheese sauce, *(Freezer Queen Family Side Dishes)*,
  4.5 oz.   48
in cheese sauce, cuts *(Green Giant* One Serving),
  5 oz..   70
in cheese sauce, cuts *(Stokely Singles)*, 4 oz.   80
in cheese-flavored sauce *(Green Giant)*, 1/2 cup   60
broccoli, w/baby carrots and water chestnuts *(Birds
  Eye* Farm Fresh), 4 oz..   45
broccoli, w/baby whole carrots and chestnuts *(Stokely
  Singles)*, 3 oz.   30
broccoli and cauliflower:
  (Frosty Acres Swiss Mix), 3 oz..   25
  (Stokely Singles), 3 oz..   20
  medley *(Green Giant Valley Combinations)*, 1/2 cup .   30
broccoli, cauliflower, and carrots:
  (Birds Eye Farm Fresh), 4 oz.   35
  no sauce *(Green Giant* One Serving), 4 oz.   25
  baby *(Stokely Singles)*, 3 oz..   25
  in butter sauce *(Birds Eye* Butter Sauce
    Combinations), 3.3 oz.   45
  in butter sauce *(Green Giant)*, 1/2 cup   30
  w/cheese sauce *(Birds Eye* Cheese Sauce
    Combinations), 4.5 oz.   110
  in cheese sauce *(Birds Eye For One)*, 5 oz.   110
  in cheese sauce *(Green Giant* One Serving), 5 oz. . . .   70
  in cheese flavored sauce *(Green Giant)*, 1/2 cup   60
  baby carrots, in cheese sauce *(Stokely Singles)*, 4 oz.   70
broccoli, cauliflower, and red peppers *(Birds Eye* Farm
  Fresh), 4 oz.   30
broccoli, corn, and red peppers *(Birds Eye* Farm
  Fresh), 4 oz.   60
broccoli fanfare *(Green Giant Valley Combinations)*,
  1/2 cup   70
broccoli, green beans, pearl onions, and red peppers
  (Birds Eye Farm Fresh), 4 oz..   35
broccoli, red peppers, bamboo shoots, and straw
  mushrooms *(Birds Eye* Farm Fresh), 4 oz.   30

Vegetables, Frozen, continued

Brussels sprouts:
(Birds Eye), 3.3 oz.	35
(Green Giant Polybag), 1/2 cup	25
(Seabrook), 3.3 oz.	35
(Southern), 3.5 oz.	37
(Stokely Singles), 3 oz.	35
baby *(Seabrook)*, 3.3 oz.	40
in butter sauce *(Green Giant)*, 1/2 cup	40
in butter sauce *(Stokely Singles)*, 4 oz.	50
w/cheese sauce, baby *(Birds Eye* Cheese Sauce Combinations), 4.5 oz.	130

Brussels sprouts, cauliflower, and carrots *(Birds Eye* Farm Fresh), 4 oz. 40

carrots:
(Birds Eye Deluxe Parisienne), 2.6 oz.	30
(Seabrook), 3.3 oz.	40
baby *(Green Giant* Harvest Fresh), 1/2 cup	18
whole *(Southern)*, 3.5 oz.	42
whole, baby *(Birds Eye* Deluxe), 3.3 oz.	40
whole, baby *(Stokely Singles)*, 3 oz.	35
sliced *(Birds Eye)*, 3.2 oz.	35
sliced *(Frosty Acres)*, 3.3 oz.	40

carrots, baby, w/sweet peas and pearl onions *(Birds Eye* Deluxe), 3.3 oz. 50

cauliflower:
(Birds Eye), 3.3 oz.	25
(Kohl's), 3 oz.	20
(Seabrook), 3.3 oz.	25
(Southern), 3.5 oz.	26
(Stokely Singles), 3 oz.	20
cuts *(Green Giant)*, 1/2 cup	12
in cheese sauce *(Birds Eye* Cheese Sauce Combinations), 5 oz.	130
in cheese sauce *(Green Giant)*, 5.5 oz.	80
in cheese sauce *(Stokely Singles)*, 4 oz.	70
in cheddar cheese sauce *(The Budget Gourmet* Side Dish), 5 oz.	110
in cheese flavor sauce *(Green Giant)*, 1/2 cup	60

cauliflower, broccoli, and carrots, in cheese sauce *(Freezer Queen* Family Side Dishes), 5 oz. 60

cauliflower, baby whole carrots, and snow pea pods
(*Birds Eye* Farm Fresh), 4 oz.   40
cauliflower, zucchini, carrots, and red peppers (*Birds
Eye* Farm Fresh), 4 oz.   30
collards, chopped (*Seabrook*), 3.3 oz.   25
collards, chopped (*Southern*), 3.5 oz.   30
corn:
   (*Health Valley*), 1/2 cup   76
   on cob (*Birds Eye*), 1 ear   120
   on cob (*Birds Eye Big Ears*), 1 ear   160
   on cob (*Birds Eye Little Ears*), 2 ears   130
   on cob (*Frosty Acres*), 1 ear   120
   on cob (*Green Giant* One Serving), 2 half ears   120
   on cob (*Green Giant Niblet Ears*, 4 ears), 1 ear   120
   on cob (*Green Giant Niblet Ears* Supersweet), 1 ear .   90
   on cob (*Green Giant Nibblers*, 6 ears), 2 ears   120
   on cob (*Green Giant Nibblers* Supersweet), 2 ears . .   90
   on cob (*Ore-Ida*), 1 ear   180
   on cob (*Seabrook*), 5" ear   120
   on cob (*Southern*), 5" ear   140
   on cob, baby (*Birds Eye* Deluxe), 2.6 oz.   25
   on cob, miniature (*Ore-Ida Mini-Gold*), 2 ears   180
   kernel (*Birds Eye* Sweet), 3.3 oz.   80
   kernel (*Birds Eye* Tender Sweet Deluxe), 3.3 oz. . . .   80
   kernel (*Green Giant Harvest Fresh Niblets*), 1/2 cup .   80
   kernel (*Green Giant Niblets*), 1/2 cup   90
   kernel (*Green Giant Niblets* Supersweet), 1/2 cup . . .   60
   kernel, cut (*Birds Eye* Portion Pack), 3 oz.   70
   kernel, cut (*Southern*), 3.5 oz.   98
   kernel, cut (*Stokely Singles*), 3 oz.   75
   kernel, cut or white (*Seabrook*), 3.3 oz.   80
   kernel, petite (*Birds Eye* Deluxe), 2.6 oz.   70
   kernel, white shoepeg (*Green Giant Harvest Fresh*),
     1/2 cup   90
   cream-style (*Green Giant*), 1/2 cup   110
   in butter sauce (*The Budget Gourmet* Side Dish),
     5.5 oz.   190
   in butter sauce (*Green Giant Niblets*), 1/2 cup   100
   in butter sauce (*Green Giant Niblets* One Serving),
     4.5 oz.   120
   in butter sauce (*Stokely Singles*), 4 oz.   110

Vegetables, Frozen, corn, continued

in butter sauce, on cob *(Stokely Singles)*, 1 ear	70
in butter sauce, golden *(Green Giant)*, 1/2 cup	100
in butter sauce, tender sweet *(Birds Eye* Butter Sauce Combinations), 3.3 oz.	90
in butter sauce, white *(Green Giant)*, 1/2 cup	100
in sauce, country style *(The Budget Gourmet* Side Dish), 5.75 oz.	140
kale, chopped *(Seabrook)*, 3.3 oz.	25
kale, chopped *(Southern)*, 3.5 oz.	30
mushrooms, whole *(Birds Eye* Deluxe), 2.6 oz.	20
mustard greens, chopped *(Seabrook)*, 3.3 oz.	20
mustard greens, chopped *(Southern)*, 3.5 oz.	25

okra:

whole *(Seabrook)*, 3.3 oz.	30
whole *(Southern)*, 3.5 oz.	35
cut *(Seabrook)*, 3.3 oz.	25
cut *(Southern)*, 3.5 oz.	31

onion:

small *(Birds Eye)*, 4 oz.	40
small *(Seabrook)*, 3.3 oz.	35
chopped *(Ore-Ida)*, 2 oz.	20
chopped *(Seabrook)*, 1 oz.	8
w/cream sauce, small *(Birds Eye* Combinations), 5 oz.	140

rings, see *"Vegetable Dishes, Frozen, onion rings,"* page 97

pea pods, Chinese:

(Chun King), 1.5 oz.	20
(Seabrook), 2 oz.	20
snow *(Birds Eye* Deluxe), 3 oz.	35
peas, crowder *(Seabrook)*, 3 oz.	130

peas, green or sweet:

(Birds Eye), 3.3 oz.	80
(Birds Eye Portion Pack), 3 oz.	70
(Health Valley), 1/2 cup	65
(Seabrook), 3.3 oz.	80
(Southern), 3.5 oz.	79
(Stokely Singles), 3 oz.	65
early, LeSueur *(Green Giant)*, 1/2 cup	60
early June *(Green Giant* Harvest Fresh), 1/2 cup	60

petite *(Southern)*, 3.5 oz.   64
sweet *(Green Giant)*, 1/2 cup   50
sweet *(Green Giant Harvest Fresh)*, 1/2 cup   50
tender tiny *(Birds Eye Deluxe)*, 3.3 oz.   60
tiny *(Seabrook)*, 3.3 oz.   60
in butter sauce, early *(Green Giant One Serving)*,
   4.5 oz.   90
in butter sauce, early *(LeSueur)*, 1/2 cup   80
in butter sauce, sweet *(Green Giant)*, 1/2 cup   80
in butter sauce, sweet *(Stokely Singles)*, 4 oz.   90
w/cream sauce *(Birds Eye Combinations)*, 5 oz. . . .   180
peas and carrots *(Seabrook)*, 3.3 oz.   60
peas and carrots *(Southern)*, 3.5 oz.   64
peas and cauliflower, in cream sauce *(The Budget
   Gourmet Side Dish)*, 5.75 oz.   170
peas, *LeSueur* style *(Green Giant Valley Combination)*,
   1/2 cup   70
peas, mini, w/pea pods and water chestnuts, in butter
   sauce *(LeSueur)*, 1/2 cup   80
peas and onions *(Seabrook)*, 3.3 oz.   70
peas, w/onions and carrots, in butter sauce *(LeSueur)*,
   1/2 cup   80
peas and pearl onions:
   (Birds Eye Combinations), 3.3 oz.   70
   w/cheese sauce *(Birds Eye Cheese Sauce
   Combinations)*, 5 oz.   140
peas and potatoes, w/cream sauce *(Birds Eye
   Combinations)*, 5 oz.   190
peas and water chestnuts Oriental *(The Budget
   Gourmet Side Dishes)*, 5 oz.   120
peas, purple hull *(Frosty Acres)*, 3.3 oz.   130
peas, snow, *see "pea pods, Chinese," page 92*
peas, sugar snap:
   (Birds Eye Deluxe), 2.6 oz.   45
   (Green Giant), 1/2 cup   30
   (Green Giant Harvest Fresh), 1/2 cup   30
peas, sugar snap, w/baby carrots and water chestnuts
   (Birds Eye Farm Fresh), 3.2 oz.   50
peppers, sweet, green *(Seabrook)*, 1 oz.   6
peppers, sweet, red *(Seabrook)*, 1 oz.   8

Vegetables, Frozen, continued
potatoes:

whole, small *(Ore-Ida)*, 3 oz.	70
whole, white *(Southern)*, 3.5 oz.	69
whole, white, boiled *(Seabrook)*, 3.2 oz.	60
diced and hash shred *(Seabrook)*, 4 oz.	80
fried *(Heinz Deep Fries)*, 3 oz.	160
fried *(MicroMagic)*, 3 oz.	290
fried *(Ore-Ida Country Style Dinner Fries)*, 3 oz.	110
fried *(Ore-Ida Crispers!)*, 3 oz.	230
fried *(Ore-Ida Crispy Crowns)*, 3 oz.	160
fried *(Ore-Ida Golden Fries)*, 3 oz.	120
fried *(Ore-Ida Lites)*, 3 oz.	90
fried *(Seabrook)*, 3 oz.	120
fried, cottage cut *(Ore-Ida)*, 3 oz.	120
fried, cottage cut *(Seabrook)*, 2.8 oz.	110
fried, crinkle cut *(Heinz Deep Fries)*, 3 oz.	150
fried, crinkle cut *(Ore-Ida Golden Crinkles)*, 3 oz.	120
fried, crinkle cut or shoestring *(Ore-Ida Lites)*, 3 oz.	90
fried, crinkle cut *(Ore-Ida Microwave)*, 3.5 oz.	180
fried, crinkle cut *(Ore-Ida Pixie Crinkles)*, 3 oz.	140
fried, crinkle cut *(Quick'n Crispy)*, 4 oz.	370
fried, crinkle cut *(Seabrook)*, 3 oz.	120
fried, w/onions *(Ore-Ida Crispy Crowns)*, 3 oz.	170
fried, shoestring *(Heinz Deep Fries)*, 3 oz.	200
fried, shoestring *(Ore-Ida)*, 3 oz.	140
fried, shoestring *(Quick'n Crispy)*, 4 oz.	390
fried, shoestring *(Seabrook)*, 3 oz.	140
fried, skinny *(MicroMagic)*, 3 oz.	350
fried, thin cuts *(Quick'n Crispy)*, 4 oz.	370
fried, wedges *(Ore-Ida Home Style Potato Wedges)*, 3 oz.	100
hash brown *(Ore-Ida Golden Patties)*, 2.5 oz.	140
hash brown *(Ore-Ida Microwave)*, 2 oz.	130
hash brown *(Ore-Ida Southern Style)*, 3 oz.	70
hash brown, w/butter and onions *(Heinz Deep Fries)*, 3 oz.	110
hash brown, w/cheddar *(Ore-Ida Cheddar Browns)*, 3 oz.	90
hash brown, shredded *(Ore-Ida)*, 3 oz.	70
O'Brien *(Ore-Ida)*, 3 oz.	60

puffs *(Ore-Ida Tater Tots),* 3 oz.	140
puffs *(Ore-Ida Tater Tots* Microwave), 4 oz.	200
puffs, w/bacon flavor or onion *(Ore-Ida Tater Tots),* 3 oz.	140
sticks *(MicroMagic* Tater Sticks), 4 oz.	390
wedges *(Quick'n Crispy),* 4 oz.	280

spinach:

(Green Giant Polybag), 1/2 cup	25
(Green Giant Harvest Fresh), 1/2 cup	25
leaf, whole *(Birds Eye* Portion Pack), 3.2 oz.	20
leaf, whole or chopped *(Birds Eye),* 3.3 oz.	20
leaf, whole or chopped *(Southern),* 3.5 oz.	25
leaf, cut or chopped *(Seabrook),* 3.3 oz.	20
creamed *(Birds Eye* Combinations), 3 oz.	60
creamed *(Green Giant),* 1/2 cup	70
creamed *(Stouffer's),* 4.5 oz.	170
in butter sauce, cut *(Green Giant),* 1/2 cup	40

squash:

crookneck, yellow *(Seabrook),* 3.3 oz.	18
crookneck, yellow *(Southern),* 3.5 oz.	21
winter, cooked *(Birds Eye),* 4 oz.	45
winter, cooked *(Seabrook),* 4 oz.	45

succotash *(Frosty Acres),* 3.3 oz.	100
succotash *(Seabrook),* 3.3 oz.	100
sweet potato, candied *(Mrs. Paul's),* 4 oz.	170
sweet potato, candied, w/apples *(Mrs. Paul's* Sweets 'n Apples), 4 oz.	160

turnip greens:

chopped *(Frosty Acres),* 3.3 oz.	20
chopped *(Southern),* 3.5 oz.	25
chopped or w/diced turnips *(Seabrook),* 3.3 oz.	20

turnips, diced *(Southern),* 3.5 oz.	17

vegetables, mixed:

(Birds Eye), 3.3 oz.	60
(Birds Eye Portion Pack), 3 oz.	50
(Green Giant/Green Giant Harvest Fresh), 1/2 cup	40
(Health Valley), 1/2 cup	68
(Seabrook), 3.3 oz.	65
(Southern), 3.5 oz.	69
(Stokely Singles), 3 oz.	60
California *(Green Giant* American Mixtures), 1/2 cup	25

Vegetables, Frozen, vegetables, mixed, continued

Chinese style *(Birds Eye Stir-Fry)*, 3.3 oz.	35
chow mein, in Oriental sauce *(Birds Eye Custom Cuisine)*, 4.6 oz.*	80
chow mein style, w/seasoned sauce *(Birds Eye International Recipes)*, 3.3 oz.	90
Dutch style *(Frosty Acres)*, 3.2 oz.	30
Heartland *(Green Giant American Mixtures)*, 1/2 cup	25
Italian style *(Frosty Acres)*, 3.2 oz.	40
Italian style, w/seasoned sauce *(Birds Eye International Recipes)*, 3.3 oz.	100
Japanese style *(Birds Eye Stir-Fry)*, 3.3 oz.	30
Japanese style, w/seasoned sauce *(Birds Eye International Recipes)*, 3.3 oz.	90
New England *(Green Giant American Mixtures)*, 1/2 cup	70
New England style, w/seasoned sauce *(Birds Eye International Recipes)*, 3.3 oz.	130
Oriental style *(Frosty Acres)*, 3.2 oz.	25
Oriental style, w/sauce for beef *(Birds Eye Custom Cuisine)*, 4.6 oz.*	90
Oriental style, w/seasoned sauce *(Birds Eye International Recipes)*, 3.3 oz.	70
pasta primavera style, w/seasoned sauce *(Birds Eye International Recipes)*, 3.3 oz.	120
San Francisco *(Green Giant American Mixtures)*, 1/2 cup	25
San Francisco style, w/seasoned sauce *(Birds Eye International Recipes)*, 3.3 oz.	100
Santa Fe *(Green Giant American Mixtures)*, 1/2 cup .	70
Seattle *(Green Giant American Mixtures)*, 1/2 cup . .	25
in butter sauce *(Finast)*, 3.3 oz.	70
in butter sauce *(Green Giant)*, 1/2 cup	60
w/herb sauce for chicken or shrimp *(Birds Eye Custom Cuisine)*, 4.6 oz.*	90
w/mushroom sauce, creamy, for beef *(Birds Eye Custom Cuisine)*, 4.6 oz.*	60
w/mustard sauce, Dijon, for chicken or fish *(Birds Eye Custom Cuisine)*, 4.6 oz.*	70
w/tomato basil sauce for chicken *(Birds Eye Custom Cuisine)*, 4.6 oz.*	110

soup mix *(Frosty Acres)*, 3 oz.   45
stew *(Frosty Acres)*, 3 oz.   42
stew *(Kohl's)*, 3.3 oz.   50
stew *(Ore-Ida)*, 3 oz.   60
'n white and wild rice pilaf *(Stokely Singles)*, 4 oz. . .   80
w/wild rice, in white wine sauce for chicken *(Birds
  Eye Custom Cuisine)*, 4.6 oz.*   100
zucchini *(Seabrook)*, 3.3 oz.   16
zucchini *(Southern)*, 3.5 oz.   18
zucchini, carrots, pearl onions, and mushrooms *(Birds
  Eye Farm Fresh)*, 4 oz.   30

* *Without added ingredients*

VEGETABLE DISHES, FROZEN
See also "Entrees, Frozen" and "Vegetables, Frozen"

	calories
asparagus pilaf *(Green Giant* Microwave Garden Gourmet), 1 pkg.	190
beans, green, and mushroom casserole *(Stouffer's)*, 4.75 oz.	160
broccoli w/cheese, in pastry *(Pepperidge Farm)*, 7¼ oz.	230
broccoli and rotini, in cheese sauce *(Green Giant* One Serving), 5.5 oz.	120
corn fritter *(Mrs. Paul's)*, 2 pieces	240
corn nuggets, breaded, fried *(Stilwell Quickkrisp)*, 3 oz.	210
corn souffle *(Stouffer's)*, 1/3 of 12-oz. pkg.	160
mushrooms, battered *(Stilwell Quick Krisp)*, 2 oz.	140

onion rings:
(Ore-Ida Onion Ringers), 2 oz.	140
battered *(Stilwell)*, 3 oz.	250
battered, precooked *(Farm Rich* Batter Dipt), 4 oz.	260
crispy *(Farm Rich Onion O's)*, 5 rings	190
crispy *(Mrs. Paul's)*, 2½ oz.	190

potatoes:
au gratin *(Birds Eye For One)*, 5.5 oz.	240
au gratin *(Freezer Queen Family Side Dish)*, 4 oz.	100
au gratin *(Green Giant* One Serving), 5.5 oz.	200
au gratin *(Stouffer's)*, 1/3 of 11½-oz. pkg.	110

Vegetable Dishes, Frozen, potatoes, continued

and broccoli, w/cheese sauce *(Freezer Queen Family
Side Dish)*, 5.5 oz.   140

and broccoli, in cheese-flavored sauce *(Green Giant
One Serving)*, 5.5 oz.   130

cheddared *(The Budget Gourmet* Side Dish), 5.5 oz.   230

cheddared, and broccoli *(The Budget Gourmet* Side
Dish), 5 oz.   130

nacho *(The Budget Gourmet* Side Dish), 5 oz.   180

new, in sour cream sauce *(The Budget Gourmet* Side
Dish), 5 oz.   120

scalloped *(Stouffer's)*, 1/3 of 11 1/2-oz. pkg.   90

shredded, 'n vegetables, in cheese sauce *(Stokely
Singles)*, 4.5 oz.   130

sliced, 'n bacon, in cheddar cheese sauce *(Stokely
Singles)*, 4.5 oz.   150

stuffed, baked, w/broccoli and cheese *(Weight
Watchers)*, 10.5 oz.   290

stuffed, baked, w/chicken divan *(Weight Watchers)*,
11 oz.   280

stuffed, baked, w/ham Lorraine topping *(Green
Giant)*, 11 oz.   250

stuffed, baked, w/sour cream and chives *(Green
Giant)*, 5 oz.   230

stuffed, w/real bacon *(Oh Boy!)*, 6 oz.   116

stuffed, w/cheddar cheese *(Oh Boy!)*, 6 oz.   142

stuffed, w/sour cream & chives *(Oh Boy!)*, 6 oz. . . .   129

three cheese *(The Budget Gourmet)*, 5.75 oz.   230

spinach au gratin *(The Budget Gourmet)*, 6 oz.   120

spinach souffle *(Stouffer's)*, 4 oz.   140

vegetable sticks, breaded *(Farm Rich)*, 4 oz.   240

vegetable sticks, breaded *(Stilwell Quickkrisp)*, 3 oz. . .   240

vegetables:

and pasta mornay, w/ham *(Lean Cuisine)*, 9 3/8 oz. . .   280

'n rice, in teriyaki sauce *(Stokely Singles)*, 4 oz.   100

'n rotini, in cheddar sauce *(Stokely Singles)*, 4 oz. . .   100

'n shells, in Italian style sauce *(Stokely Singles)*, 4 oz.   170

zucchini, breaded *(Stilwell Quickkrisp)*, 3.3 oz.   200

BEANS, BAKED & BAKED STYLE

See also "Vegetables, Canned"

	calories
(Allens), 1/2 cup	170
(Campbell's Home Style), 8 oz.	220
(Grandma Brown's), 1 cup	301
(Grandma Brown's Saucepan), 1 cup	307
(Green Giant), 1/2 cup	150
(S&W Brick Oven), 1/2 cup	160
Boston *(Health Valley* Regular/No Salt Added), 4 oz.	213
pea, small *(B&M),* 8 oz. or 7/8 cup	330
barbecue *(B&M),* 8 oz. or 7/8 cup	310
barbecue *(Campbell's),* 7 7/8 oz.	210
brown sugar *(Van Camp's),* 1 cup	284
w/franks *(Van Camp's Beanee Weenee),* 1 cup	326
honey *(B&M),* 8 oz. or 7/8 cup	280
in molasses and brown sugar sauce *(Campbell's* Old Fashioned), 8 oz.	230
w/pork:	
(Allens Extra Fancy), 1/2 cup	125
(Allens Extra Standard), 1/2 cup	90
(Allens Fancy), 1/2 cup	110
(Campbell's), 8 oz.	200
(Green Giant), 1/2 cup	90
(Joan of Arc), 1/2 cup	90
(Hormel Micro-Cup), 7.5 oz.	254
(Hunt's), 4 oz.	140
(S&W), 1/2 cup	130
(Van Camp's), 1 cup	216
tomato *(B&M),* 8 oz. or 7/8 cup	230
vegetarian:	
(Allens), 1/2 cup	110
(B&M), 8 oz. or 7/8 cup	280
(Van Camp's Vegetarian Style), 1 cup	206
w/miso *(Health Valley* Vegetarian), 4 oz.	90
western style *(Van Camp's),* 1 cup	207

TOMATO PASTE & PUREE
See also "Sauces"

	calories
tomato paste:	
(Contadina), 2 oz. or ¼ cup	50
(Del Monte Regular/No Salt Added), 6 oz.	150
(Hunt's Regular/No Salt Added), 2 oz.	45
(S&W), 6 oz.	150
Italian *(Contadina)*, 2 oz. or ¼ cup	65
tomato puree, ½ cup, except as noted:	
(Contadina)	40
(Hunt's), 4 oz.	45
(S&W)	60

PICKLES AND RELISH, one ounce, except as noted
See also "Condiments & Seasonings," "Olives," and "Vegetables, Canned"

	calories
pickles, bread and butter:	
slices *(Claussen* Bread 'n butter)	20
slices *(Claussen* Bread 'n butter), .4-oz. piece	7
slices *(Heinz* Cucumber Slices)	25
slices *(Mrs. Fanning's)*, 2 slices	16
chunks *(Vlasic* Old Fashion)	25
sweet *(Vlasic* Sweet Butter Chips)	25
sweet *(Vlasic* Sweet Butter Stix)	18
pickles, dill:	
(Vlasic Original)	4
whole *(Featherweight)*, 1 piece	4
whole, genuine or processed *(Heinz)*	2
halves *(Heinz* Deli Style)	4
spears *(Claussen)*	4
spears *(Claussen)*, 1.1-oz. piece	4
hamburger chips, half salt *(Vlasic)*	2
hamburger slices *(Heinz)*	2
kosher, whole, baby, spears, or chips *(Heinz)*	4
kosher, baby, crunchy, gherkins, or spears *(Vlasic)*	4
kosher, half salt, spears *(Vlasic)*	4

no garlic *(Claussen)*	6
no garlic *(Claussen)*, 2.9-oz. piece	17
no garlic, crunchy *(Vlasic)*	4
Polish style, whole or spears *(Heinz)*	4
zesty, spears or crunch *(Vlasic)*	4
pickles, kosher *(see also "pickles, dill," page 100):*	
whole *(Claussen)*, 2.5-oz. piece	9
whole or chips *(Heinz* Old Fashioned)	4
whole or slices *(Claussen)*	3
halves *(Claussen)*	4
halves *(Claussen)*, 2.3-oz. piece	9
halves *(Heinz* Old Fashioned Deli Halves)	4
slices *(Claussen)*, .3-oz. piece	1
pickles, mixed, garden, hot and spicy *(Vlasic)*	4
pickles, sweet:	
(Heinz Cucumber Stix)	25
whole or sliced *(Heinz)*	35
sliced *(Featherweight)*, 3–4 slices	24
sliced *(Heinz* Cucumber Slices)	20
gherkins, regular or midget *(Heinz)*	35
half salt *(Vlasic* Sweet Butter Chips)	30
mixed *(Heinz)*	40
relish:	
dill *(Vlasic)*	2
hamburger *(Heinz)*	30
hot dog *(Vlasic)*	40
hot dog or India *(Heinz)*	35
pickle *(Claussen)*	26
pickle *(Claussen)*, 1 tbsp.	14
picalilli *(Heinz)*	30
sweet *(Heinz)*	35
sweet *(Vlasic)*	30
salad cubes, sweet *(Heinz)*	30

OLIVES

	calories
green, w/pits:	
(all brands), 10 small, select or standard	33
(all brands), 10 large	45

Olives, green, w/pits, continued
(all brands), 10 giant 76
green, pitted (all brands), 1 oz. 33
ripe, Manzanillo or Mission varieties, pitted:
all sizes *(Lindsay)*, 1 oz. 32
(Lindsay), 10 small 37
(Lindsay), 10 medium 44
(Lindsay), 10 large 50
(Lindsay), 10 extra large 63
ripe, mixed varieties:
pitted *(Vlasic)*, 1 oz. 37
sliced or chopped *(Lindsay)*, 1 oz. 29
sliced *(Lindsay)*, 1/2 cup 70
ripe, salt-cured, oil-coated, Greek style:
(all brands), 10 medium 65
(all brands), 10 extra large 89
ripe, Sevillano and Ascolano varieties, pitted:
all sizes *(Lindsay)*, 1 oz. 23
(Lindsay), 10 jumbo 66
(Lindsay), 10 colossal 90
(Lindsay), 10 super colossal 122

VEGETABLE JUICES, six fluid ounces, except as
noted

	calories
carrot *(Hain)*	80
sauerkraut *(S&W)*, 5 fl. oz.	14
tomato:	
(Campbell's)	40
(Featherweight)	35
(Hunt's)	30
(S&W California/*S&W Nutradiet)*	35
(Stokely), 4 fl. oz.	20
(Welch's)	35
tomato-beef cocktail *(Beefamato)*	80
tomato-chile cocktail *(Snap-E-Tom)*	40
tomato-clam juice cocktail *(Clamato)*	96

vegetable:
("V-8"/"V-8" No Salt Added)	35
(Veryfine 100%)	32
hearty or hot and spicy *(Smucker's)*, 8 fl. oz.	58
spicy hot *("V-8")*	35

Chapter 8

VEGETARIAN FOODS

VEGETARIAN FOODS, CANNED & DRY

	calories
"beef":	
slices *(Worthington Savory Slices)*, 2 slices	100
steak *(Worthington Prime Stakes)*, 3.25-oz. piece	160
steak *(Worthington Vegetable Steaks)*, 3.2 oz.	110
stew *(Worthington Country Stew)*, 9½ oz.	220
burgers:	
(Worthington Vegetarian Burger), ½ cup	150
(Worthington Vegetarian Burger No Salt Added), ½ cup	160
mix* *(Love Natural Foods Loveburger)*, 4-oz. burger	245
mix* *(Nature's Burger Original)*, 3-oz. burger	152
mix *(Worthington Granburger)*, 6 tbsp. mix	110
mix*, barbecue *(Nature's Burger)*, 3-oz. burger	117
mix*, pizza *(Nature's Burger)*, 3-oz. burger	121
mix*, w/tofu *(Fantastic Foods)*, 3.4-oz. burger	133
"chicken":	
(Worthington FriChik), 2 pieces or 3.2 oz.	180
diced, drained *(Worthington)*, ¼ cup	90
sliced, drained *(Worthington)*, 2 slices	90
chops *(Worthington Choplets)*, 2 slices	100
cutlet:	
(Worthington), 1½ slices or 3.25 oz.	100
(Worthington Multigrain), 2 slices or 3.25 oz.	90
"eggs":	
mix *(Tofu Scrambler)*, ½ cup**	98

mix *(Tofu Scrambler)*, ½ cup***	158
"frankfurters":	
(Worthington Veja-Links), 2 links	140
(Worthington Super-Links), 1 link	100
luncheon "meat":	
(Worthington Numete), ½" slice	160
(Worthington Protose), ½" slice	180
"meat" loaf mix *(Natural Touch Loaf Mix)*, 4 oz.	180
"meatball" *(Worthington Non-Meat Balls)*, 3 pieces	100
"sausages" *(Worthington Saucettes)*, 2 links	140
"scallops":	
(Worthington Vegetable Skallops), ½ cup	90
(Worthington Vegetable Skallops No Salt), ½ cup	80
tofu spread:	
green chili *(Natural Touch Tofu Topper)*, 2 tbsp.	50
herb and spice *(Natural Touch Tofu Topper)*, 2 tbsp.	50
Mexican *(Natural Touch Tofu Topper)*, 2 tbsp.	60
"turkey":	
(Worthington Turkee Slices), 2 slices	130
(Worthington 209), 2 slices, drained	120

* *Prepared according to package directions*
** *Prepared with tofu*
*** *Prepared with tofu and butter*

VEGETARIAN FOODS, FROZEN & REFRIGERATED
See also "Dinners, Frozen" and "Entrees, Frozen"

	calories
"bacon":	
(Morningstar Farms Breakfast Strips), 3 strips	80
(Worthington Stripples), 4 strips	120
"beef":	
(Worthington Stakelets), 2.5-oz. piece	150
corned, roll *(Worthington)*, 2½ oz.	150
corned, slices *(Worthington)*, 4 slices	120
pie *(Worthington)*, 8-oz. pie	360
roll *(Worthington)*, 4 slices, 2.5 oz.	130
roll, smoked *(Worthington)*, 3 slices or 2 oz.	120

Vegetarian Foods, Frozen & Refrigerated, continued

"bologna" *(Worthington Bolono)*, 2 slices   60

breakfast dishes:

  French toast, cinnamon swirl, w/patties *(Morningstar
    Farms Country Breakfast)*, 6.5 oz.   380

  Scramblers, hash browns, and links *(Morningstar
    Farms Country Breakfast)*, 7 oz.   360

  Scramblers, pancakes, and links *(Morningstar Farms
    Country Breakfast)*, 6.8 oz.   380

burgers:

  (Morningstar Farms Grillers), 1 patty   180

  (Worthington FriPats), 2.25-oz. piece   180

"chicken":

  (Worthington Crispy Chik), 3 oz.   280

  diced *(Worthington Meatless Chicken)*, 1/2 cup   190

  nuggets, homestyle *(Morningstar Farms Country
    Crisps)*, 3 oz.   250

  nuggets, zesty *(Morningstar Farms Country Crisps)*,
    3 oz.   280

  patty *(Morningstar Farms Country Crisps)*, 1 patty . .   220

  patty *(Worthington Crispy Chik)*, 1 patty   220

  pie *(Worthington)*, 8-oz. pie   380

  roll *(Worthington Chic-ketts)*, 1/2 cup   160

  roll *(Worthington Meatless Chicken)*, 2 1/2 oz.   150

  slices *(Worthington Meatless Chicken)*, 2 slices   130

  sticks *(Worthington Chik Stiks)*, 1 piece   110

dinner patties *(Natural Touch Dinner Entree)*, 3-oz.
  patty   230

"eggs" *(see also "breakfast dishes," above)*:

  (Morningstar Farms Scramblers), 1/4 cup   60

  (Tofutti Egg Watchers), 2 oz.   50

"frankfurters":

  (Worthington Leanies), 1 link   100

  on a stick *(Worthington Dixie Dogs)*, 1 link   200

French toast, *see "breakfast dishes," above*

"ham," roll or slices *(Worthington Wham)*, 3 slices or
  2.4 oz.   120

"roast" *(Worthington Dinner Roast)*, 2 oz.   120

"salami":

  roll *(Worthington)*, 2 slices or 1.5 oz.   90

  slices *(Worthington)*, 2 slices or 1.3 oz.   80

"sausages":
  links *(Morningstar Farms* Breakfast Links), 3 links .   190
  links *(Worthington Prosage),* 3 links   190
  patties *(Morningstar Farms* Breakfast Patties),
    2 patties   190
  patties *(Worthington Prosage),* 2 patties   210
  roll *(Worthington Prosage),* 2 slices, ³/₈" each   180
tofu:
  raw, pasteurized *(Frieda* of California), 4.2 oz.   86
  flavored, Chinese 5-spice *(Nasoya),* 5 oz.   150
  flavored, French country herb *(Nasoya),* 5 oz.   150
tofu patty:
  garden *(Natural Touch),* 1 patty   90
  okara *(Natural Touch Okara),* 1 patty   160
tortellini, tofu, *see "Entrees, Frozen, tortellini,"*
    page 148
"tuna" *(Worthington Tuno),* 2 oz.   100
"turkey," smoked, roll or slices *(Worthington),* 4 slices
    or 2.7 oz.   180

VEGETARIAN (NONDAIRY) BEVERAGES, six fluid ounces, except as noted

	calories
rice beverage, chocolate *(Rice Dream)*	170
soy beverage:	
(Soy Moo), 8 fl. oz.	125
almond malted *(Westbrae Natural)*	250
carob or java malted *(Westbrae Natural)*	270
carob, chocolate, or vanilla *(Ah Soy)*	160
vanilla malted *(Westbrae Natural)*	250
soy "milk," granules *(Soyamel),* 8 fl. oz.*	130

* Prepared according to package directions

Chapter 9

SOUPS, BROTHS, AND CHOWDERS

> **SOUPS, CANNED, READY-TO-SERVE**
> *See also "Soups, Canned, Condensed," "Soups, Frozen," and "Soups, Mix"*

	calories
bean *(Grandma Brown's)*, 1 cup	190
bean, black *(Health Valley* Regular/No Salt Added), 7½ oz.	160
bean, w/ham:	
(Campbell's Chunky Old Fashioned), 11-oz. can	290
(Campbell's Chunky Old Fashioned), 9⅝ oz.	250
(Campbell's Home Cookin'), 10¾ oz.	210
chowder *(Hormel Micro-Cup* Hearty Soups), 1 cont.	191
beef:	
(Campbell's Chunky), 10¾ oz.	200
(Campbell's Chunky), 9½ oz.	170
(Progresso), 10½-oz. can	180
(Progresso), 9½ oz.	160
broth, *see "beef broth," below*	
beef, Stroganoff style *(Campbell's* Chunky), 10¾ oz.	320
beef barley *(Progresso)*, 10½-oz. can	150
beef barley *(Progresso)*, 9½ oz.	140
beef broth:	
(College Inn), 1 cup	18
(Health Valley Regular/No Salt Added), 7½ oz.	17
(Swanson), 7¼ oz.	18
seasoned *(Progresso)*, 4 oz.	10
beef cabbage *(Manischewitz)*, 1 cup	62

beef minestrone *(Progresso)*, 10½-oz. can   180
beef minestrone *(Progresso)*, 9½ oz.   170
beef noodle *(Progresso)*, 9½ oz.   170
beef vegetable:
  (Hormel Micro-Cup Hearty Soups), 1 cont.   71
  (Lipton Hearty Ones), 11-oz. cont.   229
  (Progresso), 10½-oz. can   170
  (Progresso), 9½ oz.   150
berry fruit, three *(Great Impressions)*, 6 oz.   107
blueberry fruit *(Great Impressions)*, 6 oz.   95
borscht:
  (Gold's), 8 oz.   100
  (Gold's Low Calorie), 8 oz.   20
  (Manischewitz Low Calorie), 1 cup   20
  (Rokeach), 1 cup   96
  (Rokeach Unsalted), 1 cup   103
  w/beets *(Manischewitz)*, 1 cup   80
broth, *see specific listings*
cherry fruit *(Great Impressions)*, 6 oz.   123
chickarina *(Progresso)*, 9½ oz.   130
chicken:
  (Campbell's Chunky Old Fashioned), 10¾-oz. can .   180
  (Campbell's Chunky Old Fashioned), 9½ oz.   150
  (Progresso Homestyle), 9½ oz.   110
  broth, *see "chicken broth," below*
  clear *(Manischewitz)*, 1 cup   46
  hearty *(Progresso)*, 10½-oz. can   130
  hearty *(Progresso)*, 9½ oz.   130
chicken corn chowder *(Campbell's* Chunky), 10¾ oz. .   340
chicken corn chowder *(Campbell's* Chunky), 9½ oz. . . .   300
chicken, cream of *(Progresso)*, 9½ oz.   190
chicken barley *(Manischewitz)*, 1 cup   83
chicken barley *(Progresso)*, 9¼ oz.   100
chicken broth:
  (Campbell's Low Sodium), 10½ oz.   30
  (College Inn), 1 cup   35
  (Hain), 8¾ oz.   70
  (Hain No Salt Added), 8¾ oz.   60
  (Health Valley Regular/No Salt Added), 7½ oz. . . .   35
  (Progresso), 4 oz.   8
  (Swanson), 7¼ oz.   30

Soups, Canned, Ready-to-Serve, continued

chicken gumbo w/sausage *(Campbell's* Home Cookin'), 10¾ oz.	140
chicken minestrone *(Progresso)*, 10½-oz. can	140
chicken minestrone *(Progresso)*, 9½ oz.	130
chicken mushroom, creamy *(Campbell's* Chunky), 10½-oz. can	270
chicken mushroom, creamy *(Campbell's* Chunky), 9⅜ oz.	240

chicken, w/noodles:

(Campbell's Home Cookin'), 10¾-oz. can	140
(Campbell's Home Cookin'), 9½ oz.	110
(Campbell's Low Sodium), 10¾ oz.	170

chicken noodle:

(Campbell's Chunky), 10¾-oz. can	200
(Campbell's Chunky), 9½ oz.	180
(Hain), 9½ oz.	120
(Hain No Salt Added), 9½ oz.	110
(Hormel Micro-Cup Hearty Soups), 1 pkg.	108
(Lipton Hearty Ones Homestyle), 11-oz. cont.	227
(Progresso), 10½-oz. can	120
(Progresso), 9½ oz.	120
(Weight Watchers), 10½ oz.	80

chicken nuggets, w/vegetables and noodles *(Campbell's* Chunky), 10¾-oz. can	190
chicken nuggets, w/vegetables and noodles *(Campbell's* Chunky), 9½ oz.	170
chicken, w/rice *(Campbell's* Chunky), 9½ oz.	140

chicken rice:

(Manischewitz), 1 cup	47
(Progresso), 10½-oz. can	120
(Progresso), 9½ oz.	130

chicken vegetable:

(Campbell's Chunky), 9½ oz.	170
(Health Valley Chunky, Regular/No Salt Added), 7½ oz.	125
(Manischewitz), 1 cup	55
(Progresso), 9½ oz.	140
and rice *(Hormel Micro-Cup* Hearty Soups), 1 cont.	114

chili beef *(Campbell's* Chunky), 11-oz. can	290
chili beef *(Campbell's* Chunky), 9¾ oz.	260

clam chowder, Manhattan:
   (Campbell's Chunky), 10¾-oz. can 160
   (Campbell's Chunky), 9½ oz. 150
   (Health Valley Regular/No Salt Added), 7½ oz. . . . 110
   (Progresso), 9½ oz. 120
clam chowder, New England:
   (Campbell's Chunky), 10¾-oz. can 290
   (Campbell's Chunky), 9½ oz. 260
   (Hain), 9¼ oz. 180
   (Hormel Micro-Cup Hearty Soups), 1 cont. 118
   (Progresso), 10½-oz. can 220
   (Progresso), 9¼ oz. 220
corn chowder *(Progresso),* 9¼ oz. 200
Creole style *(Campbell's* Chunky), 10¾ oz. 240
Creole style *(Campbell's* Chunky), 9½ oz. 220
escarole, in chicken broth *(Progresso),* 9¼ oz. 30
ham and bean *(Progresso),* 9½ oz. 140
ham and butter bean *(Campbell's* Chunky), 10¾ oz. . . . 280
lemon fruit *(Great Impressions),* 6 oz. 90
lentil:
   (Health Valley Regular/No Salt Added), 7½ oz. . . . 170
   (Progresso), 10½-oz. can 140
   (Progresso), 9½ oz. 140
   hearty *(Campbell's* Home Cookin'), 10¾-oz. can . . . 170
   hearty *(Campbell's* Home Cookin'), 9½ oz. 140
   vegetarian *(Hain* Regular/No Salt Added), 9½ oz. . 160
lentil, w/sausage *(Progresso),* 9½ oz. 170
macaroni and bean *(Progresso),* 10½-oz. can 150
macaroni and bean *(Progresso),* 9½ oz. 140
minestrone:
   (Campbell's Chunky), 9½ oz. 160
   (Campbell's Home Cookin'), 10¾-oz. can 140
   (Campbell's Home Cookin'), 9½ oz. 120
   (Hain), 9½ oz. 170
   (Hain No Salt Added), 9½ oz. 160
   (Health Valley Regular/No Salt Added), 7½ oz. . . . 130
   (Hormel Micro-Cup Hearty Soups), 1 pkg. 104
   (Lipton Hearty Ones), 11-oz. cont. 189
   (Progresso), 10½-oz. can 120
   (Progresso), 9½ oz. 130
   zesty *(Progresso),* 9½ oz. 150

Soups, Canned, Ready-to-Serve, continued

mushroom:

cream of *(Campbell's* Low Sodium), 10½ oz. 210

cream of *(Progresso),* 9¼ oz. 160

cream of *(Weight Watchers),* 10½ oz. 90

creamy *(Hain),* 9¼ oz. 110

mushroom barley:

(Hain), 9½ oz. 100

(Health Valley Regular/No Salt Added), 7½ oz. . . . 100

(Manischewitz), 1 cup 72

pea, split:

(Campbell's Low Sodium), 10½ oz. 230

(Grandma Brown's), 1 cup 208

(Hain Regular/No Salt Added), 9½ oz. 170

(Manischewitz), 1 cup 133

green *(Health Valley* Regular/No Salt Added),

7½ oz. 190

green *(Progresso),* 10½-oz. can 201

green *(Progresso),* 9½ oz. 160

pea, split, w/ham:

(Campbell's Chunky), 10¾-oz. can 230

(Campbell's Chunky), 9½ oz. 210

(Campbell's Home Cookin'), 10¾-oz. can 230

(Campbell's Home Cookin'), 9½ oz. 200

(Progresso), 10½-oz. can 160

(Progresso), 9½ oz. 150

pepper steak *(Campbell's* Chunky), 10¾-oz. can 180

pepper steak *(Campbell's* Chunky), 9½ oz. 160

potato leek *(Health Valley* Regular/No Salt Added),

7½ oz. 130

schav *(Gold's),* 8 oz. 25

schav *(Manischewitz),* 1 cup 11

sirloin burger *(Campbell's* Chunky), 10¾-oz. can 220

sirloin burger *(Campbell's* Chunky), 9½ oz. 200

steak and potato *(Campbell's* Chunky), 10¾-oz. can . . 200

steak and potato *(Campbell's* Chunky), 9½ oz. 170

tomato:

(Health Valley Regular/No Salt Added), 7½ oz. . . . 100

(Manischewitz), 1 cup 60

(Progresso), 9½ oz. 120

garden *(Campbell's* Home Cookin'), 10¾-oz. can . . 150

garden *(Campbell's* Home Cookin'), 9½ oz. 130
w/tomato pieces *(Campbell's* Low Sodium), 10½ oz. 190
w/tortellini *(Progresso)*, 9¼ oz. 130
tomato beef, w/rotini *(Progresso)*, 9½ oz. 170
tortellini *(Progresso)*, 9½ oz. 90
tortellini, creamy *(Progresso)*, 9¼ oz. 240
turkey rice *(Hain* Regular/No Salt Added), 9½ oz. . . 100
turkey vegetable *(Campbell's* Chunky), 9⅜ oz. 150
turkey vegetable *(Weight Watchers)*, 10½ oz. 70
vegetable:
    (Campbell's Chunky), 10¾-oz. can 160
    (Campbell's Chunky), 9½ oz. 150
    (Health Valley Regular/No Salt Added), 7½ oz. . . . 110
    (Manischewitz), 1 cup 63
    (Progresso), 9½ oz. 80
    w/beef stock *(Weight Watchers)*, 10½ oz. 90
    country *(Campbell's* Home Cookin'), 10¾ oz. 120
    country *(Campbell's* Home Cookin'), 9½ oz. 100
    country *(Hormel Micro-Cup* Hearty Soups), 1 cont. . 89
    five bean, chunky *(Health Valley* Regular/No Salt
        Added), 7½ oz. 110
    Mediterranean *(Campbell's* Chunky), 9½ oz. 170
    vegetarian *(Hain)*, 9½ oz. 140
    vegetarian *(Hain* No Salt Added), 9½ oz. 150
    vegetarian, chunky *(Weight Watchers)*, 10½ oz. 100
vegetable beef:
    (Campbell's Chunky Old Fashioned), 10¾-oz. can . 190
    (Campbell's Chunky Old Fashioned), 9½ oz. 160
    (Campbell's Home Cookin'), 10¾-oz. can 140
    (Campbell's Home Cookin'), 9½ oz. 120
vegetable chicken *(Hain* Regular/No Salt Added),
    9½ oz. 120
vegetable pasta, Italian *(Hain)*, 9½ oz. 160
vegetable pasta, Italian *(Hain* Low Sodium), 9½ oz. . . 140

> **SOUPS, CANNED, CONDENSED***
> *See also "Soups, Canned, Ready-to-Serve," "Soups,
> Frozen," and "Soups, Mixes"*

	calories
asparagus, cream of *(Campbell's)*, 8 oz.	80
barley and mushroom *(Rokeach)*, 1 cup	85
bean, w/bacon *(Campbell's)*, 8 oz.	140
bean, w/bacon *(Campbell's Special Request)*, 8 oz. . . .	140
beef *(Campbell's)*, 8 oz.	80
beef broth or bouillon *(Campbell's)*, 8 oz.	16
beef consommé, w/gelatin *(Campbell's)*, 8 oz.	25
beef noodle *(Campbell's)*, 8 oz.	70
beef noodle *(Campbell's* Homestyle), 8 oz.	80
broccoli, cream of *(Campbell's)*, 8 oz.	80
broccoli, cream of *(Campbell's)*, 8 oz.**	140
celery, cream of *(Campbell's)*, 8 oz.	100
cheese:	
cheddar *(Campbell's)*, 8 oz.	110
nacho *(Campbell's)*, 8 oz.	110
nacho *(Campbell's)*, 8 oz.**	180
chicken alphabet *(Campbell's)*, 8 oz.	80
chicken barley *(Campbell's)*, 8 oz.	70
chicken broth *(Campbell's)*, 8 oz.	30
chicken broth and noodles *(Campbell's)*, 8 oz.	45
chicken, cream of *(Campbell's/Campbell's Special Request)*, 8 oz.	110
chicken 'n dumplings *(Campbell's)*, 8 oz.	80
chicken gumbo *(Campbell's)*, 8 oz.	60
chicken mushroom, creamy *(Campbell's)*, 8 oz.	120
chicken noodle:	
(Campbell's), 8 oz.	60
(Campbell's Noodle-O's), 8 oz.	70
(Campbell's Special Request), 8 oz.	60
chicken rice *(Campbell's/Campbell's Special Request)*, 8 oz.	60
chicken and stars *(Campbell's)*, 8 oz.	60
chicken vegetable *(Campbell's)*, 8 oz.	70
chili beef *(Campbell's)*, 8 oz.	140
clam chowder, Manhattan:	
(Campbell's), 8 oz.	70

(Doxsee), 7.5 oz.	70
(Snow's), 7.5 oz.	70
clam chowder, New England:	
(Campbell's), 8 oz.	80
(Campbell's), 8 oz.**	150
(Gorton's), 1/4 can**	140
(Snow's), 7.5 oz.**	140
corn chowder *(Snow's)*, 7.5 oz.**	150
fish chowder *(Snow's)*, 7.5 oz.**	130
minestrone *(Campbell's)*, 8 oz.	80
mushroom, beefy *(Campbell's)*, 8 oz.	60
mushroom, cream of *(Campbell's/Campbell's Special Request)*, 8 oz.	100
mushroom, golden *(Campbell's)*, 8 oz.	70
noodle, curly, w/chicken *(Campbell's)*, 8 oz.	80
noodle and ground beef *(Campbell's)*, 8 oz.	90
onion, cream of *(Campbell's)*, 8 oz.	100
onion, cream of *(Campbell's)*, 8 oz.***	140
onion, French *(Campbell's)*, 8 oz.	60
oyster stew *(Campbell's)*, 8 oz.	70
oyster stew *(Campbell's)*, 8 oz.**	140
pea, green *(Campbell's)*, 8 oz.	160
pea, split, w/egg barley *(Rokeach)*, 1 cup	132
pea, split, w/ham and bacon *(Campbell's)*, 8 oz.	160
pepper pot *(Campbell's)*, 8 oz.	90
potato, cream of *(Campbell's)*, 8 oz.	80
potato, cream of *(Campbell's)*, 8 oz.***	120
Scotch broth *(Campbell's)*, 8 oz.	80
seafood chowder *(Snow's)*, 7.5 oz.**	140
shrimp, cream of *(Campbell's)*, 8 oz.	90
shrimp, cream of *(Campbell's)*, 8 oz.**	160
tomato:	
(Campbell's), 8 oz.	90
(Campbell's), 8 oz.**	150
(Campbell's Zesty), 8 oz.	100
(Campbell's Special Request), 8 oz.	90
tomato, cream of *(Campbell's Homestyle)*, 8 oz.	110
tomato, cream of *(Campbell's Homestyle)*, 8 oz.**	180
tomato bisque *(Campbell's)*, 8 oz.	120
tomato rice *(Campbell's Old Fashioned)*, 8 oz.	110
turkey noodle *(Campbell's)*, 8 oz.	70

Soups, Canned, Condensed*, continued

turkey vegetable *(Campbell's)*, 8 oz.	70
vegetable:	
(Campbell's), 8 oz.	90
(Campbell's Homestyle/Old Fashioned), 8 oz.	60
w/beef stock *(Campbell's Special Request)*, 8 oz. . . .	90
vegetable, vegetarian *(Campbell's)*, 8 oz.	80
vegetable beef *(Campbell's/Campbell's Special Request)*,	
8 oz.	70
won ton *(Campbell's)*, 8 oz.	40

* *Prepared according to package directions, with water, except as noted*
** *Prepared with whole milk*
*** *Prepared with 4 oz. soup, 2 oz. whole milk and 2 oz. water*

SOUPS, FROZEN, six fluid ounces, except as noted

	calories
asparagus, cream of *(Kettle Ready)*	62
asparagus, cream of *(Myers)*, 9.75 oz.	152
bean, black, w/ham *(Kettle Ready)*	154
bean, savory, w/ham *(Kettle Ready)*	113
beef, hearty, vegetable *(Kettle Ready)*	85
broccoli, cream of *(Kettle Ready)*	94
broccoli, cream of *(Myers)*, 9.75 oz.	174
cauliflower, cream of *(Kettle Ready)*	93
cheese:	
and broccoli *(Myers)*, 9.75 oz.	325
cheddar, cream of *(Kettle Ready)*	158
cheddar, and broccoli, cream of *(Kettle Ready)*	137
chicken:	
cream of *(Kettle Ready)*	98
gumbo *(Kettle Ready)*	94
noodle *(Kettle Ready)*	94
noodle *(Myers)*, 9.75 oz.	87
chili, traditional *(Kettle Ready)*	161
chili, jalapeño *(Kettle Ready)*	173
clam chowder:	
Boston *(Kettle Ready)*	131
Manhattan *(Kettle Ready)*	69

New England *(Kettle Ready)* 116
New England *(Myers)*, 9.75 oz. 152
New England *(Stouffer's)*, 8 oz. 180
corn and broccoli chowder *(Kettle Ready)* 102
minestrone, hearty *(Kettle Ready)* 104
mushroom, cream of *(Kettle Ready)* 85
onion, French *(Kettle Ready)* 42
pea, split, w/ham *(Kettle Ready)* 155
pea, tortellini, in tomato *(Kettle Ready)* 122
seafood bisque *(Myers)*, 9.75 oz. 163
spinach, cream of *(Myers)*, 9.75 oz. 174
spinach, cream of *(Stouffer's)*, 8 oz. 210
vegetable, garden *(Kettle Ready)* 85
vegetable beef *(Myers)*, 9.75 oz. 120

SOUPS, MIXES*, six fluid ounces, except as noted

	calories
beef or beef flavor:	
(Lipton Cup-a-Soup)	44
base *(Tone's)*, 1 tsp.	11
bouillon, *see "bouillon," below*	
hearty, and noodles *(Lipton)*, 7 fl. oz.	107
noodle *(Estee)*, 6 oz.	20
bouillon, dry mix or cube:	
beef *(Featherweight)*, 1 tsp.	18
beef *(Lite-Line* Low Sodium), 1 tsp.	12
beef *(Steero)*, 1 tsp.	6
beef *(Steero)*, 1 cube	6
beef *(Weight Watchers* Broth Mix), 1 pkt.	8
beef *(Wyler's)*, 1 tsp.	6
beef *(Wyler's)*, 1 cube	6
brown *(G. Washington's* Seasoning & Broth Regular/ Kosher), 1 pkt.	6
chicken *(Featherweight)*, 1 tsp.	18
chicken *(Lite-Line* Low Sodium), 1 tsp.	12
chicken *(Steero)*, 1 tsp.	8
chicken *(Steero)*, 1 cube	8
chicken *(Weight Watchers* Broth Mix), 1 pkt.	8
chicken *(Wyler's)*, 1 tsp.	8

Soups, Mixes*, bouillon, dry mix or cube, continued

chicken *(Wyler's)*, 1 cube 8
golden *(G. Washington's* Seasoning & Broth Regular/
   Kosher), 1 pkt. 6
onion *(G. Washington's* Seasoning & Broth), 1 pkt. . 12
onion *(Wyler's)*, 1 tsp. 10
vegetable *(G. Washington's* Seasoning & Broth), 1
   pkt. 12
vegetable *(Wyler's)*, 1 tsp. 6
broccoli:
creamy *(Lipton Cup-a-Soup)* 62
creamy, and cheese *(Lipton Cup-a-Soup)* 70
golden *(Lipton Cup-a-Soup* Lite) 42
cheddar, creamy, w/noodles *(Fantastic Noodles)*, 7 oz. . 178
cheese *(Hain* Savory Soup & Sauce Mix) 250
cheese and broccoli *(Hain* Soup & Recipe Mix) 310
chicken or chicken flavor:
bouillon, *see "bouillon," page 117*
broth *(Lipton Cup-a-Soup)* 20
cream of *(Lipton Cup-a-Soup)* 84
creamy, w/vegetables *(Lipton Cup-a-Soup)* 93
creamy, w/white meat *(Campbell's* Cup 2 Minute
   Soup) 90
w/sweet corn *(Lipton Cup-a-Soup* Country Style) . . 133
Florentine *(Lipton Cup-a-Soup* Lite) 42
hearty *(Lipton Cup-a-Soup* Country Style) 69
hearty, supreme *(Lipton Cup-a-Soup)* 107
lemon *(Lipton Cup-a-Soup* Lite) 48
supreme *(Lipton Cup-a-Soup* Country Style) 107
chicken noodle:
(Campbell's Quality Soup & Recipe), 1 cup 100
(Estee Instant), 6 oz. 25
(Lipton), 1 cup 81
(Lipton Cup-a-Soup) 48
(Mrs. Grass Chickeny Rich), 1/4 pkg. 70
hearty *(Lipton)*, 1 cup 83
hearty *(Lipton Lots-a-Noodles Cup-a-Soup)*, 7 fl. oz. . 110
hearty, creamy *(Lipton Lots-a-Noodles Cup-a-Soup)*,
   7 fl. oz. 179
w/meat *(Lipton Cup-a-Soup)* 46
w/white meat *(Campbell's* Cup 2 Minute Soup) . . . 90

w/white meat, diced *(Lipton),* 1 cup 81
w/vegetables, hearty *(Lipton),* 1 cup 75
chicken 'n rice *(Lipton Cup-a-Soup)* 47
chicken vegetable *(Lipton Cup-a-Soup)* 47
clam chowder, Manhattan *(Golden Dipt),* 1/4 pkg. 80
clam chowder, New England *(Golden Dipt),* 1/4 pkg. . . 70
lentil *(Hain Savory Soup Mix)* 130
lobster bisque *(Golden Dipt),* 1/4 pkg. 30
minestrone *(Hain Savory Soup Mix)* 110
minestrone *(Manischewitz)* 50
mushroom:
   (Estee Instant), 6 oz. 40
   (Hain Savory Soup & Recipe Mix) 210
   (Hain Savory Soup & Recipe Mix No Salt Added) . 250
   beef flavor *(Lipton),* 1 cup 38
   cream of *(Lipton Cup-a-Soup)* 71
noodle:
   (Campbell's Quality Soup & Recipe), 1 cup 110
   (Lipton Cup-a-Soup Ring Noodle) 47
   beef *(Cup O'Noodles),* 1 cup 290
   beef flavor *(Oodles of Noodles/Top Ramen),* 1 cup . . 390
   beefy, hearty, w/vegetables *(Lipton),* 1 cup 85
   chicken flavor *(Cup O'Noodles),* 1 cup 300
   chicken flavor *(Oodles of Noodles/Top Ramen),*
    1 cup 400
   chicken flavor, country *(Cup O'Noodles Hearty),*
    1 cup 300
   w/chicken broth *(Campbell's Cup 2 Minute Soup)* . 90
   w/chicken broth *(Lipton Giggle Noodle)* 1 cup 77
   w/chicken broth *(Lipton Ring-O-Noodle),* 1 cup . . . 71
   hearty, w/vegetables *(Lipton),* 1 cup 75
   Oriental *(Oodles of Noodles/Top Ramen),* 1 cup . . . 390
   pork *(Oodles of Noodles/Top Ramen),* 1 cup 390
   seafood, savory *(Cup O'Noodles Hearty),* 1 cup 300
   shrimp *(Cup O'Noodles),* 1 cup 300
   vegetable, old fashioned *(Cup O'Noodles Hearty),* 1
    cup. 290
   vegetable beef *(Cup O'Noodles Hearty),* 1 cup 290
onion:
   (Campbell's Quality Soup & Recipe), 1 cup 30
   (Estee), 6 oz. 25

Soups, Mixes*, onion, continued

(Hain Savory Soup, Dip & Recipe Mix Regular/No
  Salt Added)........................ 50
(Lipton), 1 cup 20
(Lipton Cup-a-Soup) 27
(Mrs. Grass Soup & Dip Mix), ¼ pkg. 35
beefy *(Lipton)*, 1 cup 29
bouillon, *see "bouillon," above*
creamy *(Lipton Cup-a-Soup)* 70
golden, w/chicken broth *(Lipton)*, 1 cup 62
mushroom *(Lipton)*, 1 cup 41
Oriental *(Lipton Cup-a-Soup Lite)* 45
pea:
  green *(Lipton Cup-a-Soup)* 113
  split *(Hain* Savory Soup Mix) 310
  split *(Manischewitz)* 45
  Virginia *(Lipton Cup-a-Soup Country Style)* 148
potato leek *(Hain* Savory Soup Mix) 260
seafood chowder *(Golden Dipt)*, ¼ pkg. dry 70
shrimp bisque *(Golden Dipt)*, ¼ pkg. dry 30
tomato:
  (Estee Instant), 6 oz....................... 40
  (Hain Savory Soup & Recipe Mix) 220
  (Lipton Cup-a-Soup) 103
  creamy, and herb *(Lipton Cup-a-Soup Lite)* 66
vegetable:
  (Hain Savory Soup Mix Regular/No Salt Added) .. 80
  (Lipton), 1 cup 39
  (Manischewitz) 50
  bouillon, *see "bouillon," page 117*
  country *(Lipton)*, 1 cup 80
  curry, w/noodles *(Fantastic Noodles)*, 7 oz. 150
  garden *(Lipton Lots-a-Noodles Cup-a-Soup)*, 7 fl. oz. 123
  harvest *(Lipton Cup-a-Soup Country Style)* 91
  miso, w/noodles *(Fantastic Noodles)*, 7 oz. 152
  noodle, w/meatballs, *(Lipton Cup-a-Soup Country
    Style)* 95
  spring *(Lipton Cup-a-Soup)* 33
  tomato, w/noodles *(Fantastic Noodles)*, 7 oz. 158

* *Prepared according to package directions, with water, except as noted*

Chapter 10

DIPS AND
APPETIZERS

DIPS, two tablespoons, except as noted
See also "Cheese Spreads" and "Sauces"

---

	calories
Acapulco *(Ortega)*, 1 oz.	8
avocado *(Kraft)*	50
bacon and horseradish *(Kraft)*	60
bacon and horseradish *(Kraft* Premium)	50
bacon and onion *(Kraft* Premium)	50
blue cheese *(Kraft* Premium)	45
chili *(La Victoria)*, 1 tbsp.	6
clam *(Kraft)*	50
clam *(Kraft* Premium)	45
cucumber, creamy *(Kraft* Premium)	50
dill, creamy *(Nasoya Vegi-Dip)*, 1 oz.	60
garlic, w/tofu *(Life* All Natural), 1 tbsp.	70
garlic and herb *(Nasoya Vegi-Dip)*, 1 oz.	50
hummus, dip mix *(Fantastic Foods)*, 2 oz. or ¼ cup	111
hummus, mix *(Casbah)*, 1 oz. dry	110
jalapeño bean *(Wise)*	25
jalapeño bean, medium *(Hain)*, 4 tbsp.	70
jalapeño pepper *(Kraft/Kraft* Premium)	50
jalapeño pepper, nacho *(Price's)*, 1 oz.	80
Mexican bean *(Hain)*, 4 tbsp.	60
mushroom and herb *(Breakstone's* Gourmet)	50
nacho cheese *(Kraft* Premium)	50
onion:	
bean *(Hain)*, 4 tbsp.	70
creamy *(Kraft* Premium)	45

Dips, onion, continued

French *(Bison)*, 1 oz.	60
French *(Kraft)*	60
French *(Kraft* Premium)	45
French *(Nasoya Vegi-Dip)*, 1 oz.	50
green *(Kraft)*	60
salad, egg-free *(Nasoya Vegi-Dip)*, 1 oz.	45
salsa, *see "Sauces, salsa" page 210*	
taco *(Hain)*, 4 tbsp.	25
taco *(Wise)*	12

APPETIZERS & SNACKS, CANNED OR DRIED
See also "Appetizers & Snacks, Frozen" and "Meat, Fish & Poultry Spreads"

---

	calories
anchovies, flat *(Reese)*, 2-oz. can	100
beef jerky *(see also "sausage sticks," page 123)*:	
(Frito-Lay's), .21 oz.	25
(Frito-Lay's Tender), .7 oz.	120
(Hormel Lumberjack), 1 oz.	101
(Pemmican Arrowhead), .7-oz. piece	70
(Pemmican Steakers), 1 pouch	80
(Pemmican Steakers), 1 strip	40
(Pemmican Tender Brave/Chief/Trail/Tribe Packs), 1 oz.	80
(Pemmican Tender Tomahawk), .25-oz. piece	20
(Slim Jim), 1 piece	20
(Slim Jim Big Jerk), 1 piece	25
(Slim Jim Giant Jerk), 1 piece	60
natural, peppered, jalapeño, or *Tabasco (Pemmican)*, 1.1 oz.	90
natural style *(Pemmican)*, 1 oz.	80
regular or *Tabasco (Slim Jim Super Jerk)*, 1 piece	30
teriyaki, natural style *(Pemmican)*, 1 oz.	80
caviar:	
black sturgeon *(Northland Queen)*, 1 oz.	74
black sturgeon *(Romanoff)*, 1 oz.	74
red salmon *(Romanoff)*, 1 oz.	68
red salmon *(Romar Brand)*, 1 oz.	68

clam cocktail, w/sauce *(Sau-Sea)*, 4-oz. jar   99
crab cocktail, w/sauce *(Sau-Sea)*, 4-oz. jar   107
egg, pickled *(Penrose)*, 1 egg   80
eggplant *(Progresso* Caponata)*, ½ can   70
frankfurters, cocktail *(Oscar Mayer* Little Wieners),
  .3-oz. link   28
herring snacks, kippered *(King Oscar* Kippered
  Snacks), 3¾-oz. can   205
mushrooms, cocktail *(Reese* Buttons), 4-oz. jar, drained   25
nachos, microwave:
  cheese sauce *(Tio Sancho* Snacks), 3.5 oz.   247
  chips *(Tio Sancho* Snacks), 4 oz.   567
olive appetizer *(Progresso)*, ½ cup   180
olive condite *(Progresso)*, ½ cup   130
onions, cocktail, lightly spiced *(Vlasic)*, 1 oz.   4
peppers, sweet, fried *(Progresso)*, ½ jar   37
pate, liver *(Hormel)*, 1 tbsp.   33
sardines, see *"Fish & Shellfish, Canned or in Jars,*
  sardines," page 176
sardines, kippered *(Brunswick* Kippered Snacks),
  3½ oz.   185
sausage sticks *(see also "beef jerky," page 122)*, 1 stick:
  beef, pepperoni *(Pemmican)*, 1.1 oz.   170
  beef, *Tabasco (Pemmican)*, 1.1 oz.   120
  beef, teriyaki *(Pemmican)*, 1.1 oz.   150
  smoked *(Slim Jim Big Slim)*, .52 oz.   80
  smoked *(Slim Jim Giant Slim)*, 1.1 oz.   180
  smoked *(Slim Jim Jumbo Jim)*, 1 oz.   150
  smoked, all types *(Slim Jim* Handi-Paks), .31 oz. . .   50
  smoked, nacho *(Slim Jim Super Slim)*, .7 oz.   100
  smoked, *Tabasco (Slim Jim Super Slim/Super Slim)*,
    .7 oz.   110
  summer sausage, regular or teriyaki *(Pemmican)*,
    .8 oz.   110
  summer sausage, smoked *(Slim Jim)*, .5 oz.   80
sausages, pickled:
  (Penrose Firecracker), 1.5-oz. link   120
  giant *(Penrose* Firecracker), 2.1-oz. link   170
  hot, red hot, Polish, beer, or firecracker *(Penrose)*,
    .5-oz. link   40

Appetizers & Snacks, continued

sausages, Vienna:

in barbecue sauce *(Libby's)*, 2½ oz.	180
in beef broth *(Libby's)*, 3½ links	160
no broth *(Hormel)*, 4 links	200
shrimp cocktail, w/sauce *(Sau-Sea)*, 4 oz.	113

APPETIZERS & SNACKS, FROZEN
See also "Appetizers & Snacks, Canned, Dried, or in Jars"

---

calories

cheese, *see "Cheese Dishes, Frozen," page 59*

egg rolls:

chicken *(Chun King)*, 3.6 oz.	220
chicken *(Jeno's Snacks)*, 3 oz. or 6 rolls	190
meat and shrimp *(Chun King)*, 3.6 oz.	220
meat and shrimp *(Jeno's Snacks)*, 3 oz. or 6 rolls	200
pork *(Chun King Restaurant Style)*, 3 oz.	180
shrimp *(Chun King)*, 3.6 oz.	200
shrimp and cheese *(Jeno's Snacks)*, 3 oz. or 6 rolls	190
vegetarian *(Worthington)*, 3-oz. roll	160
franks in pastry *(Durkey Franks-N-Blankets)*, 1 piece	45

pizza rolls, 3 oz. or 6 rolls:

cheese or hamburger *(Jeno's)*	240
pepperoni and cheese *(Jeno's)*	230
pepperoni and cheese *(Jeno's Microwave)*	240
sausage and cheese *(Jeno's Microwave)*	250
sausage and pepperoni *(Jeno's)*	230

DINNERS, ENTREES, AND POT PIES

DINNERS, FROZEN, one complete dinner
See also "Entrees, Frozen"

---

	calories
beans and frankfurter:	
(Banquet), 10 oz.	520
(Morton), 10 oz.	350
(Swanson), 10.5 oz.	440
beef:	
(Banquet Extra Helping), 16 oz.	870
(Swanson), 11.25 oz.	310
in barbecue sauce *(Swanson),* 11 oz.	460
chopped *(Banquet),* 11 oz.	420
chopped steak *(Swanson Hungry-Man),* 16.75 oz.	640
enchilada, see "enchilada," page 127	
meat loaf, see "meat loaf," page 128	
Mexicana *(The Budget Gourmet),* 12.8 oz.	560
patty, charbroiled *(Freezer Queen),* 10 oz.	300
pepper steak *(Armour Classics Lite),* 11.25 oz.	220
pepper steak *(Healthy Choice),* 11 oz.	290
pepper steak *(Le Menu),* 11.5 oz.	370
pot roast, Yankee *(Armour Classics),* 10 oz.	310
pot roast, Yankee *(The Budget Gourmet),* 11 oz.	380
pot roast, Yankee *(Healthy Choice),* 11 oz.	260
pot roast, Yankee *(Le Menu),* 10 oz.	330
short ribs, boneless *(Armour Classics),* 9.75 oz.	380
sirloin, chopped *(Le Menu),* 12.25 oz.	430
sirloin, chopped *(Swanson),* 10.75 oz.	340
sirloin, roast *(Armour Classics),* 10.45 oz.	190

Dinners, Frozen, beef, continued

sirloin tips *(Armour Classics)*, 10.25 oz.	230
sirloin tips *(Healthy Choice)*, 11.75 oz.	290
sirloin tips *(Le Menu)*, 11.5 oz.	400
sirloin tips, in Burgundy sauce *(The Budget Gourmet)*, 11 oz.	310
sliced *(Morton)*, 10 oz.	220
sliced *(Swanson Hungry-Man)*, 15.25 oz.	450
sliced, gravy and *(Freezer Queen)*, 10 oz.	210
steak Diane *(Armour Classics Lite)*, 10 oz.	290
Stroganoff *(Armour Classics Lite)*, 11.25 oz.	250
Stroganoff *(Le Menu)*, 10 oz.	430
Swiss steak *(The Budget Gourmet)*, 11.2 oz.	450
Swiss steak *(Swanson)*, 10 oz.	350
burrito *(Patio)*, 12 oz.	517
burrito, beef and bean *(Old El Paso Festive Dinners)*, 11 oz.	470

chicken:

à la king *(Armour Classics Lite)*, 11.25 oz.	290
à la king *(Le Menu)*, 10.25 oz.	330
barbecue-style *(Stouffer's Dinner Supreme)*, 10.5 oz. .	390
boneless *(Swanson Hungry-Man)*, 17.75 oz.	700
breast, baked, w/gravy *(Stouffer's Dinner Supreme)*, 10 oz.	300
breast, glazed *(Le Menu LightStyle)*, 10 oz.	230
breast, Marsala *(Armour Classics Lite)*, 10.5 oz.	250
Burgundy *(Armour Classics Lite)*, 10 oz.	210
cacciatore *(The Budget Gourmet)*, 11 oz.	300
casserole *(Pillsbury Microwave Classic)*, 1 pkg.	400
and cheese, casserole *(Pillsbury Microwave Classic)*, 1 pkg.	480
Cordon Bleu *(Le Menu)*, 11 oz.	460
and dumplings *(Banquet)*, 10 oz.	430
fettuccine *(Armour Classics)*, 11 oz.	260
Florentine *(Stouffer's Dinner Supreme)*, 11 oz.	430
fried *(Banquet)*, 10 oz.	400
fried *(Banquet Extra Helping)*, 16 oz.	570
fried *(Kid Cuisine)*, 7.25 oz.	420
fried *(Stouffer's Dinner Supreme)*, 10⅝ oz.	450
fried, barbecue flavored *(Swanson)*, 10 oz.	540
fried, dark meat *(Swanson)*, 1 pkg.	560

fried, dark meat *(Swanson Hungry-Man)*, 1 pkg. . . .   860
fried, white meat *(Banquet Extra Helping)*, 16 oz. . .   570
fried, white meat *(Swanson)*, 1 pkg.   550
fried, white meat *(Swanson Hungry-Man)*, 1 pkg. . .   870
glazed *(Armour Classics)*, 10.75 oz.   300
herb roasted *(Healthy Choice)*, 11 oz.   260
herb roasted *(Le Menu* LightStyle), 10 oz.   240
mesquite *(Armour Classics)*, 9.5 oz.   370
mesquite *(Healthy Choice)*, 10.5 oz.   310
Mexicana *(The Budget Gourmet)*, 12.8 oz.   510
and noodles *(Armour Classics)*, 11 oz.   230
nuggets *(Swanson)*, 8.75 oz.   470
nuggets, w/barbecue sauce *(Banquet Extra Helping)*,
    10 oz.   640
nuggets, platter *(Freezer Queen)*, 6 oz.   410
nuggets, w/sweet and sour sauce *(Banquet Extra
    Helping)*, 10 oz.   650
Oriental *(Armour Classics Lite)*, 10 oz.   180
Oriental *(Healthy Choice)*, 11.25 oz.   220
parmigiana *(Armour Classics)*, 11.5 oz.   370
parmigiana *(Healthy Choice)*, 11.5 oz.   280
parmigiana *(Le Menu)*, 11.75 oz.   410
parmigiana *(Stouffer's Dinner Supreme)*, 11.5 oz. . . .   360
and pasta divan *(Healthy Choice)*, 11.5 oz.   310
pattie platter *(Freezer Queen)*, 7.5 oz.   360
roast *(The Budget Gourmet)*, 11.2 oz.   280
w/supreme sauce *(Stouffer's Dinner Supreme)*,
    11⅜ oz.   360
sweet and sour *(Armour Classics Lite)*, 11 oz.   240
sweet and sour *(Healthy Choice)*, 11.5 oz.   280
sweet and sour *(Le Menu)*, 11.25 oz.   400
teriyaki *(The Budget Gourmet)*, 12 oz.   360
in wine sauce *(Le Menu)*, 10 oz.   280
w/wine and mushroom sauce *(Armour Classics)*,
    10.75 oz.   280
chimichanga, beef *(Old El Paso* Festive Dinners),
    11 oz.   540
chimichanga, beef and cheese *(Old El Paso* Festive
    Dinners), 11 oz.   510
enchilada:
beef *(Banquet)*, 12 oz.   500

Dinners, Frozen, enchilada, continued

beef *(Old El Paso* Festive Dinners), 11 oz.	390
beef *(Patio)*, 13.25 oz.	520
beef *(Swanson)*, 13.75 oz.	480
beef *(Van de Kamp's* Mexican Dinner), ½ pkg.	200
cheese *(Banquet)*, 12 oz.	550
cheese *(Old El Paso* Festive Dinners), 11 oz.	590
cheese *(Patio)*, 12.25 oz.	380
cheese *(Van de Kamp's* Mexican Dinner), ½ pkg.	220
chicken *(Old El Paso* Festive Dinners), 11 oz.	460
fish *(see also specific fish listings):*	
(Morton), 9.75 oz.	370
'n' chips *(Swanson)*, 10 oz.	500
ham *(Morton)*, 10 oz.	290
ham steak:	
(Armour Classics), 10.75 oz.	270
(Le Menu), 10 oz.	300
glazed *(Stouffer's Dinner Supreme)*, 10.5 oz.	380
lasagna *(Banquet Extra Helping)*, 16.5 oz.	645
macaroni and beef *(Swanson)*, 12 oz.	370
macaroni and cheese *(Banquet)*, 10 oz.	420
macaroni and cheese *(Swanson)*, 12.25 oz.	370
manicotti, w/three cheeses *(Le Menu)*, 11.75 oz.	390
meat loaf:	
(Armour Classics), 11.25 oz.	360
(Banquet), 11 oz.	440
(Freezer Queen), 10 oz.	350
(Morton), 10 oz.	310
(Swanson), 10.75 oz.	360
homestyle *(Stouffer's Dinner Supreme)*, 12⅛ oz.	410
meatballs, Swedish *(Armour Classics)*, 11.25 oz.	330
Mexican or Mexican style:	
(Banquet), 12 oz.	490
(Morton), 10 oz.	300
(Patio), 13.25 oz.	540
(Patio Fiesta), 12.25 oz.	470
(Swanson Hungry-Man), 20.25 oz.	820
combination *(Banquet)*, 12 oz.	520
combination *(Swanson)*, 14.25 oz.	490
pork, loin of *(Swanson)*, 10.75 oz.	280
pot roast, *see "beef," page 125*	

ravioli, mini cheese *(Kid Cuisine)*, 8.75 oz.   250
Salisbury steak:
    (Armour Classics), 11.25 oz.   350
    (Armour Classics Lite), 11.5 oz.   300
    (Banquet), 11 oz.   500
    (Banquet Extra Helping), 18 oz.   910
    (Freezer Queen), 10 oz.   380
    (Healthy Choice), 11.5 oz.   300
    (Le Menu LightStyle), 10 oz.   280
    (Morton), 10 oz.   300
    (Swanson), 10.75 oz.   400
    (Swanson Hungry-Man), 16.5 oz.   680
    w/gravy and mushrooms *(Stouffer's Dinner
       Supreme)*, 11⅝ oz.   400
    w/mushroom gravy *(Banquet Extra Helping)*, 18 oz.   890
    parmigiana *(Armour Classics)*, 11.5 oz.   410
    sirloin *(The Budget Gourmet)*, 11.5 oz.   410
scallop and shrimp Mariner *(The Budget Gourmet)*,
    11.5 oz.   320
seafood, w/natural herbs *(Armour Classics Lite)*, 10 oz.   190
shrimp:
    baby bay *(Armour Classics Lite)*, 9.75 oz.   220
    Creole *(Armour Classics Lite)*, 11.25 oz.   260
    Creole *(Healthy Choice)*, 11.25 oz.   210
    marinara *(Healthy Choice)*, 10.5 oz.   220
sole au gratin *(Healthy Choice)*, 11 oz.   270
spaghetti and meatballs:
    (Banquet), 10 oz.   290
    (Morton), 10 oz.   200
    (Swanson), 12.5 oz.   390
Swiss steak, *see "beef," page 126*
tamale *(Patio)*, 13 oz.   470
tortellini, w/meat *(Dinner Classics Lite)*, 10 oz.   250
turkey:
    (Banquet), 10.5 oz.   390
    (Banquet Extra Helping), 19 oz.   750
    (Morton), 10 oz.   230
    (Swanson), 11.5 oz.   350
    (Swanson Hungry-Man), 17 oz.   550
turkey breast:
    (Healthy Choice), 10.5 oz.   290

Dinners, Frozen, turkey breast, continued

Dijon *(The Budget Gourmet)*, 11.2 oz.	340
Divan *(Le Menu* LightStyle), 10 oz.	260
roast *(Stouffer's Dinner Supreme)*, 10.75 oz.	330
sliced *(The Budget Gourmet)*, 11.1 oz.	290
sliced *(Freezer Queen)*, 10 oz.	280
sliced, w/mushroom gravy *(Le Menu)*, 10.5 oz.	300
sliced, in mushroom sauce *(Lean Cuisine)*, 8 oz. . . .	240
w/dressing and gravy *(Armour Classics)*, 11.5 oz. . .	320
veal marsala *(Le Menu* LightStyle), 10 oz.	230
veal parmigiana:	
(Armour Classics), 11.25 oz.	400
(Morton), 10 oz.	260
(Stouffer's Dinner Supreme), 11.25 oz.	350
(Swanson), 12.25 oz.	430
(Swanson Hungry-Man), 18.25 oz.	590
breaded *(Freezer Queen)*, 5 oz.	220
platter *(Freezer Queen)*, 10 oz.	400
Western:	
(Banquet), 11 oz.	630
(Morton), 10 oz.	290
style *(Swanson)*, 11.5 oz.	430

ENTREES, CANNED & PACKAGED
See also "Macaroni Dishes, Canned," "Noodle Dishes, Canned," and "Pasta Dishes, Canned"

---

	calories
amaranth, w/garden vegetables *(Health Valley Fast Menu)*, 7.5 oz.	120
beef:	
chow mein *(La Choy* Bi-Pack), 3/4 cup	70
pepper Oriental *(La Choy* Bi-Pack), 3/4 cup	80
pepper steak, Oriental *(Hormel Top Shelf)*, 1 serving	290
ribs, boneless *(Hormel Top Shelf)*, 1 serving	440
roast, tender *(Hormel Top Shelf)*, 1 serving	240
Salisbury steak, w/potatoes *(Hormel Top Shelf)*, 1 serving	254
Stroganoff *(Hormel Top Shelf)*, 1 serving	320
sukiyaki *(Hormel Top Shelf)*, 1 serving	330

beef, corned, hash:
    (Dinty Moore), 2 oz. 130
    (Libby's, 24 oz.), 8 oz. 420
    (Libby's, 15 oz.), 7.5 oz. 400
    (Mary Kitchen, 25 oz.), 8.33 oz. 400
    (Mary Kitchen, 15 oz.), 7.5 oz. 360
beef, roast, hash *(Mary Kitchen)*, 7.5 oz. 350
beef stew:
    (Dinty Moore, 40 oz.), 8 oz. 210
    (Dinty Moore, 24 oz.), 8 oz. 220
    (Estee), 7.5 oz. 210
    (Featherweight), 7.5 oz. 160
    (Hormel/Dinty Moore Micro-Cup), 7.5 oz. 190
    (Libby's, 24 oz.), 8 oz. 170
    (Libby's, 15 oz.), 7.5 oz. 160
    (Wolf Brand), scant cup, 7.5 oz. 179
black bean, Western, w/garden vegetables *(Health
    Valley Fast Menu)*, 7.5 oz. 120
cannelloni, mini *(Chef Boyardee)*, 7.5 oz. 230
chicken:
    à la king *(Swanson)*, 5.25 oz. 190
    Acapulco *(Hormel Top Shelf)*, 1 serving 390
    breast of, glazed *(Hormel Top Shelf)*, 1 serving 210
    chow mein *(La Choy* Bi-Pack), 3/4 cup 80
    and dumplings *(Featherweight)*, 7.5 oz. 160
    and dumplings *(Luck's)*, 7.25 oz. 240
    and dumplings *(Swanson)*, 7.5 oz. 220
    Oriental *(La Choy* Bi-Pack), 3/4 cup 240
    stew *(Swanson)*, 75/8 oz. 160
    stew, w/wild rice *(Featherweight)*, 7.5 oz. 140
    sweet and sour *(Hormel Top Shelf)* 270
chili, w/beans:
    (Dennison's, 15 oz.), 7.5 oz. 310
    (Dennison's Cook-Off), 7.5 oz. 340
    (Estee), 7.5 oz. 370
    (Featherweight), 7.5 oz. 280
    (Hormel, 15 oz.), 7.5 oz. 310
    (Hormel Micro-Cup), 7.5 oz. 250
    (Libby's, 15 oz.), 7.5 oz. 270
    (Van Camp's), 1 cup 352
    (Wolf Brand), 1 cup 345

Entrees, Canned & Packaged, chili, w/beans, continued

beef *(Chef Boyardee)*, 7.5 oz.	330
chunky *(Dennison's)*, 7.5 oz.	310
extra spicy *(Wolf* Brand), 7.5 oz.	324
hot *(Dennison's,* 15 oz.), 7.5 oz.	310
hot *(Gebhardt)*, 4 oz.	189
hot *(Heinz)*, 7.75 oz.	330
hot *(Hormel,* 15 oz.), 7.5 oz.	310
chili, w/out beans:	
(Dennison's, 15 oz.), 7.5 oz.	300
(Hormel, 15 oz.), 7.5 oz.	370
(Libby's), 7.5 oz.	390
(Van Camp's), 1 cup	412
(Wolf Brand), 1 cup	387
extra spicy *(Wolf* Brand), 7.5 oz.	363
w/franks *(Van Camp's Chilee Weenee)*, 1 cup	309
hot *(Hormel,* 15 oz.), 7.5 oz.	370
chili, w/chicken, spicy *(Hain)*, 7.5 oz.	130
chili, vegetarian:	
(Gebhardt), 4 oz.	219
(Worthington), 2/3 cup	190
w/beans, mild or spicy *(Health Valley* Regular/No Salt Added), 4 oz.	130
w/lentils, mild *(Health Valley* Regular/No Salt Added), 4 oz.	130
spicy *(Hain)*, 7.5 oz.	160
spicy *(Hain* Reduced Sodium), 7.5 oz.	170
spicy *(Natural Touch)*, 2/3 cup	230
tempeh, spicy *(Hain)*, 7.5 oz.	160
chili con carne suprema *(Hormel Top Shelf)*, 1 serving	320
chili mac *(Heinz)*, 7.5 oz.	250
chili mac *(Wolf* Brand), 7.5 oz.	317
lasagna, Italian style *(Hormel Top Shelf)*, 1 serving	360
lasagna, vegetable *(Hormel Top Shelf)*, 10.6 oz.	275
lentil, w/garden vegetables *(Health Valley Fast Menu)*, 7.5 oz.	160
linguine, w/clam sauce *(Hormel Top Shelf)*, 1 serving	330
oat bran pilaf, w/garden vegetables *(Health Valley Fast Menu)*, 7.5 oz.	210
pork chow mein *(La Choy* Bi-Pack), 3/4 cup	80
shrimp chow mein *(La Choy* Bi-Pack), 3/4 cup	50

spaghettini *(Hormel Top Shelf)*, 1 serving   240
tamale:
   (Old El Paso), 2 pieces   190
   (Wolf Brand), scant cup, 7.5 oz.   328
   beef *(Hormel/Hormel* Hot'N Spicy), 2 pieces   140
   w/sauce *(Van Camp's)*, 1 cup   293
tamalito, in chili gravy *(Dennison's)*, 7.5 oz.   310

ENTREES, FROZEN, one serving
See also "Dinners, Frozen," "Pot Pies, Frozen," and
"Pasta Dishes, Frozen"

---

                                                          calories
beef:
   (Banquet Platter), 10 oz.   460
   and broccoli, w/rice *(La Choy Fresh & Lite)*, 11 oz.   260
   burrito, *see "burrito," page 135*
   casserole *(Pillsbury Microwave Classic)*, 1 pkg.   430
   Champignon *(Tyson Gourmet Selection)*, 10.5 oz. . . .   370
   chop suey, w/rice *(Stouffer's)*, 12 oz.   300
   creamed, chipped *(Banquet Cookin' Bag)*, 4 oz.   100
   creamed, chipped *(Freezer Queen Cook-In-Pouch)*,
     5 oz.   80
   creamed, chipped *(Stouffer's)*, 5.5 oz.   230
   Dijon, w/pasta and vegetables *(Right Course)*, 9.5 oz.   290
   enchilada, *see "enchilada," page 141*
   fiesta, w/corn pasta *(Right Course)*, 8⅞ oz.   270
   London broil, in mushroom sauce *(Weight Watchers)*,
     7.37 oz.   140
   meat loaf, *see "meat loaf," page 145*
   Oriental *(The Budget Gourmet* Slim Selects), 10 oz. .   290
   Oriental, w/vegetables and rice *(Lean Cuisine)*,
     8⅝ oz.   250
   patty, mushroom gravy and *(Banquet Cookin' Bag)*,
     5 oz.   210
   patty, mushroom gravy and *(Banquet Family*
     Entree), 8 oz.   290
   patty, mushroom gravy and *(Freezer Queen Cook-In-*
     Pouch), 5 oz.   90

Entrees, Frozen, beef, continued

patty, mushroom gravy and *(Freezer Queen Family Supper)*, 7 oz.	180
patty, onion gravy and *(Banquet Family Entree)*, 8 oz.	300
patty, onion gravy and *(Freezer Queen Family Supper)*, 7 oz.	200
and peppers, in sauce, w/rice *(Freezer Queen Single Serve)*, 9 oz.	260
pepper Oriental *(Chun King)*, 13 oz.	310
pepper steak *(Dining Lite)*, 9 oz.	260
pepper steak *(Healthy Choice)*, 9.5 oz.	250
pepper steak *(Tyson Gourmet Selection)*, 11.25 oz.	330
pepper steak, green, w/rice *(Stouffer's)*, 10.5 oz.	330
pepper steak, w/rice *(The Budget Gourmet)*, 10 oz.	300
pepper steak, w/rice and vegetables *(La Choy Fresh & Lite)*, 10 oz.	280
pot roast, homestyle *(Right Course)*, 9.25 oz.	220
ragout, w/rice pilaf *(Right Course)*, 10 oz.	300
roast, hash *(Stouffer's)*, 10 oz.	380
Salisbury steak, *see "Salisbury steak," page 146*	
short ribs *(Tyson Gourmet Selection)*, 11 oz.	470
short ribs, in gravy *(Stouffer's)*, 9 oz.	350
sirloin, in herb sauce *(The Budget Gourmet Slim Selects)*, 10 oz.	290
sirloin, roast *(The Budget Gourmet)*, 9.5 oz.	330
sirloin tips, in Burgundy sauce *(Swanson Homestyle Recipe)*, 7 oz.	160
sirloin tips, w/country style vegetables *(The Budget Gourmet)*, 10 oz.	310
sirloin tips, and mushrooms, in wine sauce *(Weight Watchers)*, 7.5 oz.	220
sliced, barbecue sauce and *(Banquet Cookin' Bag)*, 4 oz.	100
sliced, gravy and *(Banquet Cookin' Bag)*, 4 oz.	100
sliced, gravy and *(Banquet Family Entree)*, 8 oz.	160
sliced, gravy and *(Freezer Queen Cook-In-Pouch)*, 4 oz.	60
sliced, gravy and *(Freezer Queen Deluxe Family Supper)*, 7 oz.	130
steak, breaded *(Hormel)*, 4 oz.	370

steak, Ranchero *(Lean Cuisine)*, 9.25 oz.. 270
stew *(Banquet Family Entree)*, 7 oz. 140
stew *(Freezer Queen Family Supper)*, 7 oz. 150
Stroganoff *(The Budget Gourmet* Slim Selects),
    8.75 oz.. 280
Stroganoff *(Weight Watchers)*, 8.5 oz. 290
Stroganoff, w/parsley noodles *(Stouffer's)*, 9.75 oz. . . 390
Stroganoff sauce with, and noodles *(Banquet Family
    Entree)*, 7 oz. 190
Szechuan *(Chun King)*, 13 oz. 340
Szechwan, w/noodles and vegetables *(Lean Cuisine)*,
    9.25 oz.. 260
teriyaki *(Chun King)*, 13 oz. 380
teriyaki *(Dining Lite)*, 9 oz. 270
teriyaki, w/rice and vegetables *(La Choy Fresh &
    Lite)*, 10 oz. 240
teriyaki, in sauce, w/rice and vegetables *(Stouffer's)*,
    9.75 oz.. 290
tortellini, *see "tortellini," page 148*
burrito:
    (Hormel Burrito Grande), 5.5 oz. 380
    bean and cheese *(Old El Paso)*, 1 pkg. 340
    beef *(Hormel)*, 1 piece 205
    beef and bean *(Patio)*, 5-oz. pkg. 370
    beef and bean *(Patio Britos)*, 3.63 oz. 250
    beef and bean, green chili *(Patio)*, 5-oz. pkg. 330
    beef and bean, hot *(Old El Paso)*, 1 pkg.. 340
    beef and bean, medium or mild *(Old El Paso)*, 1 pkg. 330
    beef and bean, red chili *(Patio)*, 5-oz. pkg. 340
    beef, nacho *(Patio Britos)*, 3.63 oz. 270
    cheese *(Hormel)*, 1 piece 210
    cheese, nacho *(Patio Britos)*, 3.63 oz. 250
    chicken *(Weight Watchers)*, 7.62 oz. 330
    chicken, spicy *(Patio Britos)*, 3.63 oz. 250
    chicken and rice *(Hormel)*, 1 piece 200
    chili, green *(Patio Britos)*, 3.63 oz. 250
    chili, hot *(Hormel)*, 1 piece 240
    chili, red *(Patio Britos)*, 3.63 oz. 240
    red hot *(Patio)*, 5-oz. pkg. 360
cabbage, stuffed, w/meat, in tomato sauce *(Lean
    Cuisine)*, 10.75 oz. 220

Entrees, Frozen, continued

cannelloni:

beef and pork, w/mornay sauce *(Lean Cuisine)*, 9⅝ oz.	260
cheese *(Dining Lite)*, 9 oz.	310
cheese, w/tomato sauce *(Lean Cuisine)*, 9⅛ oz. . . .	260
Florentine *(Celentano)*, 12 oz.	350

cavatelli *(Celentano)*, 3.2 oz. 250

cheese enchilada, see *"enchilada," page 141*

cheeseburger, see *"Sandwiches, Frozen, cheeseburger,"*
    page 196

chili:

con carne *(Swanson* Homestyle Recipe), 8.25 oz. . . .	270
con carne, w/beans *(Stouffer's)*, 8.75 oz.	260
vegetarian *(Right Course)*, 9.75 oz.	280

chicken:

à la king *(Banquet Cookin' Bag)*, 4 oz.	110
à la king *(Dining Lite)*, 9 oz.	240
à la king *(Freezer Queen Cook-In-Pouch)*, 4 oz.	70
à la king *(Weight Watchers)*, 9 oz.	240
à la king, w/rice *(Freezer Queen* Single Serve), 9 oz.	270
à la king, w/rice *(Stouffer's)*, 9.5 oz.	290
à la king, w/seasoned rice *(Le Menu* Light Style), 8.25 oz.	240
almond, w/rice and vegetables *(La Choy Fresh & Lite)*, 9.75 oz.	270
à l'orange *(Healthy Choice)*, 9 oz.	260
à l'orange *(Tyson Gourmet Selection)*, 9.5 oz.	300
à l'orange, w/almond rice *(Lean Cuisine)*, 8 oz.	260
au gratin *(The Budget Gourmet* Slim Selects), 9.1 oz.	260
breast, see *"chicken breast," page 139*	
and broccoli *(Green Giant* Entree), 9.5 oz.	340
cacciatore *(Freezer Queen* Single Serve), 9 oz.	270
cacciatore *(Swanson* Homestyle Recipe), 11 oz.	260
cacciatore, w/vermicelli *(Lean Cuisine)*, 10⅞ oz. . .	250
Cajun style *(Pilgrim's Pride)*, 3 oz.*	241
cannelloni, see *"cannelloni," above*	
cashew, in sauce, w/rice *(Stouffer's)*, 9.5 oz.	380
w/cheddar *(Tyson* Chick'n Cheddar), 2.6 oz.	220
chow mein *(Chun King)*, 13 oz.	370
chow mein *(Dining Lite)*, 9 oz.	180

chow mein *(Healthy Choice)*, 8.5 oz.   220
chow mein, w/out noodles *(Stouffer's)*, 8 oz.   130
chow mein, w/rice *(Lean Cuisine)*, 11.25 oz.   250
chunks *(Country Pride)*, 3 oz.   240
chunks *(Tyson* Chick'n Chunks), 2.6 oz.   220
chunks, Southern fried *(Country Pride)*, 3 oz.   280
Cordon Bleu *(Swift International)*, 6 oz.   360
Cordon Bleu, breaded *(Weight Watchers)*, 8 oz.   220
creamed *(Stouffer's)*, 6.5 oz.   300
croquettes, breaded, gravy and *(Freezer Queen*
    Family Supper), 7 oz.   240
diced *(Tyson)*, 3 oz.   150
Dijon *(Tyson Gourmet Selection)*, 8.5 oz.   310
Dijon, w/pasta and vegetables *(Le Menu* LightStyle),
    8.5 oz.   240
divan *(Stouffer's)*, 8.5 oz.   320
drumsnackers *(Banquet* Chicken Hot Bites), 2.63 oz.   220
drumsnackers *(Banquet* Platters), 7 oz.   430
drumsters *(Pilgrim's Pride)*, 3 oz.   200
and dumplings *(Banquet Family Entree)*, 7 oz.   280
and egg noodles, w/broccoli *(The Budget Gourmet)*,
    10 oz.   450
empress, w/seasoned rice *(Le Menu* LightStyle),
    8.25 oz.   210
enchilada, see "enchilada," page 141
escalloped, and noodles *(Stouffer's)*, 10 oz.   420
w/fettuccine *(The Budget Gourmet)*, 10 oz.   400
fettuccini *(Weight Watchers)*, 8.25 oz.   280
fiesta *(Healthy Choice)*, 8.5 oz.   250
Francais *(Tyson Gourmet Selection)*, 9.5 oz.   280
French recipe *(The Budget Gourmet* Slim Selects),
    10 oz.   260
fried *(Banquet/Banquet* Hot'n Spicy), 6.4 oz.   330
fried *(Pilgrim's Pride)*, 3 oz.*   255
fried *(Swanson* Homestyle Recipe), 7 oz.*   390
fried, breast *(Banquet)*, 5.75 oz.   220
fried, breast *(Swanson* Plump & Juicy), 4.5 oz.* . . .   360
fried, thighs and drumsticks *(Banquet)*, 6.25 oz. . . .   250
fried, white meat *(Banquet* Platter), 9 oz.   430
fried, white meat, hot'n spicy *(Banquet* Platter),
    9 oz.   430

Entrees, Frozen, chicken, continued

glazed *(Dining Lite)*, 9 oz.   220
glazed *(Healthy Choice)*, 8.5 oz.   220
glazed, w/vegetable rice *(Lean Cuisine)*, 8.5 oz.   270
hot'n spicy *(Banquet* Snack'n), 3.75 oz.   140
Imperial *(Chun King)*, 13 oz.   300
Imperial *(Weight Watchers)*, 9.25 oz.   240
Imperial, w/rice *(La Choy Fresh & Lite)*, 11 oz. . . .   260
Italiano, w/fettuccini and vegetables *(Right Course)*,
9⅝ oz.   280
Kiev *(Swift International)*, 6 oz.   420
Kiev *(Tyson Gourmet Selection)*, 9.25 oz.   520
Mandarin *(The Budget Gourmet* Slim Selects), 10 oz.   290
Marsala *(The Budget Gourmet)*, 10 oz.   250
Marsala *(Tyson Gourmet Selection)*, 10.5 oz.   300
mesquite *(Tyson Gourmet Selection)*, 9.5 oz.   320
nibbles *(Swanson* Homestyle Recipe), 4.25 oz.*   340
nibbles *(Swanson* Plump & Juicy), 3.25 oz.*   300
and noodles *(Dining Lite)*, 9 oz.   240
and noodles, homestyle *(Stouffer's)*, 10 oz.   310
nuggets, *see "chicken nuggets," page 140*
Oriental *(Lean Cuisine)*, 9⅜ oz.   230
Oriental *(Tyson Gourmet Selection)*, 10.25 oz.   270
Oriental, spicy *(La Choy Fresh & Lite)*, 9.75 oz. . . .   270
parmigiana *(Celentano)*, 9 oz.   330
parmigiana *(Tyson Gourmet Selection)*, 11.25 oz. . . .   380
patties, *see "chicken patties," page 140*
picatta *(Tyson Gourmet Selection)*, 9 oz.   240
pie, *see "Pot Pies, Frozen, pot pies, chicken,"*
page 154
primavera *(Celentano)*, 11.5 oz.   270
primavera *(Banquet Cookin' Bag)*, 4 oz.   100
primavera *(Banquet Family Entree)*, 7 oz.   140
sesame *(Right Course)*, 10 oz.   320
sliced, gravy and *(Freezer Queen Cook-In-Pouch)*,
5 oz.   80
steaks, chicken fried *(Pilgrim's Pride)*, 3 oz.   183
sticks *(Banquet* Chicken Hot Bites), 2.63 oz.   220
sticks *(Country Pride)*, 3 oz.   240
sweet and sour *(Banquet Cookin' Bag)*, 4 oz.   130
sweet and sour *(Tyson Gourmet Selection)*, 11 oz. . .   420

sweet and sour, w/rice *(The Budget Gourmet)*, 10 oz. ... 350

sweet and sour, w/rice *(Freezer Queen* Single Serve),
9 oz. 300

sweet and sour, w/rice and vegetables *(La Choy
Fresh & Lite)*, 10 oz. 260

tenderloins, in barbecue sauce *(Right Course)*,
8.75 oz. 270

tenderloins, in peanut sauce *(Right Course)*, 9.25 oz. 330

tenders *(Tyson* Microwave), 3.5 oz. 230

thighs and drumsticks *(Swanson* Plump & Juicy),
3.25 oz.* 290

and vegetables, w/vermicelli *(Lean Cuisine)*,
11.75 oz. 270

walnut, crunchy *(Chun King)*, 13 oz. 310

wings *(Pilgrim's Pride* Wing Zappers), 3 oz.* 187

wings, all varieties *(Tyson Flyers)*, 3.5 oz. or
6–7 wings 220

wings, Southern fried *(Pilgrim's Pride)*, 3 oz.* 228

chicken beef luau *(Tyson Gourmet Selection)*, 10.5 oz. .. 330

chicken breast:

barbecue marinated *(Tyson)*, 3.75 oz. 120

butter garlic marinated *(Tyson)*, 3.75 oz. 160

chunks *(Tyson)*, 3 oz. 240

fillets *(Pilgrim's Pride)*, 3 oz. 195

fillets *(Tyson)*, 3 oz. 190

in herb cream sauce *(Lean Cuisine)*, 9.5 oz. 260

herb roasted, w/rice and vegetables *(Le Menu
LightStyle)*, 7.75 oz. 260

Italian marinated *(Tyson)*, 3.75 oz. 130

lemon pepper marinated *(Tyson)*, 3.75 oz. 120

Marsala, w/vegetables *(Lean Cuisine)*, 8¹/₈ oz. 190

Parmesan *(Lean Cuisine)*, 10 oz. 260

patties, see *"chicken patties,"* page 140

tenders *(Banquet* Chicken Hot Bites), 2.25 oz. 150

tenders *(Banquet* Chicken Hot Bites Microwave),
4 oz. 260

tenders *(Pilgrim's Pride)*, 3 oz. 181

tenders, Southern fried *(Banquet* Chicken Hot Bites),
2.25 oz. 160

tenders, Southern fried *(Tyson)*, 3 oz. 220

teriyaki marinated *(Tyson)*, 3.75 oz. 130

Entrees, Frozen, continued

chicken nuggets:
(Banquet Chicken Hot Bites), 2.63 oz.	210
(Banquet Platter), 6.4 oz.	430
(Country Pride), 3 oz.	250
(Freezer Queen Deluxe Family Supper), 3 oz.	270
(Pilgrim's Pride), 3 oz.	202
(Tyson Microwave), 3.5 oz.	220
(Weight Watchers), 5.9 oz.	270
breast, Southern fried, w/barbecue sauce *(Banquet Microwave Chicken Hot Bites)*, 4.5 oz.	370
w/cheddar *(Banquet Chicken Hot Bites)*, 2.63 oz. . .	250
hot'n spicy *(Banquet Chicken Hot Bites)*, 2.63 oz. . .	250
hot'n spicy, w/barbecue sauce *(Banquet Microwave Chicken Hot Bites)*, 4.5 oz.	360
Southern fried *(Banquet Chicken Hot Bites)*, 2.63 oz.	220
Southern fried, w/barbecue sauce *(Banquet Microwave Chicken Hot Bites)*, 4.5 oz.	370
w/sweet and sour sauce *(Banquet Microwave Chicken Hot Bites)*, 4.5 oz.	360

chicken patties:
(Banquet Platter), 7.5 oz.	380
(Country Pride), 3 oz.	250
(Pilgrim's Pride), 3 oz.	205
(Tyson), 2.6 oz.	220
(Tyson Thick & Crispy), 2.6 oz.	220
breast *(Banquet Chicken Hot Bites)*, 2.63 oz.	210
breast, and bun *(Banquet Microwave Chicken Hot Bites)*, 4-oz. pkg.	310
breast, Southern fried *(Country Pride)*, 3 oz.	240
breast, Southern fried *(Banquet Chicken Hot Bites)*, 2.63 oz.	210
breast, Southern fried *(Tyson)*, 2.6 oz.	220
breast, Southern fried, and biscuit *(Banquet Microwave Chicken Hot Bites)*, 4 oz.	320
breast, Southern fried *(Weight Watchers)*, 6.5 oz. . . .	320

chimichanga, 1 pkg.:
bean and cheese *(Old El Paso)*	350
beef *(Old El Paso)*	380
beef and pork *(Old El Paso)*	340
chicken *(Old El Paso)*	370

clam strips, crunchy *(Gorton's* Microwave Specialty),
    3.5 oz.   330
clams, battered, fried *(Mrs. Paul's),* 2.5 oz.   200
crab, deviled *(Mrs. Paul's),* 1 cake   180
crab, deviled, miniature *(Mrs. Paul's),* 3.5 oz.   240
eggplant parmigiana:
    (Celentano), 8 oz.   280
    (Celentano), 10 oz.   350
    (Mrs. Paul's), 4 oz.   240
eggplant rollettes *(Celentano),* 11 oz.   320
enchilada, beef:
    (Hormel), 1 piece   140
    (Old El Paso), 1 pkg.   210
    (Van de Kamp's Mexican Entrees), 1 pkg.   270
    (Van De Kamp's Mexican Entrees Family Pack),
        1/4 pkg.   150
    and bean *(Lean Cuisine* Enchanadas), 9.25 oz.   280
    chili gravy and *(Banquet Family Entree),* 7 oz.   270
    Ranchero *(Weight Watchers),* 9.12 oz.   230
    shredded *(Van de Kamp's* Mexican Entrees), 1 pkg. .   360
    sirloin Ranchero *(The Budget Gourmet* Slim Selects),
        9 oz.   290
enchilada, cheese:
    (Hormel), 1 piece   151
    (Old El Paso), 1 pkg.   250
    (Stouffer's), 10 1/8 oz.   590
    (Van de Kamp's Mexican Entrees), 1 pkg.   300
    (Van de Kamp's Mexican Entrees Family Pack),
        1/4 pkg.   200
    Ranchero *(Van de Kamp's* Mexican Entrees), 1/2 pkg.   260
    Ranchero *(Weight Watchers),* 8.87 oz.   360
enchilada, chicken:
    (Lean Cuisine Enchanadas), 9 7/8 oz.   270
    (Old El Paso), 1 pkg.   220
    (Stouffer's), 10 oz.   490
    (Van de Kamp's Mexican Entrees), 1 pkg.   260
    w/sour cream sauce *(Old El Paso),* 1 pkg.   280
    Suiza *(The Budget Gourmet* Slim Selects), 9 oz.   270
    Suiza *(Van de Kamp's* Mexican Entrees), 1 pkg. . . .   230
    Suiza *(Weight Watchers),* 9 oz.   280

Entrees, Frozen, continued

enchilada, vegetable, w/tofu and sauce *(Legume* Mexican)*, 11 oz.	270
fajita, beef *(Weight Watchers)*, 6.75 oz.	250
fajita, chicken *(Weight Watchers)*, 6.75 oz.	280

fettuccini:

Alfredo *(Healthy Choice)*, 8 oz.	240
Alfredo *(Stouffer's)*, 1/2 of 10-oz. pkg.	270
Alfredo *(Weight Watchers)*, 9 oz.	210
w/broccoli *(Dining Lite)*, 9 oz.	290
w/meat sauce *(The Budget Gourmet)*, 10 oz.	290
primavera *(Green Giant)*, 1 pkg.	230
primavera *(Green Giant* Microwave Garden Gourmet)*, 1 pkg.	260

fish *(see also specific fish listings)*:

(Banquet Platters)*, 8.75 oz.	450
almondine *(Gorton's)*, 1 pkg.	340
cakes *(Mrs. Paul's)*, 2 pieces	190
coated, fillets, ranch *(Gorton's* Specialty Microwave, Large)*, 1 piece	330
Dijon *(Mrs. Paul's* Light)*, 8.75 oz.	200
Divan *(Lean Cuisine)*, 12 3/8 oz.	260
fillets, *see "fish fillets," below*	
Florentine *(Lean Cuisine)*, 9 oz.	230
Florentine *(Mrs. Paul's* Light)*, 8 oz.	220
'n' fries *(Swanson* Homestyle Recipe)*, 6.5 oz.	340
gems, fancy style *(Wakefield)*, 4 oz.	80
gems, salad style *(Wakefield)*, 3 oz.	70
in herb butter *(Gorton's)*, 1 pkg.	190
jardinière, w/potatoes *(Lean Cuisine)*, 11.25 oz.	290
Mornay *(Mrs. Paul's* Light)*, 9 oz.	230
sticks, *see "fish sticks," page 143*	

fish fillets, battered:

(Gorton's Crispy Batter)*, 2 pieces	300
(Gorton's Crispy Batter, Large)*, 1 piece	320
(Gorton's Crunchy)*, 2 pieces	320
(Gorton's Crunchy Microwave)*, 2 pieces	340
(Gorton's Crunchy Microwave, Large)*, 1 piece	320
(Gorton's Potato Crisp)*, 2 pieces	310
(Gorton's Value Pack)*, 1 piece	180
(Mrs. Paul's), 2 pieces	330

(Mrs. Paul's Crunchy), 2 pieces   280
(Van de Kamp's), 1 piece   170
minced *(Mrs. Paul's* Portions), 2 pieces   300
tempura *(Gorton's Light Recipe)*, 1 piece   200
fish fillets, breaded:
   (Gorton's Light Recipe), 1 piece   180
   (Mrs. Paul's Crispy Crunchy), 2 pieces   220
   (Van de Kamp's), 2 pieces   260
   crispy *(Van de Kamp's* Microwave), 1 piece   130
   minced *(Mrs. Paul's* Crispy Crunchy), 2 pieces   230
fish sticks, battered:
   (Gorton's Crispy Batter), 4 pieces   260
   (Gorton's Crunchy), 4 pieces   220
   (Gorton's Crunchy Microwave), 6 pieces   340
   (Gorton's Potato Crisp), 4 pieces   260
   (Gorton's Value Pack), 4 pieces   210
   (Van de Kamp's), 4 pieces   170
   minced *(Mrs. Paul's)*, 4 pieces   210
fish sticks, breaded:
   (Frionor Bunch O' Crunch), 4 pieces or 2.7 oz.   210
   (Mrs. Paul's Crispy Crunchy), 4 pieces   190
   (Van de Kamp's), 4 pieces   190
   crispy *(Van de Kamp's* Microwave), 3 pieces   150
   minced *(Mrs. Paul's* Crispy Crunchy), 4 pieces   140
   whole wheat *(Booth* Microwave), 2 oz.   150
flounder:
   battered *(Mrs. Paul's* Crunchy), 2 pieces   220
   breaded *(Van de Kamp's* Light), 1 piece   240
   stuffed *(Gorton's Microwave Entrees)*, 1 pkg.   350
haddock:
   battered *(Mrs. Paul's* Crunchy), 2 pieces   190
   battered *(Van de Kamp's)*, 2 pieces   250
   breaded *(Van de Kamp's)*, 2 pieces   260
   breaded *(Van de Kamp's* Light), 1 piece   250
   in lemon butter *(Gorton's Microwave Entrees)*, 1 pkg.   360
halibut fillets, battered *(Van de Kamp's)*, 2 pieces   180
halibut steaks, w/out seasoning mix *(SeaPak)*, 6 oz. . .   160
ham:
   (Banquet Platter), 10 oz.   400
   and asparagus bake *(Stouffer's)*, 9.5 oz.   510

Entrees, Frozen, ham, continued

scalloped potatoes and *(Swanson* Homestyle Recipe), 9 oz.	300
ham and cheese casserole *(Pillsbury Microwave Classic),* 1 pkg.	470

hamburger, *see "Sandwiches, Frozen, hamburger," page 197*

lasagna:

(Celentano), 8 oz.	370
(Celentano), 10 oz.	460
(Green Giant Entree), 12 oz.	490
(Stouffer's), 10.5-oz. pkg.	360
(Stouffer's 21 oz.), 10.5 oz.	360
(Tyson Gourmet Selection), 11.5 oz.	380
cheese *(Dining Lite),* 9 oz.	260
cheese, Italian *(Weight Watchers),* 11 oz.	350
cheese, three *(The Budget Gourmet),* 10 oz.	400
fiesta *(Stouffer's),* 10.25 oz.	430
garden *(Weight Watchers),* 11 oz.	290
meat *(Buitoni* Single Serving), 9 oz.	580
w/meat and sauce *(Lean Cuisine),* 10.25 oz.	270
w/meat sauce *(Banquet Family Entree),* 7 oz.	270
w/meat sauce *(The Budget Gourmet* Slim Selects), 10 oz.	290
w/meat sauce *(Dining Lite),* 9 oz.	240
w/meat sauce *(Freezer Queen Deluxe Family Supper),* 7 oz.	200
w/meat sauce *(Healthy Choice),* 9 oz.	260
w/meat sauce *(Swanson* Homestyle Recipe), 10.5 oz.	400
w/meat sauce *(Weight Watchers),* 11 oz.	320
primavera *(Celentano),* 11 oz.	330
in sauce *(Buitoni* Family Style), 7.3 oz.	370
sausage, Italian *(The Budget Gourmet),* 10 oz.	420
seafood *(Mrs. Paul's* Light), 9.5 oz.	290
w/tofu and sauce *(Legume* Classic), 8 oz.	210
tuna, w/spinach noodles and vegetables *(Lean Cuisine),* 9.75 oz.	270
vegetable *(Stouffer's),* 10.5 oz.	420
vegetable, garden *(Le Menu* LightStyle), 10.5 oz.	260
vegetable, w/tofu and sauce *(Legume),* 12 oz.	240
zucchini *(Lean Cuisine),* 11 oz.	260

lentil rice loaf *(Harvest Bake)*, 4 oz.   190
linguine:
  w/clam sauce *(Lean Cuisine)*, 9⅝ oz.   270
  w/scallops and clams *(The Budget Gourmet* Slim
    Selects), 9.5 oz.   280
  w/shrimp *(The Budget Gourmet)*, 10 oz.   330
  w/shrimp *(Healthy Choice)*, 9.5 oz.   230
lobster Newburg *(Stouffer's)*, 6.5 oz.   380
macaroni and beef, w/tomatoes *(Stouffer's)*, ½ pkg. . . .   170
macaroni and cheese:
  (Banquet Casserole), 8 oz.   350
  (Banquet Family Entree), 8 oz.   290
  (The Budget Gourmet Side Dish), 5.3 oz.   210
  (Freezer Queen Family Side Dish), 4 oz.   110
  (Green Giant One Serving), 5.7 oz.   230
  (Stouffer's), ½ of 12-oz. pkg.   250
  (Stouffer's), ¼ of 20-oz. pkg.   210
  (Swanson Homestyle Recipe), 10 oz.   390
manicotti:
  (Buitoni Single Serving), 9-oz. pkg.   470
  (Celentano), 8 oz.   300
  (Celentano), 10 oz.   380
  cheese *(Weight Watchers)*, 9.25 oz.   280
  cheese, w/meat sauce *(The Budget Gourmet)*, 10 oz.   450
  w/spinach, tofu and sauce *(Legume* Florentine),
    11 oz.   260
  w/tofu and sauce *(Legume* Classic), 8 oz.   220
meat loaf *(Banquet Cookin' Bag)*, 4 oz.   200
meat loaf, tomato sauce and *(Freezer Queen Family
  Supper)*, 7 oz.   230
meatballs:
  Italian style, w/noodles and peppers *(The Budget
    Gourmet)*, 10 oz.   310
  stew *(Lean Cuisine)*, 10 oz.   250
  Swedish *(Swanson* Homestyle Recipe), 8.5 oz.   360
  Swedish, in gravy, w/parsley noodles *(Stouffer's)*,
    11 oz.   480
  Swedish, w/noodles *(The Budget Gourmet)*, 10 oz. .   600
  Swedish, sauce and *(Dining Lite)*, 9 oz.   280
  Swedish, in sauce, w/pasta and vegetables *(Le Menu*
    LightStyle), 8.5 oz.   260

Entrees, Frozen, continued

Mexican *(Van de Kamp's)*, 1/2 pkg.	220
mostaccioli and meat sauce *(Banquet Family Entree)*, 7 oz.	170
noodles:	
and beef, w/gravy *(Banquet Family Entree)*, 8 oz.	200
and julienne beef, w/sauce *(Banquet Family Entree)*, 7 oz.	170
Romanoff *(Stouffer's)*, 1/3 of 12-oz. pkg.	170
pasta *(see also specific pasta listings):*	
baked, and cheese *(Celentano)*, 6 oz.	290
carbonara *(Stouffer's)*, 9.75-oz. pkg.	620
casino *(Stouffer's)*, 9.25-oz. pkg.	300
Dijon *(Green Giant Microwave Garden Gourmet)*, 1 pkg.	300
Mexicali *(Stouffer's)*, 10-oz. pkg.	490
Oriental *(Stouffer's)*, 9 7/8-oz. pkg.	300
primavera *(Stouffer's)*, 10 5/8-oz. pkg.	540
primavera *(Weight Watchers)*, 8.5 oz.	260
rigati *(Weight Watchers)*, 10.6 oz.	300
trio *(Tyson Gourmet Selection)*, 11 oz.	450
pepper, green, stuffed, w/beef, in tomato sauce *(Stouffer's)*, 7.75 oz.	200
pepper, sweet red, stuffed *(Celentano)*, 13 oz.	350
pepper steak, *see "beef," page 134*	
pork, sweet and sour *(Chun King)*, 13 oz.	400
pork steak, breaded *(Hormel)*, 3 oz.	220
ravioli:	
(Celentano), 6.5 oz.	380
cheese *(The Budget Gourmet Slim Selects)*, 10 oz.	260
cheese *(Buitoni)*, 1/4 pkg. or 4 oz.	360
cheese, baked *(Weight Watchers)*, 9 oz.	290
mini *(Celentano)*, 4 oz.	250
rigatoni bake, w/meat sauce and cheese *(Lean Cuisine)*, 9.75 oz.	260
rotini, cheddar *(Green Giant Microwave Garden Gourmet)*, 1 pkg.	230
Salisbury steak:	
(Dining Lite), 9 oz.	200
(Swanson Homestyle Recipe), 10 oz.	320

charbroiled, w/vegetable medley *(Freezer Queen*
Single Serve), 9 oz. 330
gravy and *(Banquet Cookin' Bag)*, 5 oz. 190
gravy and *(Banquet Family Entree)*, 8 oz. 300
gravy and *(Freezer Queen Cook-In-Pouch)*, 5 oz. ... 160
gravy and *(Freezer Queen Family Supper)*, 7 oz. ... 200
in gravy *(Stouffer's)*, 9⅞ oz. 250
w/Italian style sauce and vegetables *(Lean Cuisine)*,
9.5 oz. 280
Romana *(Weight Watchers)*, 8.75 oz............. 190
sirloin *(The Budget Gourmet* Slim Selects), 9 oz. ... 280
supreme *(Tyson Gourmet Selection)*, 10 oz. 430
scallop, fried *(Mrs. Paul's)*, 3 oz. 160
seafood *(see also specific fish listings):*
casserole *(Pillsbury Microwave Classic)*, 1 pkg...... 420
combination platter, breaded *(Mrs. Paul's)*, 9 oz. ... 600
Creole, w/rice *(Swanson* Homestyle Recipe), 9 oz. .. 240
Newberg *(The Budget Gourmet)*, 10 oz. 350
Newburg *(Healthy Choice)*, 8 oz. 200
rotini *(Mrs. Paul's* Light), 9 oz. 240
shells, stuffed:
(Buitoni Single Serving), 9 oz. 460
(Celentano), 8 oz. 330
(Celentano), 10 oz. 410
w/vegetables, tofu, and sauce *(Legume* Provencale),
11 oz. 240
shells and beef *(The Budget Gourmet)*, 10 oz. 340
shells and cheese, w/tomato sauce *(Stouffer's)*, 9.25 oz. 330
shrimp:
(SeaPak Super Valu Heat and Serve), 4 oz. 210
'n batter *(SeaPak)*, 4 oz. 260
'n batter, w/crabmeat stuffing *(SeaPak)*, 4 oz. 260
breaded, butterfly *(SeaPak* Mikado), 4 oz......... 160
breaded, butterfly/round *(SeaPak)*, 4 oz.......... 150
and chicken Cantonese, w/noodles *(Lean Cuisine)*,
10⅛ oz. 270
crisps *(Gorton's* Specialty), 4 oz................ 280
crunchy, whole *(Gorton's* Microwave Specialty), 5 oz. 380
and fettuccini *(The Budget Gourmet)*, 9.5 oz. 375
fettuccine Alfredo *(Booth)*, 10 oz............... 260

Entrees, Frozen, shrimp, continued

w/garlic butter sauce and vegetable rice *(Booth)*, 10 oz.	400
w/lobster sauce *(La Choy Fresh & Lite)*, 10 oz.	240
New Orleans, w/wild rice *(Booth)*, 10 oz.	230
Oriental, w/pineapple rice *(Booth)*, 10 oz.	190
primavera *(Right Course)*, 9⅝ oz.	240
primavera, w/fettuccine *(Booth)*, 10 oz.	200
scampi *(Gorton's Microwave Entrees)*, 1 pkg.	470
shrimp and clams, w/linguini *(Mrs. Paul's* Light), 10 oz.	240
sole:	
in lemon butter *(Gorton's Microwave Entrees)*, 1 pkg.	380
w/lemon butter sauce *(Healthy Choice)*, 8.25 oz.	230
fillets, breaded *(Van de Kamp's* Light), 1 piece	240
in wine sauce *(Gorton's Microwave Entrees)*, 1 pkg.	180
spaghetti:	
w/beef *(Dining Lite)*, 9 oz.	220
w/beef and mushroom sauce *(Lean Cuisine)*, 11.5 oz.	280
w/beef sauce and mushrooms *(Le Menu* LightStyle), 9.5 oz.	280
w/Italian style meatballs *(Swanson* Homestyle Recipe), 13 oz.	490
w/meat sauce *(Banquet* Casserole), 8 oz.	270
w/meat sauce *(Freezer Queen* Single Serve), 10 oz.	350
w/meat sauce *(Healthy Choice)*, 10 oz.	310
w/meat sauce *(Stouffer's)*, 12⅞ oz.	370
w/meat sauce *(Weight Watchers)*, 10.5 oz.	280
w/meatballs *(Stouffer's)*, 12⅝ oz.	380
tamale, beef *(Hormel)*, 1 piece	140
tortellini:	
beef, w/marinara sauce *(Stouffer's)*, 10 oz.	360
cheese *(The Budget Gourmet* Side Dish), 5.5 oz.	180
cheese, in Alfredo sauce *(Stouffer's)*, 8⅞ oz.	600
cheese, marinara *(Green Giant* One Serving), 5.5 oz.	260
meat sauce and cheese *(Le Menu* LightStyle), 8.25 oz.	250
cheese, in tomato sauce *(Birds Eye For One)*, 5.5 oz.	210
cheese, w/tomato sauce *(Stouffer's)*, 9⅝ oz.	360
cheese, w/vinaigrette dressing *(Stouffer's)*, 6⅞ oz.	400
meatless *(Tofutti)*, 2 oz.	220

nondairy, regular or spinach *(Tofutti)*, 2 oz. 210
Provençale *(Green Giant* Microwave Garden
    Gourmet)*, 1 pkg. 260
veal, in Alfredo sauce *(Stouffer's)*, 8⅝ oz. 500
tortilla *(Stouffer's* Grande), 9⅝ oz. 530
tuna noodle casserole *(Stouffer's)*, 10 oz. 310
turkey:
    (Tyson Gourmet Selection), 11.5 oz. 380
    à la king, w/rice *(The Budget Gourmet)*, 10 oz. 390
    breast, stuffed *(Weight Watchers)*, 8.5 oz. 270
    casserole *(Pillsbury Microwave Classic)*, 1 pkg. 430
    casserole, w/dressing *(Stouffer's)*, 9.75 oz. 360
    croquettes, breaded, gravy and *(Freezer Queen*
      Family Supper), 7 oz. 250
    Dijon *(Lean Cuisine)*, 9.5 oz. 270
    w/dressing and potatoes *(Swanson* Homestyle
      Recipe), 9 oz. 290
    glazed *(The Budget Gourmet* Slim Selects), 9 oz. . . . 270
    and gravy, w/dressing *(Freezer Queen Deluxe Family*
      Supper), 7 oz. 160
    sliced, breast, in mushroom sauce *(Lean Cuisine)*,
      8 oz. 240
    sliced, gravy and *(Banquet Cookin' Bag)*, 5 oz. 100
    sliced, gravy and *(Banquet Family Entree)*, 8 oz. . . . 150
    sliced, gravy and *(Freezer Queen Cook-In-Pouch)*,
      5 oz. 70
    sliced, gravy and *(Freezer Queen Family Supper)*,
      7 oz. 110
    sliced, and gravy, w/dressing *(Freezer Queen* Single
      Serve), 9 oz. 230
    sliced, in mild curry sauce, w/rice pilaf *(Right*
      Course), 8.75 oz. 320
    tetrazzini *(Stouffer's)*, 10 oz. 380
    white meat, w/gravy and stuffing *(Le Menu*
      LightStyle Traditional), 8.25 oz. 200
veal parmigiana:
    (Swanson Homestyle Recipe), 10 oz. 330
    breaded *(Banquet Cookin' Bag)*, 4 oz. 230
    breaded *(Freezer Queen Cook-In-Pouch)*, 5 oz. 220
    breaded *(Freezer Queen Deluxe Family Supper)*, 7 oz. 300
    patty, breaded *(Banquet Family Entree)*, 8 oz. 370

Entrees, Frozen, veal parmigiana, continued

patty, breaded *(Weight Watchers)*, 8.44 oz.	190
veal primavera *(Lean Cuisine)*, 9¹/8 oz.	250
veal steak *(Hormel)*, 4 oz.	130
veal steak, breaded *(Hormel)*, 4 oz.	240
Welsh rarebit *(Stouffer's)*, 10 oz.	350

* *Edible portion*

ENTREES, REFRIGERATED, one serving
See also "Meat & Poultry, Frozen & Refrigerated"

calories

chicken, 5 oz.:

bleu cheese, Italian *(Chicken By George)*	190
Cajun *(Chicken By George)*	200
fajita *(Chicken By George)*	170
lemon herb *(Chicken By George)*	150
mesquite barbecue *(Chicken By George)*	170
mustard, country, and dill *(Chicken By George)*	180
teriyaki *(Chicken By George)*	180
tomato herb and basil *(Chicken By George)*	190

pork, barbecued:

back ribs *(John Morrell Pork Classics)*, 4.75 oz.	240
chops, center cut *(John Morrell Pork Classics)*, 4.5 oz.	230
loin, thin sliced *(John Morrell Pork Classics)*, 5 slices or 3 oz.	150
spare ribs *(John Morrell Pork Classics)*, 4.5 oz.	250
tenderloin *(John Morrell Pork Classics)*, 3 oz.	130

ENTREES, MIXES*
See also "Macaroni Dishes, Mixes," "Noodle Dishes, Mixes," "Pasta Dishes, Mixes," and "Rice Dishes, Mixes"

calories

beef:

meat loaf, *see "meat loaf," page 152*
noodle *(Hamburger Helper)*, ¹/5 pkg. dry   140

noodle *(Hamburger Helper)*, 1 cup   320
Romanoff *(Hamburger Helper)*, 1/5 pkg. dry   180
Romanoff *(Hamburger Helper)*, 1 cup   350
stew, hearty *(Lipton Microeasy)*, 1/4 pkg. dry   70
stew, hearty *(Lipton Microeasy)*, 1/4 pkg.   370
burrito dinner kit:
  seasoning mix *(Tio Sancho)*, 3.25 oz.   265
  tortilla *(Tio Sancho)*, 1 piece   125
cheeseburger macaroni *(Hamburger Helper)*, 1/5 pkg.
  dry   190
cheeseburger macaroni *(Hamburger Helper)*, 1 cup . . .   370
chicken:
  barbecue, and scalloped potatoes, oven bake
    (Chicken Applause! Dinner), 1/5 box   380
  barbecue style *(Lipton Microeasy)*, 1/4 pkg. dry   110
  barbecue style *(Lipton Microeasy)*, 1/4 pkg.   220
  country style *(Lipton Microeasy)*, 1/4 pkg. dry   80
  country style *(Lipton Microeasy)*, 1/4 pkg.   190
  mushroom, and rice, oven bake *(Chicken Applause!*
    Dinner), 1/5 box   380
  sweet and sour, and rice, oven bake *(Chicken
    Applause!* Dinner), 1/5 box   360
  three cheese, and rice, oven bake *(Chicken Applause!*
    Dinner), 1/5 box   430
chili:
  w/beans *(Good Times* Chili Fixin's Original), 4 oz. .   80
  w/beans *(Hamburger Helper)*, 1/4 pkg. dry   130
  w/beans *(Hamburger Helper)*, 1 1/4 cup   350
  w/beans, Texas style *(Good Times* Chili Fixin's),
    4 oz.   90
  w/beans, vegetarian *(Fantastic Foods)*, 1/2 cup   104
  w/out beans *(Good Times* Chili Fixin's Original),
    4 oz.   50
  w/out beans, Texas style *(Good Times* Chili Fixin's),
    4 oz.   60
  tomato *(Hamburger Helper)*, 1/5 pkg. dry   150
  tomato *(Hamburger Helper)*, 1 cup   330
chow mein, meatless:
  Mandarin *(Tofu Classics)*, 1/2 cup**   110
  Mandarin *(Tofu Classics)*, 1/2 cup***   134
egg foo young *(La Choy)*, 8.8 oz.   164

Entrees, Mixes*, continued

enchilada dinner kit:

sauce mix *(Tio Sancho)*, 3 oz.	278
shell *(Tio Sancho)*, 1 piece	80

fettucini Alfredo *(Tuna Helper)*, 1/5 pkg. dry 160
fettucini Alfredo *(Tuna Helper)*, 7 oz. 300

hamburger:

hash *(Hamburger Helper)*, 1/5 pkg. dry	140
hash *(Hamburger Helper)*, 1 cup	320
stew *(Hamburger Helper)*, 1/5 pkg. dry	120
stew *(Hamburger Helper)*, 1 cup	300

Italian:

cheesy *(Hamburger Helper)*, 1/5 pkg. dry	160
cheesy *(Hamburger Helper)*, 1 cup	360
zesty *(Hamburger Helper)*, 1/5 pkg. dry	170
zesty *(Hamburger Helper)*, 1 cup	340

lasagna *(Hamburger Helper)*, 1/5 pkg. dry 160
lasagna *(Hamburger Helper)*, 1 cup 340

meat loaf:

(Hamburger Helper), 1/5 pkg. dry	70
(Hamburger Helper), 1 cup	360
homestyle *(Lipton Microeasy)*, 1/4 pkg. dry	90
homestyle *(Lipton Microeasy)*, 1/4 pkg.	390

mushroom, creamy *(Tuna Helper)*, 1/5 pkg. dry 140
mushroom, creamy *(Tuna Helper)*, 7 oz. 220

noodle:

cheesy *(Tuna Helper)*, 1/5 pkg. dry	160
cheesy *(Tuna Helper)*, 7.75 oz.	250
creamy *(Tuna Helper)*, 1/5 pkg. dry	210
creamy *(Tuna Helper)*, 8 oz.	300

pizza style:

(Hamburger Helper Pizzabake), 1/6 pkg. dry	150
(Hamburger Helper Pizzabake), 4.5 oz.	320
dish *(Hamburger Helper)*, 1/5 pkg. dry	180
dish *(Hamburger Helper)*, 1 cup	360

potato:

au gratin *(Hamburger Helper)*, 1/5 pkg. dry	150
au gratin *(Hamburger Helper)*, 1 cup	320
Stroganoff *(Hamburger Helper)*, 1/5 pkg. dry	140
Stroganoff *(Hamburger Helper)*, 1 cup	320

rice, buttery *(Tuna Helper)*, 1/5 pkg. dry 160

rice, buttery *(Tuna Helper)*, 6 oz.   280
rice Oriental *(Hamburger Helper)*, 1/5 pkg. dry   180
rice Oriental *(Hamburger Helper)*, 1 cup   340
sloppy Joe *(Hamburger Helper Sloppy Joe Bake)*,
    1/6 pkg. dry   180
sloppy Joe *(Hamburger Helper Sloppy Joe Bake)*, 5 oz.   340
spaghetti *(Hamburger Helper)*, 1/5 pkg. dry   170
spaghetti *(Hamburger Helper)*, 1 cup   340
Stroganoff:
    creamy *(Hamburger Helper)*, 1/5 pkg. dry   190
    creamy *(Hamburger Helper)*, 1 cup   390
    meatless, creamy *(Tofu Classics)*, 1/2 cup**   94
    meatless, creamy *(Tofu Classics)*, 1/2 cup****   127
taco dinner kit:
    taco sauce *(Tio Sancho)*, 2 oz.   62
    taco seasoning *(Tio Sancho)*, 1.25 oz.   104
    taco shell *(Tio Sancho)*, 1 piece   64
taco style:
    (Hamburger Helper Tacobake), 1/6 pkg. dry   170
    (Hamburger Helper Tacobake), 5.75 oz.   320
    (Old El Paso), 1 taco   67
    meatless *(Natural Touch)*, 2 tbsp.   90
tamale pie *(Hamburger Helper)*, 1/5 pkg. dry   200
tamale pie *(Hamburger Helper)*, 1 cup   380
tuna *(see also specific listings)*:
    au gratin *(Tuna Helper)*, 1/5 pkg. dry   180
    au gratin *(Tuna Helper)*, 6 oz.   280
    pot pie *(Tuna Helper)*, 1/6 pkg. dry   290
    pot pie *(Tuna Helper)*, 5.1 oz.   420
    salad *(Tuna Helper)*, 1/5 pkg. dry   140
    salad *(Tuna Helper)*, 5.5 oz.   420
    tetrazzini *(Tuna Helper)*, 1/5 pkg. dry   160
    tetrazzini *(Tuna Helper)*, 6 oz.   240

    * *Prepared according to package directions, except as noted*
   ** *Prepared with tofu*
 *** *Prepared with tofu and oil*
**** *Prepared with tofu and butter*

POT PIES, FROZEN, one whole pie
See also "Dinners, Frozen" and "Entrees, Frozen"

---

calories

beef:
   (Banquet), 7 oz. 510
   (Banquet Supreme Microwave), 7 oz. 440
   (Morton), 7 oz. 430
   (Myers), 3.5 oz. 123
   (Stouffer's), 10 oz. 500
   (Swanson Pot Pie), 7 oz. 370
   (Swanson Hungry-Man), 16 oz. 610
chicken:
   (Banquet), 7 oz. 550
   (Banquet Supreme Microwave), 7 oz. 430
   (Morton), 7 oz. 420
   (Myers), 3.5 oz. 129
   (Stouffer's), 10 oz. 530
   (Swanson Homestyle Recipe), 8 oz. 410
   (Swanson Pot Pie), 7 oz. 380
   (Swanson Hungry-Man), 16 oz. 630
macaroni and cheese *(Swanson* Pot Pie), 7 oz. 200
tuna *(Banquet)*, 7 oz. 540
turkey:
   (Banquet), 7 oz. 510
   (Banquet Supreme Microwave), 7 oz. 430
   (Morton), 7 oz. 420
   (Stouffer's), 10 oz. 540
   (Swanson Pot Pie), 7 oz. 380
   (Swanson Hungry-Man), 16 oz. 650

Chapter 12

MEAT, FISH,
AND POULTRY

MEAT & POULTRY, CANNED
See also "Entrees, Canned"

---

	calories
chicken:	
breast, chunk *(Hormel)*, 6¾ oz.	350
dark, chunk *(Hormel)*, 6¾ oz.	327
chunk *(Featherweight)*, 3 oz.	90
chunk style *(Swanson* Mixin' Chicken), 2½ oz.	130
loaf *(Hormel)*, 2 oz.	130
white and dark, chunk *(Hormel)*, 6¾ oz.	340
white and dark, chunk *(Hormel* Unsalted), 6¾ oz.	330
white or white and dark *(Swanson)*, 2½ oz.	100
ham:	
(Black Label, 3 lb./5 lb.), 4 oz.	140
(Black Label 1½ lb.), 4 oz.	150
(EXL), 4 oz.	120
(EXL Deli Ham, 10 lb.), 4 oz.	130
(Holiday Glaze, 3 lb.), 4 oz.	130
(Hormel Bone-In), 4 oz.	210
(Hormel Cure 81), 4 oz.	160
(Hormel Curemaster), 4 oz.	140
(JM 95% Fat Free), 2 oz.	60
(Light & Lean Boneless), 2 oz.	60
(Oscar Mayer Jubilee), 1 oz.	29
chopped *(Hormel)*, 3 oz.	240
chunk *(Hormel)*, 6¾ oz.	310

Meat & Poultry, Canned, ham, continued

· hickory smoked *(Rath Black Hawk)*, 2 oz.	60
roll *(Hormel)*, 4 oz.	170
spiced *(Hormel)*, 3 oz.	240
ham patty *(Hormel)*, 1 patty	180
ham and cheese patty *(Hormel)*, 1 patty	190
pig's feet, pickled *(Penrose)*, 6-oz. piece	220
pig's knuckles, pickled *(Penrose)*, 6-oz. piece	290
pork *(Hormel)*, 3 oz.	240
pork, chopped *(Hormel)*, 3 oz.	200
turkey, chunk *(Hormel)*, 6¾ oz.	230
turkey, white *(Swanson)*, 2½ oz.	80

MEAT & POULTRY, FROZEN & REFRIGERATED
See also "Dinners, Frozen," "Entrees, Frozen," and "Entrees, Refrigerated"

---

	calories
ham patty *(Swift Premium* Brown 'N Serve), 1 patty . .	130
pork:	
chop, boneless *(JM* America's Cut), 6-oz. chop	330
ground *(JM)*, 3 oz.	190
loin, whole or half, center cut, boneless *(JM)*, 3 oz. .	190
shoulder butt, boneless *(JM)*, 3 oz.	210
spareribs, raw *(JM Gourmet)*, 4½ oz.	250
tenderloin, boneless *(JM)*, 3 oz.	120
turkey:	
breast, *see "turkey breast," page 157*	
cutlets, raw *(Norbest Tasti-Lean)*, 4 oz.	135
dark meat, skinless, roasted *(Swift Butterball)*,	
3.5 oz.	195
drumsticks *(Land O'Lakes)*, 3 oz.	120
drumsticks *(Louis Rich)*, 1 oz. cooked	56
w/gravy, raw *(Norbest)*, 4 oz.	115
ground, *see "turkey, ground," page 157*	
hindquarter roast *(Land O'Lakes)*, 3 oz.	140
thigh *(Land O'Lakes)*, 3 oz.	150
thigh *(Louis Rich)*, 1 oz. cooked	64
white meat, skinless, roasted *(Swift Butterball)*,	
3.5 oz.	160

white and dark meat, w/skin, roasted *(Swift Butterball)*, 3.5 oz.   195
whole, boneless *(Norbest)*, 1 oz. cooked   42
whole, boneless, smoked *(Norbest)*, 1 oz. cooked . . .   42
whole, w/out giblets *(Louis Rich)*, 1 oz. cooked   . . .   52
wings *(Land O'Lakes)*, 3 oz.   120
wings *(Louis Rich)*, 1 oz. cooked   54
wings *(Louis Rich* Drumettes), 1 oz. cooked   51
young *(Land O'Lakes)*, 3 oz.   130
young, butter basted *(Land O'Lakes)*, 3 oz.   140
young, self-basting broth *(Land O'Lakes)*, 3 oz.   120
turkey, ground:
raw *(Norbest)*, 1 oz.   45
(Longacre), 1 oz.   60
(Louis Rich), 1 oz. cooked   60
(Louis Rich 90% Lean), 1 oz. cooked   52
(Mr. Turkey), 1 oz.   54
(Hudson's), 1 oz.   55
turkey breast, raw:
(Longacre Cook-N-Bag), 1 oz.   27
(Longacre Ready-to-Cook), 1 oz.   39
w/gravy *(Norbest)*, 4 oz.   115
steaks, cubed *(Norbest)*, 4-oz. steak   135
strips and tips *(Norbest Tasti-Lean)*, 4 oz.   135
tenderloin *(Norbest Tasti-Lean* Tenders), 4 oz.   135
turkey breast, cooked:
(Land O'Lakes), 3 oz.   100
(Longacre Cook-N-Bag), 1 oz.   38
(Louis Rich), 1 oz.   47
barbecued *(Louis Rich)*, 1 oz.   33
barbecue, quarter *(Mr. Turkey* Chub), 1 oz.   34
hickory smoked or honey roasted *(Louis Rich)*, 1 oz.   33
oven prepared, quarter *(Mr. Turkey* Chub), 1 oz. . . .   34
oven roasted *(Louis Rich)*, 1 oz.   31
smoked, quarter *(Mr. Turkey* Chub), 1 oz.   35
steaks or tenderloin (Louis Rich), 1 oz.   39
turkey nuggets, cooked* *(Louis Rich)*, .7-oz. piece . . .   62
turkey patty, cooked* *(Louis Rich)*, 2.8-oz. patty   209
turkey sticks, cooked* *(Louis Rich)*, 1 stick   81

* *Prepared according to package directions*

> **FRANKFURTERS,** one link, except as noted
> *See also "Sausages"*

	calories
(Eckrich, 12 oz.)	110
(Eckrich, 1 lb.)	160
(Eckrich Bunsize/Jumbo)	190
(Eckrich Jumbo Lean Supreme)	140
(Hillshire Farm Bun Size Wieners), 2 oz.	180
(JM), 1.2-oz. link	110
(JM, 10/lb.), 1.6-oz. link	140
(JM German Brand)	160
(JM Jumbo)	190
(Kahn's Bun Size, Frank or Jumbo)	190
(Kahn's Wieners)	140
(OHSE Wieners), 1 oz.	90
(Oscar Mayer Bun-Length Wieners)	184
(Oscar Mayer Wieners), 1.6-oz. link	144
(Pilgrim's Pride, 1 lb.), 2-oz. link	118
(Pilgrim's Pride, 12 oz.), 1.5-oz. link	88
bacon and cheddar cheese *(Oscar Mayer* Hot Dogs)	137
batter-wrapped, frozen *(Hormel* Corn Dogs)	220
batter-wrapped, frozen *(Hormel* Tater Dogs)	210
beef:	
(Boar's Head), 1 oz.	80
(Eckrich, 12 oz.)	110
(Eckrich, 1 lb.)	150
(Eckrich Bunsize/Jumbo)	190
(Hebrew National)	149
(Hillshire Farm Bun Size Wieners), 2 oz.	180
(Hormel 12 oz.)	100
(Hormel 1 lb.)	140
(JM), 1.2-oz. link	100
(JM, 10/lb.), 1.6-oz. link	140
(JM Jumbo), 2-oz. link	180
(Kahn's)	140
(Kahn's Bun Size/Bun Size Franks/Jumbo)	190
(King Kold), 2 oz.	173
(OHSE), 1 oz.	85
(Oscar Mayer Bun-Length Franks)	182
(Oscar Mayer Franks), 1.6-oz. link	143

(Oscar Mayer Light Franks), 2-oz. link 131
w/cheddar *(Kahn's* Beef n'Cheddar) 180
w/cheddar *(Oscar Mayer* Franks), 1.6-oz. link 136
cheese:
   (Eckrich) 180
   (Hillshire Farm Bun Size Wieners), 2 oz. 180
   (JM Cheese Franks) 140
   (JM German Brand) 160
   (Kahn's Cheese Wiener) 150
   (Oscar Mayer Hot Dogs), 1.6-oz. link 143
chicken:
   (Health Valley Weiners) 96
   (Longacre), 1 oz. 63
   batter-wrapped *(Tyson* Corn Dogs), 3.5 oz. 280
chicken, beef, and pork *(OHSE)*, 1 oz. 85
chili *(Hormel* Frank 'n Stuff) 165
cocktail, see *"Appetizers & Snacks, Canned or Dried,*
   frankfurters, cocktail," page 123
hot, regular or beef *(Hillshire Farm* Hot Links), 2 oz. . 190
meat *(Hormel*, 12 oz.) 110
meat *(Hormel*, 1 lb.) 140
Mexacali *(Hormel* Mexacali Dogs), 5 oz. 400
natural casing *(Hillshire Farm* Wieners), 2 oz. 180
pork and beef *(Boar's Head)*, 1 oz. 80
smoked:
   (Hormel Range Brand Wranglers) 170
   (Kahn's Big Red Smokey) 170
   (Kahn's Bun Size Smokey) 180
   beef *(Hormel* Wranglers) 170
   beef *(Kahn's* Bun Size Beef Smokey) 190
   w/cheese *(Hormel* Wranglers) 180
turkey:
   (Butterball) 140
   (Health Valley Weiners) 96
   (Longacre), 1 oz. 66
   (Louis Rich) 101
   (Louis Rich Bun Length) 128
   (Mr. Turkey), 1.6 oz. 106
   cheese *(Mr. Turkey)*, 1.6 oz. 109

> **LUNCHEON MEATS,** one ounce, except as noted
> *See also "Meat & Poultry, Canned," "Meat &*
> *Poultry, Frozen & Refrigerated," "Meat, Fish &*
> *Poultry Spreads," and "Sausages"*

	calories
barbecue loaf *(Oscar Mayer)*	46
beef:	
(Eckrich Slender Sliced)	35
corned *(Eckrich* Slender Sliced)	40
corned *(Healthy Deli)*	35
corned *(Healthy Deli* St. Paddy's)	24
corned *(Hillshire Farm)*	31
corned *(Oscar Mayer)*, .6-oz. slice	17
loaf, jellied *(Hormel* Perma-Fresh), 2 slices	90
roast *(Healthy Deli)*	30
roast *(Oscar Mayer* Thin Sliced), .42-oz. slice	14
roast, Italian *(Healthy Deli)*	31
roast, oven-roasted, cured *(Hillshire Farm* Deli Select)	31
roast, top round, oven-roasted *(Boar's Head)*	40
roast, top round, oven-roasted *(Boar's Head* Deluxe)	45
sandwich steak *(Steak-Umm)*, 2 oz.	180
smoked *(Hillshire Farm* Deli Select)	31
smoked *(Oscar Mayer)*, .5-oz. slice	14
smoked, cured *(Hormel)*	50
smoked, cured, dried *(Hormel)*	45
beef jerky or beef sticks, *see "Appetizers & Snacks, Canned or Dried, beef jerky," page 122*	
bologna:	
(Boar's Head Lower Salt)	80
(Eckrich German Brand)	80
(Eckrich Lean Supreme)	70
(Eckrich/Eckrich Smorgas Pac/Sandwich)	100
(Eckrich Thick Sliced, 1 lb.), 1.8-oz. slice	170
(Hillshire Farm Large)	90
(Hillshire Farm Ring)	89
(Hormel Coarse Ground, 1 lb.), 2 oz.	160
(Hormel Fine Ground, 1 lb.), 2 oz.	170
(Hormel Perma-Fresh), 2 slices	180
(JM)	90

(JM German Brand)	70
(Kahn's Deluxe Club/Giant Deluxe), 1 slice	90
(Kahn's Deluxe Club Family Pack), 1 slice	70
(Kahn's Giant Thick Deluxe), 1 slice	110
(Kahn's Thick Deluxe), 1 slice	140
(Kahn's Thin Sliced Deluxe), 1 slice	60
(Light & Lean), 2 slices	140
(Light & Lean Thin Sliced), 2 slices	70
(OHSE)	75
(OHSE 15% Chicken)	90
(Oscar Mayer)	90
(Oscar Mayer Lite)	64
(Pilgrim's Pride)	59
w/cheese *(Eckrich)*	90
w/cheese *(Oscar Mayer),* .8-oz. slice	74
beef *(Boar's Head)*	74
beef *(Eckrich)*	90
beef *(Eckrich* Thick Sliced), 1.5-oz. slice	130
beef *(Hebrew National* Original Deli Style)	90
beef *(Hormel* Coarse Ground, 1 lb.), 2 oz.	160
beef *(Hormel* Perma-Fresh), 2 slices	170
beef *(JM)*	90
beef *(Kahn's/Kahn's* Giant/*Kahn's* Pounder), 1 slice	90
beef *(Kahn's* Family Pack), 1 slice	70
beef *(OHSE)*	85
beef *(Oscar Mayer)*	89
beef *(Oscar Mayer* Light)	64
beef, garlic flavored *(Oscar Mayer)*	90
beef, Lebanon *(Oscar Mayer),* .8-oz. slice	46
beef and cheddar *(Kahn's),* 1 slice	90
beef and pork *(Healthy Deli)*	41
garlic *(Eckrich)*	90
garlic *(JM)*	90
garlic or ham *(Kahn's),* 1 slice	90
ham *(Boar's Head)*	40
pork and beef *(Boar's Head)*	80
turkey, see "turkey bologna," page 167	
bratwurst, *see "Sausages, bratwurst," page 170*	
braunschweiger:	
(Hormel)	80
(JM)	80

Luncheon Meats, braunschweiger, continued
   (Oscar Mayer German Brand) 96
   (Oscar Mayer Slices/Tube) 97
capoccolo *(Hormel)* 80
cervelat, *see "thuringer cervelat," page 167*
cheddarwurst, *see "Sausages, cheddarwurst," page 170*
chicken:
   breast *(Longacre Premium)* 45
   breast *(Mr. Turkey)* 32
   breast, hickory smoked *(Louis Rich)* 30
   breast, oven-roasted *(Louis Rich Deluxe)* 30
   breast, oven-roasted *(Oscar Mayer)* 25
   breast, smoked *(Hillshire Farm Deli Select)* 31
   breast, smoked *(Oscar Mayer)* 26
   roll *(Pilgrim's Pride)* 35
   roll, sliced *(Longacre)* 60
   white meat, oven-roasted *(Louis Rich)* 35
chicken bologna *(Health Valley)*, 1 slice 85
chicken ham *(Pilgrim's Pride)* 35
Dutch brand loaf:
   (Eckrich/Eckrich Smorgas Pac) 70
   (Eckrich Lean Supreme) 60
   (Kahn's), 1 slice 80
frankfurter, *see "Frankfurters," page 158*
gourmet loaf *(Eckrich)* 30
ham:
   (Boar's Head Lower Salt) 28
   (Healthy Deli Deluxe/Taverne) 31
   (Healthy Deli Lessalt) 32
   (Healthy Deli Light AM) 27
   (JM Slice'n Eat 93% Fat Free), 2 oz. 70
   (JM Slice'n Eat 95% Fat Free Presliced), 2 slices . . 60
   (Jones Dairy Farm), 1 slice 50
   (Jones Dairy Farm Family Ham) 35
   (Kahn's Low Salt), 1 slice 30
   (Oscar Mayer Breakfast Ham), 1.5-oz. slice 47
   (Oscar Mayer Jubilee) 43
   (Oscar Mayer Jubilee), 8-oz. slice 29
   (Oscar Mayer Lower Salt), .75-oz. slice 23
   (Oscar Mayer Thin Sliced), .42-oz. slice 13
   (Swift Premium Hostess/Sugar Plum) 30

baked *(Oscar Mayer)*, .75-oz. slice   21
baked, Virginia *(Healthy Deli)*   34
baked, Virginia *(Healthy Deli* Lessalt)   32
barbecue *(Light & Lean)*, 2 slices   50
Black Forest *(Healthy Deli)*   32
boiled *(Boar's Head* Deluxe)   28
boiled *(Oscar Mayer)*, .75-oz. slice   23
Cajun *(Hillshire Farm* Deli Select)   31
chopped *(Eckrich)*   45
chopped *(Eckrich* Lean Supreme)   35
chopped *(Hormel* Perma-Fresh), 2 slices   88
chopped *(JM)*   80
chopped *(Kahn's)*, 1 slice   50
chopped *(Light & Lean)*, 2 slices   70
chopped *(OHSE)*   65
chopped *(Oscar Mayer)*   41
cooked *(JM)*   30
cooked *(OHSE)*   30
cooked, fresh *(Healthy Deli)*   33
cooked, sliced *(Kahn's)*, 1 slice   30
cooked or glazed *(Light & Lean)*, 2 slices   50
honey *(Healthy Deli* Honey Valley)   31
honey *(Hillshire Farm* Deli Select)   31
honey *(Oscar Mayer)*, .75-oz. slice   23
jalapeño *(Healthy Deli)*   25
loaf *(Eckrich)*   50
peppered, black or red *(Light & Lean)*, 2 slices   50
peppered, black, cracked *(Oscar Mayer)*, .75-oz. slice   22
peppered, chopped *(Oscar Mayer)*   55
pit *(OHSE)*   40
smoked *(Eckrich* Slender Sliced)   40
smoked *(Hillshire Farm* Deli Select)   31
smoked *(OHSE* 95% Fat Free)   30
smoked, cooked *(Light & Lean)*, 2 slices   50
smoked, cooked *(Oscar Mayer)*, .75-oz. slice   22
smoked, golden *(JM)*, 2 oz.   80
smoked, golden, and water *(JM)*, 2 oz.   70
turkey, *see "turkey ham," page 169*
ham and cheese loaf:
  (Eckrich)   50
  (Hormel Perma-Fresh), 2 slices 110

Luncheon Meats, ham and cheese loaf, continued

(Kahn's), 1 slice	70
(Light & Lean), 2 slices	90
(OHSE)	65
(Oscar Mayer)	66
head cheese *(Oscar Mayer)*	54

honey loaf:

(Eckrich/Eckrich Smorgas Pac)	35
(Hormel Perma-Fresh), 2 slices	90
(Kahn's), 1 slice	40
(Oscar Mayer)	34
Iowa brand loaf *(Hormel* Perma-Fresh), 2 slices	90
jalapeño loaf *(Kahn's)*, 1 slice	70
kielbasa, *see "Sausages, kielbasa," page 171*	
knockwurst, *see "Sausages, knockwurst," page 171*	
liver cheese *(JM)*	70
liver cheese *(Oscar Mayer)*, 1 slice, 6 per 8-oz. pkg.	116
liver loaf *(Hormel* Perma-Fresh), 2 slices	160
liver loaf *(Kahn's)*, 1 slice	170
liverwurst *(Jones Dairy Farm* Chub)	80
liverwurst *(Jones Dairy Farm* Slices), 1 slice	75

luncheon meat:

(Oscar Mayer)	94
loaf, spiced *(JM)*	70
loaf *(OHSE)*	75
spiced *(Hormel* Perma-Fresh), 2 slices	118
spiced *(Kahn's* Luncheon Loaf), 1 slice	80
spiced *(Light & Lean)*, 2 slices	120
macaroni and cheese loaf *(Eckrich)*	75
macaroni and cheese loaf *(OHSE)*	60

New England brand sausage:

(Eckrich), 1 oz. or 1 slice	35
(Light & Lean), 2 slices	90
(Oscar Mayer), .8-oz. slice	29
old fashioned loaf *(Oscar Mayer)*	62

olive loaf:

(Boar's Head)	60
(Eckrich)	80
(Hormel Perma-Fresh), 2 slices	110
(Oscar Mayer)	63
P&B loaf *(Kahn's)*, 1 slice	40

P&B loaf *(JM)* 70
pastrami:
  (Boar's Head Round) 40
  (Healthy Deli Round) 34
  (Hillshire Farm Deli Select) 31
  (Oscar Mayer), .6-oz. slice 16
  turkey, *see "turkey pastrami," page 169*
peppered loaf:
  (Eckrich) 35
  (Kahn's), 1 slice 40
  (Oscar Mayer) 39
pepperoni:
  (Hormel/Hormel Chunk) 140
  (Hormel Leoni Brand) 130
  (Hormel Perma-Fresh), 2 slices 80
  (Hormel Rosa/Rosa Grande) 140
  (JM), 8 slices, approx. .5 oz. 70
pickle loaf:
  (Eckrich/Eckrich Smorgas Pac) 80
  (Hormel Perma-Fresh), 2 slices 102
  (Kahn's), 1 slice 80
  (Kahn's Family Pack), 1 slice 70
  (Light & Lean), 2 slices 100
  (OHSE) 60
  beef *(Kahn's* Family Pack), 1 slice 60
pickle and pimento loaf *(Oscar Mayer)* 66
picnic loaf *(Oscar Mayer)* 61
Polish sausage, *see "Sausages, Polish," page 171*
pork luncheon meat *(Eckrich* Slender Sliced) 45
prosciutto, boneless *(Hormel)* 90
salami:
  (Hormel Party) 90
  beef *(Boar's Head)* 60
  beef *(Hebrew National* Original Deli Style) 80
  beef *(Hormel* Perma-Fresh), 2 slices 50
  beef *(Kahn's)*, 1 slice 70
  beef *(Kahn's* Family Pack), 1 slice 60
  beer *(Eckrich)* 70
  beer *(Oscar Mayer* Salami for Beer), .8-oz. slice 50
  beer, beef *(Oscar Mayer* Salami for Beer), .8-oz. slice ... 63
  cooked *(Kahn's)*, 1 slice 60

Luncheon Meats, salami, continued

cooked *(OHSE)*	65
cotto *(Eckrich)*	70
cotto *(Hormel* Chub)	100
cotto *(Hormel* Perma-Fresh), 2 slices	105
cotto *(JM)*	80
cotto *(Kahn's* Family Pack), 1 slice	45
cotto *(Light & Lean)*, 2 slices	80
cotto *(Oscar Mayer)*, .8-oz. slice	52
cotto, beef *(Eckrich)*, 1.3 oz.	100
cotto, beef *(Oscar Mayer)*, .8-oz. slice	45
dry or hard *(Hormel/Hormel* Sliced)	110
dry or hard *(Hormel* National Brand)	120
dry or hard *(Hormel* Perma-Fresh), 2 slices	80
dry or hard *(JM)*	110
dry or hard *(Oscar Mayer* Hard), .3-oz. slice	33
Genoa *(Hormel/Hormel* Gran Valore)	110
Genoa *(Hormel DiLusso)*	100
Genoa *(Hormel* San Remo Brand)	118
Genoa *(JM)*	100
Genoa *(Oscar Mayer)*, .3-oz. slice	34
piccolo *(Hormel* Stick)	120
turkey, *see "turkey salami," page 169*	
sausage, *see "Sausages," page 170*	
scrapple *(Jones Dairy Farm)*, 1 slice	65
souse loaf *(Kahn's)*, 1 slice	90
summer sausage *(see also "thuringer cervelat," page 167):*	
(Eckrich)	80
(Hillshire Farm), 2 oz.	180
(Hormel Perma-Fresh), 2 slices	140
(Hormel Tangy Chub/Thuringer)	90
(Lean & Lite)	43
(Light & Lean), 2 slices	100
(OHSE)	75
(Oscar Mayer), 1 slice, 10 per 8-oz. pkg.	69
beef *(Hillshire Farm)*, 2 oz.	190
beef *(Hormel* Beefy)	100
beef *(OHSE)*	80
beef *(Oscar Mayer)*, 1 slice, 10 per 8-oz. pkg.	70
w/cheese *(Hillshire Farm)*, 2 oz.	200

thuringer cervelat *(see also "summer sausage,"*
   page 166):
  (Hillshire Farm), 2 oz. 180
  (Hormel Old Smokehouse) 90
  (Hormel Old Smokehouse Chub/Sliced) 100
  (Hormel Viking Chub Cervelat) 90
  (JM Cervalot) 70
  beef *(JM* Thuringer) 80
turkey:
  breast, *see "turkey breast," below*
  diced, white meat *(Norbest)* 31
  ham, *see "turkey ham," page 169*
  ham flavor, hickory smoked, dark meat *(Norbest*
    Gourmet Cured) 39
  loaf *(Louis Rich)* 45
  luncheon loaf, spiced *(Mr. Turkey)* 51
  oven cooked *(OHSE)* 30
  pastrami, *see "turkey pastrami," page 169*
  roll, white meat *(Norbest* Orange Label) 29
  roll, white and dark meat *(Norbest* Orange Label) . . 36
  salami, *see "turkey salami," page 169*
  smoked *(Butterball* Cold Cuts) 35
  smoked *(Butterball Turkey Variety Pak)*, .75 oz. . . . 25
  smoked *(Louis Rich)* 32
  summer sausage, *see "turkey summer sausage,"*
    page 170
turkey bologna:
  *(Butterball Deli/Slice 'n Serve/*Cold Cuts) 70
  (Butterball Turkey Variety Pak), .75 oz. 50
  (Louis Rich) 61
  (Norbest Blue Label, 2–2.5 lb.) 68
  (OHSE) 70
  mild *(Louis Rich)* 59
  sliced *(Longacre)* 61
turkey breast:
  (Butterball Cold Cuts) 30
  (Butterball Deli No Salt Added) 45
  (Butterball Slice 'n Serve) 35
  (Healthy Deli Gourmet) 28
  (Healthy Deli Lessalt) 25
  (Hormel Perma-Fresh), 2 slices 60

Luncheon Meats, turkey breast, continued

(Light & Lean), 2 slices	60
(Longacre Catering/Gourmet)	35
(Longacre Gourmet Low Salt/Premium)	30
(Longacre Salt Watchers)	32
(Louis Rich)	45
(Mr. Turkey)	31
barbecue seasoned *(Butterball Slice 'n Serve* BBQ)	40
browned, glazed or roasted *(Longacre* Gourmet)	35
browned, glazed or roasted *(Longacre* Premium)	30
honey *(Healthy Deli)*	28
honey-roasted *(Louis Rich)*	32
golden *(Boar's Head)*	35
golden, skinless *(Boar's Head)*	30
lite, regular, skinless, or smoked *(Longacre* Deli)	35
oven cooked *(Healthy Deli)*	26
oven roasted *(Hillshire Farm* Deli Select)	31
oven roasted *(Louis Rich)*	31
oven roasted *(Oscar Mayer)*, 1 slice, 8 per 6-oz. pkg.	23
roast *(Louis Rich)*	40
w/skin *(Norbest* Blue or Orange Label)	28
w/skin, prebrowned *(Norbest* Orange Label)	29
w/skin, salt free *(Norbest* Blue Label)	35
w/skin, smoked *(Norbest* Orange Label)	30
skinless *(Longacre* Catering)	35
skinless *(Longacre* Gourmet/Premium)	30
skinless *(Norbest* Blue, Orange, or Yellow Label)	26
skinless, salt-free *(Norbest* Blue Label)	33
sliced *(Longacre)*	30
sliced *(Louis Rich)*	40
smoked *(Butterball* Cold Cuts)	35
smoked *(Healthy Deli,* 3 lb.)	29
smoked *(Healthy Deli* Gourmet)	31
smoked *(Hillshire Farm* Deli Select)	31
smoked *(Hormel* Perma-Fresh), 2 slices	60
smoked *(Longacre)*	35
smoked *(Louis Rich)*, .7-oz. slice	21
smoked *(Mr. Turkey)*	31
smoked *(Norbest* Gold Label)	29
smoked *(OHSE)*	30
smoked *(Oscar Mayer)*, 1 slice, 8 per 6-oz. pkg.	20

smoked, hickory *(Butterball Slice 'n Serve)*   35
smoked, sliced *(Longacre)*   26
and white *(Longacre Deli Chef)*   35
and white, browned and roasted or skinless
   (Longacre Deli Chef)   40
and thigh *(Norbest* Blue Label)   31
turkey and corned beef *(Healthy Deli* Doubledecker) . .   30
turkey frankfurter, *see "Frankfurters, turkey," page 159*
turkey ham:
  (Butterball Slice n' Serve /Cold Cuts)   35
  (Louis Rich Round).   34
  (Louis Rich Square), .75-oz. slice   24
  (OHSE)   30
  breakfast, smoked *(Mr. Turkey)*   33
  buffet style, smoked *(Mr. Turkey)*   32
  chopped *(Louis Rich)*   46
  chopped *(Mr. Turkey)*   37
  chunk *(Longacre)*   37
  cured, thigh *(Norbest* Tavern, 2–2.5 lb. Half)   29
  cured, thigh, Canadian style *(Norbest)*   35
  honey cured *(Butterball* Cold Cuts)   35
  honey cured *(Butterball Slice 'n Serve)*   40
  honey cured *(Louis Rich),* .75-oz. slice   25
  lean lite *(Longacre* Deli)   37
  roll *(Norbest)*   31
  sliced *(Butterball* Deli Thin)   35
  sliced *(Longacre)*.   33
  smoked *(Mr. Turkey* Regular/Chub).   32
turkey and ham *(Healthy Deli* Doubledecker)   30
turkey pastrami:
  (Butterball Cold Cuts)   30
  (Butterball Slice 'n Serve)   35
  (Louis Rich Round).   32
  (Louis Rich Square), .8-oz. slice   24
  (Mr. Turkey)   28
  (Norbest)   29
  sliced *(Longacre)*   32
turkey salami:
  (Butterball Deli/Slice 'n Serve Cold Cuts)   50
  (Butterball Turkey Variety Pak), .75 oz.   40
  (Louis Rich)   54

Luncheon Meats, turkey salami, continued
   (Norbest Blue Label, 2–2.5 lb.)   45
   (OHSE)   50
   cotto *(Louis Rich)*   53
   cotto *(Mr. Turkey)*   45
   sliced *(Longacre)*   52
turkey sausage, *see "Sausages, turkey," page 172*
turkey summer sausage *(Louis Rich)*   55

SAUSAGES
See also "Frankfurters" and "Luncheon Meats"

	calories
(Eckrich Lean Supreme Heat 'n Serve), 2 links	120
(Hormel Brown & Serve), 2 links	140
(Jones Dairy Farm Light Brown & Serve), 1 link	60
(Swift Premium Brown 'N Serve Country Recipe),	
1 patty or link	130
(Swift Premium Brown 'N Serve Microwave), 1 link . .	120
(Swift Premium Original Brown 'N Serve), 1 link	130
(Swift Premium Original Brown 'N Serve), 1 patty . . .	120
w/bacon *(Swift Premium* Brown 'N Serve), 1 link	120
beef *(Jones Dairy Farm* Golden Brown), 1 link	75
beef *(Swift Premium* Brown 'N Serve), 1 link	120
beef and cheddar *(Hillshire Farm* Flavorseal), 2 oz. . . .	190
bratwurst:	
(Eckrich), 1 link	310
(Hillshire Farm Fully Cooked), 2 oz.	170
(Kahn's), 1 link	190
fresh or smoked *(Hillshire Farm),* 2 oz.	190
spicy *(Hillshire Farm),* 2 oz.	180
cheddarwurst *(Hillshire Farm* Bun Size), 2 oz.	200
cheddarwurst *(Hillshire Farm* Links), 2 oz.	190
country *(Hillshire Farm* Country Recipe), 2 oz.	180
w/ham *(Swift Premium* Brown 'N Serve), 1 link	130
hot *(OHSE* Hot Links), 1 oz.	80
hot or mild, canned *(Hormel),* 1 patty	150
Italian:	
hot *(Hillshire Farm* Links), 2 oz.	180
mild *(Hillshire Farm* Links), 2 oz.	190

smoked *(Hillshire Farm* Flavorseal), 2 oz.   200
kielbasa *(see also "Polish sausage," below):*
   (Eckrich Lean Supreme Polska), 1 oz.   72
   (Hillshire Farm Bun Size), 2 oz.   180
   (Hillshire Farm Polska Flavorseal/Links), 2 oz.   190
   (Hillshire Farm Polska Flavorseal Lite), 2 oz.   160
   (Hormel Kolbase), 3 oz.   220
   beef *(Hillshire Farm* Polska Flavorseal), 2 oz.   190
   mild *(Hillshire Farm* Polska Flavorseal), 2 oz.   190
   skinless *(Eckrich* Polska), 1 link   180
   skinless *(Hormel),* ½ link   180
knockwurst *(Hillshire Farm* Links), 2 oz.   180
knockwurst, beef *(Hebrew National),* 3-oz. link   263
maple flavor *(Swift Premium* Brown 'N Serve), 1 link .   120
minced roll *(Eckrich),* 1-oz. slice   80
New England, *see "Luncheon Meats, New England*
   brand sausage," page 164
pickled, *see "Appetizers & Snacks, Canned or Dried,*
   sausages, pickled," page 123
Polish *(see also "kielbasa," above):*
   (Hillshire Farm Links), 2 oz.   190
   (Hormel), 2 links   170
   (OHSE), 1 oz.   80
   (Pilgrim's Pride), 3 oz.   131
   hot *(OHSE),* 1 oz.   70
pork:
   (Hormel Little Sizzlers), 2 links   103
   (Hormel Midget Links), 2 links   143
   (JM Tasty Link), 2 raw links   260
   (JM Tasty Link), 2 cooked links   190
   (Jones Dairy Farm), 1 link   140
   (Jones Dairy Farm Golden Brown Light), 1 link . . .   55
   (Jones Dairy Farm Light), 1 link   70
   (Jones Dairy Farm Regular/Golden Brown), 1 patty   155
   (Oscar Mayer Little Friers), 1 cooked link   82
   mild *(Jones Dairy Farm* Golden Brown), 1 link   100
   regular or hot *(JM),* 1-oz. raw patty   130
   regular or hot *(JM),* 1 cooked patty, .5 oz.   70
   roll *(Jones Dairy Farm* Cello Roll), 1 slice   105
   spicy *(Jones Dairy Farm* Golden Brown), 1 link . . .   100
pork and bacon *(JM* Tasty Link), 2 raw links   220

Sausages, continued

pork and bacon *(JM* Tasty Link), 2 cooked links	100
smoked:	
(*Eckrich* Lean Supreme), 1 oz.	70
(*Eckrich* Skinless), 1 link	180
(*Hillshire Farm* Bun Size), 2 oz.	180
(*Hillshire Farm* Flavorseal/Links), 2 oz.	190
(*Hillshire Farm* Lite), 2 oz.	160
(*Hormel* Smokies), 2 links	160
(*OHSE*), 1 oz.	80
(*Oscar Mayer* Little Smokies), .3-oz. link	27
(*Oscar Mayer* Smokie Links), 1.5-oz. link	126
(*Pilgrim's Pride*), 3 oz.	144
all varieties, except hot (*Eckrich Smok-Y-Links*),	
2 links	160
beef (*Eckrich*), 1 oz.	100
beef (*Eckrich* Lean Supreme), 1 oz.	80
beef (*Hillshire Farm* Bun Size/Flavorseal), 2 oz.	180
beef (*Oscar Mayer* Smokies), 1.5-oz. link	124
cheese (*Hormel* Smokie Cheezers), 2 links	168
cheese (*Oscar Mayer* Smokies), 1.5-oz. link	126
flavor (*Swift Premium* Brown 'N Serve), 1 link	120
hot (*Eckrich Smok-Y-Links*), 2 links	150
hot (*Hillshire Farm* Flavorseal), 2 oz.	180
pork (*Hormel*), 3 oz.	290
summer, *see "Luncheon Meats, summer sausage,"*	
page 166	
Swedish (*Hickory Farms*), 1 oz.	100
turkey, 1 oz.:	
(*Butterball*)	50
(*Norbest Tasti-Lean,* Chub or Links)	53
breakfast (*Mr. Turkey*)	58
breakfast, ground (*Hudson's*)	65
breakfast, ground, cooked (*Louis Rich*)	56
breakfast links, cooked (*Louis Rich*), 1 link	46
Polish (*Louis Rich* Polska Kielbasa)	40
Polish (*Mr. Turkey* Polska Kielbasa)	59
smoked (*Louis Rich*)	43
smoked (*Mr. Turkey*)	47

smoked, w/cheese *(Louis Rich)*   47
Vienna, *see "Appetizers & Snacks, Canned or Dried,*
    sausages, Vienna," page 124

BACON, cooked, except as noted

	calories
(Black Label Sliced), 2 slices	60
(JM), 2 slices	100
(JM Lower Sodium), 2 slices	100
(Jones Dairy Farm), 1 raw slice	165
(Kahn's American Beauty), 2 slices	100
(Oscar Mayer/Oscar Mayer Lower Salt), 1 slice	33
(Oscar Mayer Center Cut), 1 slice	25
(Range Brand Sliced), 2 slices	110
(Red Label), 3 slices	110
thick sliced *(Oscar Mayer)*, 1 slice	58
Canadian-style:	
(Hormel Sliced), 1 oz.	45
(Jones Dairy Farm), 1 unheated slice	25
(Light & Lean), 2 slices	35
(Oscar Mayer), .8-oz. slice	28
substitute *(see also "Vegetarian Foods, Frozen &*	
Refrigerated, 'bacon,' " page 105):	
beef *(JM)*, 2 slices	100
beef *(Sizzlean)*, 2 strips	70
pork *(Sizzlean)*, 2 strips	90
pork, brown sugar cured *(Sizzlean)*, 2 strips	110
turkey *(Louis Rich)*, 1 slice	32

MEAT, FISH & POULTRY SPREADS
See also "Fish & Shellfish, Canned or in Jars,"
"Luncheon Meats," and "Meat & Poultry, Canned"

	calories
anchovy paste *(Crosse & Blackwell)*, 1 tbsp.	20
corned beef spread *(Hormel)*, .5 oz.	35
corned beef spread *(Underwood)*, 1/2 can or 2.25 oz. . . .	120
roast beef spread *(Hormel)*, .5 oz.	31

Meat, Fish & Poultry Spreads, continued

roast beef spread *(Underwood)*, ½ can or 2.4 oz.   140
chicken salad *(Longacre)*, 1 oz.   64
chicken salad *(Longacre* Saladfest), 1 oz.   47
chicken spread:
   (Hormel), .5 oz.   30
   chunky *(Swanson)*, 1 oz.   60
   chunky *(Underwood)*, ½ can or 2.4 oz.   150
ham spread, deviled *(Hormel)*, 1 tbsp.   35
ham spread, deviled *(Underwood)*, ½ can or 2.25 oz. .   220
liverwurst spread *(Hormel)*, .5 oz.   35
liverwurst spread *(Underwood)*, ½ can or 2.25 oz. . . .   190
luncheon meat:
   all styles, except deviled *(Spam)*, 2 oz.   170
   deviled *(Spam)*, 1 tbsp.   35
   spiced *(Hormel)*, 3 oz.   280
meat, potted *(Hormel* Food Product), 1 tbsp.   30
sandwich spread *(Oscar Mayer* Chub), 1 oz.   67
seafood and crabmeat salad *(Longacre* Saladfest), 1 oz.   45
shrimp salad *(Longacre* Saladfest), 1 oz.   45
tuna salad *(Longacre)*, 1 oz.   58
tuna salad *(Longacre* Saladfest), 1 oz.   52
turkey salad *(Longacre)*, 1 oz.   70
turkey salad *(Longacre* Saladfest), 1 oz.   68
turkey ham salad *(Longacre)*, 1 oz.   53
turkey ham salad *(Longacre* Saladfest), 1 oz.   58

FISH & SHELLFISH, CANNED OR IN JARS
*See also "Appetizers & Snacks, Canned or Dried,"
"Fish & Shellfish, Frozen," and "Meat, Fish & Poultry
Spreads"*

                                   calories

clam juice *(Doxsee)*, 3 fl. oz.   4
clam juice *(Snow's)*, 3 fl. oz.   4
clams, chopped or minced:
   (Gorton's), ½ can   70
   w/liquid *(Doxsee)*, 6.5 oz.   100
   w/liquid *(Orleans)*, 6.5 oz.   100

gefilte fish, 1 piece:
   (Manischewitz, 12/24 oz.)   53
   (Manischewitz Homestyle, 12/24 oz.)   55
   (Manischewitz Unsalted)   45
   sweet *(Manischewitz, 12/24 oz.)*   65
   whitefish and pike *(Manischewitz, 12/24 oz.)*   49
   whitefish and pike, sweet *(Manischewitz 12/24 oz.)* . .   64
gefilte fish, in jelled broth, 1 piece, except as noted:
   (Mother's Old Fashioned, 12 oz.)   54
   (Mother's Old Fashioned, 24 oz.)   70
   (Mother's Unsalted)   45
   (Rokeach Old Vienna, 12 oz.), 2 oz.   54
   (Rokeach Old Vienna, 24 oz.), 2.6 oz.   70
   (Rokeach Redi-Jelled), 2 oz.   46
   (Rokeach Redi-Jelled), 3 oz.   65
   (Rokeach Redi-Jelled), 4 oz.   92
   whitefish *(Mother's, 24/31 oz.)*   60
   whitefish or whitefish and pike *(Mother's, 12 oz.)* . .   46
   whitefish and pike *(Mother's, 24/31 oz.)*   60
   whitefish and pike *(Mother's* Old World, 12 oz.) . . .   54
   whitefish and pike *(Mother's* Old World, 24 oz.) . . .   70
   whitefish and pike *(Rokeach, 24/31 oz.),* 2.6 oz.   60
   whitefish and pike *(Rokeach,* 12 oz.), 2 oz.   46
gefilte fish, in liquid, 1 piece, except as noted:
   (Mother's Old Fashioned, 12 oz.)   54
   (Mother's Old Fashioned, 24/31 oz.)   70
   natural broth *(Rokeach,* 24 oz.), 4 oz.   60
   natural broth *(Rokeach,* 24 oz.), 2.6 oz.   50
   sweet *(Mother's* Old World)   54
   whitefish *(Mother's,* 12 oz.)   54
   whitefish *(Mother's,* 24/31 oz.)   70
   whitefish and pike *(Mother's)*   70
oysters *(Bumble Bee),* 1 cup   218
oysters, whole *(S&W* Fancy), 2 oz.   95
salmon:
   blueback *(S&W/Nutradiet),* 1/2 cup   188
   chum, keta *(Bumble Bee),* 1 cup   306
   coho, Alaska *(Deming's),* 1/2 cup   140
   pink *(Bumble Bee),* 1 cup   310
   pink *(Del Monte),* 1/2 cup   160
   pink *(Featherweight),* 2 oz.   70

Fish & Shellfish, canned or in jars, salmon, continued

pink *(Libby's)*, 7.75 oz.	310
pink, Alaska *(Deming's)*, 1/2 cup	140
pink chunk, in water *(Deming's)*, 3.25 oz.	120
red, w/liquid *(Del Monte)*, 1/2 cup	180
red, blueback *(S&W Fancy)*, 1/2 cup	190
red, sockeye *(Bumble Bee)*, 1 cup	376
red, sockeye *(Libby's)*, 7.75 oz.	380
red, sockeye *(S&W/Nutradiet)*, 1/2 cup	188
red, sockeye, Alaska *(Deming's)*, 1/2 cup	170
red, sockeye, Alaska, medium *(Deming's)*, 1/2 cup	150
sardines:	
Norway, in oil, w/liquid *(Empress)*, 3.75-oz. can	460
Norway, in oil, drained *(Empress)*, 3.75-oz. can	260
Norwegian brisling *(S&W)*, 1.5 oz.	130
in water *(Featherweight)*, 1⅞ oz.	95
in oil *(Featherweight)*, 1⅞ oz.	130
in tomato sauce *(Del Monte)*, 1/2 cup	360
kippered *(Brunswick Kippered Snacks)*, 3.5 oz.	185
shrimp *(Louisiana Brand)*, 2 oz.	58
shrimp, large *(ShopRite)*, 2 oz.	50
tuna, in oil, 2 oz.:	
chunk light *(S&W Fancy)*	140
chunk light *(Star-Kist)*	150
chunk light or white *(Bumble Bee)*	110
chunk white *(Star-Kist)*	140
solid light *(Star-Kist Prime Catch)*	150
solid white, Albacore *(Bumble Bee)*	100
solid white, Albacore *(Star-Kist)*	140
solid white, Albacore *(S&W Fancy)*	160
tuna, in water, 2 oz.:	
chunk light *(Bumble Bee)*	50
chunk light *(Featherweight)*	60
chunk light *(S&W Fancy)*	60
chunk light, in spring water *(Star-Kist)*	60
chunk light, in spring water *(Star-Kist Select–60% Less Salt)*	65
chunk light, diet, in distilled water *(Star-Kist)*	65
chunk white *(Bumble Bee)*	60
chunk white, in spring water *(Star-Kist Select–60% Less Salt)*	70

chunk white, diet, in distilled water *(Star-Kist)*   70
light *(Empress)*   60
solid light, in spring water *(Star-Kist/Star-Kist* Prime
    Catch)   60
solid white, Albacore *(Bumble Bee)*   60
solid white, Albacore, in spring water *(Star-Kist)* . . .   70

FISH & SHELLFISH, FROZEN
See also "Dinners, Frozen" and "Entrees, Frozen"

	calories
catfish, fillets *(Delta Pride)*, 4 oz.	132
catfish, ocean *(Booth)*, 4 oz.	115
cod:	
(Booth), 4 oz.	89
(Booth Individually Wrapped), 4 oz.	90
(Gorton's Fishmarket Fresh), 5 oz.	110
(SeaPak), 4 oz.	90
(Van de Kamp's Natural), 4 oz.	90
crab, imitation *(Icicle Brand)*, 3.5 oz.	99
flounder:	
(Booth Individually Wrapped), 4 oz.	90
(Gorton's Fishmarket Fresh), 5 oz.	110
(SeaPak), 4 oz.	90
(Van de Kamp's Natural), 4 oz.	80
Atlantic *(Booth)*, 4 oz.	90
haddock:	
(Booth Individually Wrapped), 4 oz.	90
(Gorton's Fishmarket Fresh), 5 oz.	110
(SeaPak), 4 oz.	90
(Van de Kamp's Natural), 4 oz.	90
halibut, steaks, w/out seasoning mix *(SeaPak)*, 6 oz. . .	160
ocean perch:	
(Booth), 4 oz.	100
(Gorton's Fishmarket Fresh), 5 oz.	140
(Van de Kamp's Natural), 4 oz.	110
perch *(Booth)*, 4 oz.	100
perch *(SeaPak)*, 4 oz.	100
shrimp *(SeaPak* PDQ), 3.5 oz.	60
shrimp, butterfly *(Gorton's* Specialty), 4 oz.	160

Fish & Shellfish, Frozen, continued
sole:
   (Gorton's Fishmarket Fresh), 5 oz.   110
   Atlantic *(Booth)*, 4 oz.   90
   fillets *(SeaPak)*, 4 oz.   90
   fillets *(Van de Kamp's* Natural), 4 oz.   80
tuna, steak, w/out seasoning mix *(SeaPak)*, 6-oz. pkg. .   180
whiting *(Booth)*, 4 oz.   100
whiting *(Booth* Individually Wrapped), 4 oz.   80

Chapter 13

PASTA, NOODLES, AND RICE

MACARONI, NOODLES, & PASTA, plain, uncooked, two ounces

	calories
macaroni (all brands)	210
noodles, egg:	
(Creamette)	221
(Gioia)	220
(Goodman's Country Style)	220
(Mrs. Grass)	220
(Mueller's)	220
(P&R)	220
(Prince)	210
(San Giorgio)	220
pasta:	
(Antoine's Penne Rigati)	210
(Creamette)	210
(Ronzoni)	210
all varieties, except whole wheat *(Al Dente)*	220
all varieties, except tomato basil, tri-color, or whole wheat *(De Boles)*	210
amaranth *(Health Valley* Spaghetti)	170
w/egg *(Creamette)*	221
oat bran *(Health Valley* Spaghetti)	120
spicy *(Antoine's* Spirals)	210
spinach, w/egg *(Creamette)*	220
tomato basil, tri-color, or whole wheat *(De Boles)*	200
tri-color *(Antoine's* Fusilli)	210

Macaroni, Noodles, & Pasta, pasta, continued

tri-color *(Creamette)* 210
whole wheat *(Al Dente* Fettucine) 210
whole wheat *(Health Valley* Lasagna/Spaghetti) 170
whole wheat, w/bran *(Misura)* 197
whole-wheat spinach *(Health Valley)* 170

MACARONI DISHES, CANNED
*See also "Entrees, Canned & Packaged," "Noodle
Dishes, Canned," and "Pasta Dishes, Canned"*

                                                      calories
and beef:
  (Chef Boyardee Beefaroni), 7.5 oz. 220
  in tomato sauce *(Franco-American* Hearty Pasta),
    7.5 oz. 200
  in tomato sauce *(Heinz)*, 7.25 oz. 200
and cheese *(Heinz)*, 7.5 oz. 190
and cheese *(Hormel Micro Cup)*, 7.5-oz. cont. 189
shells, and cheddar *(Lipton Hearty Ones)*, 11 oz. 367
shells, in tomato sauce *(Chef Boyardee)*, 7.5 oz. 150

MACARONI DISHES, MIXES*
*See also "Noodle Dishes, Mixes" and "Pasta Dishes,
Mixes"*

                                                      calories
and cheese:
  (Golden Grain), 1.81 oz. dry 190
  (Golden Grain), 1 serving.................... 310
  (Kraft/Kraft Family Size Dinner), ¾ cup 290
  (Kraft Deluxe Dinner), ¾ cup 260
  cheddar *(Fantastic Foods* Traditional), ½ cup 112
  Parmesan and herbs *(Fantastic Foods)*, ½ cup 109
  shells *(Velveeta* Dinner), ¾ cup 260
  spirals *(Kraft* Dinner), ¾ cup 330

shells 'n curry *(Tofu Classics)*, 1/2 cup**   103
shells 'n curry *(Tofu Classics)*, 1/2 cup***   143

   * *Prepared according to package directions, except as noted*
  ** *Prepared with tofu*
*** *Prepared with tofu and butter*

NOODLE DISHES, CANNED
See also "Entrees, Canned & Packaged," "Macaroni Dishes, Canned," and "Pasta Dishes, Canned"

---

	calories
and beef, in sauce *(Heinz)*, 7.5 oz.	170
and chicken *(Hormel/Dinty Moore Micro Cup)*, 7.5 oz.	180
w/franks *(Van Camp's Noodle Weenee)*, 1 cup	245

NOODLE DISHES, MIXES*
See also "Entrees, Mixes," "Macaroni Dishes, Mixes," and "Pasta Dishes, Mixes"

---

	calories
Alfredo *(see also "carbonara Alfredo," below)*:	
(Lipton Noodles & Sauce), 1/4 pkg. dry	150
(Lipton Noodles & Sauce), 1/2 cup**	220
(Minute Microwave Family Size), 1/2 cup	170
(Minute Microwave Single Size), 1/2 cup	160
(Mueller's Chef's Series), 1/2 cup	190
beef *(Lipton* Noodles & Sauce), 1/4 pkg. dry	120
beef *(Lipton* Noodles & Sauce), 1/2 cup***	180
butter *(Lipton* Noodles & Sauce), 1/4 pkg. dry	150
butter *(Lipton* Noodles & Sauce), 1/2 cup***	200
butter and herb:	
(Lipton Noodles & Sauce), 1/4 pkg. dry	140
(Lipton Noodles & Sauce), 1/2 cup***	190
carbonara Alfredo:	
(Lipton Noodles & Sauce), 1/4 pkg. dry	140
(Lipton Noodles & Sauce), 1/2 cup**	210
cheese *(see also "Parmesan," page 182)*:	
(Kraft Dinner), 3/4 cup	340

Noodle Dishes, Mixes*, cheese, continued

    (Lipton Noodles & Sauce), 1/4 pkg. dry   140
    (Lipton Noodles & Sauce), 1/2 cup***   190
chicken or chicken flavor:
    (Kraft Dinner), 3/4 cup   240
    (Lipton Noodles & Sauce), 1/4 pkg. dry   130
    (Lipton Noodles & Sauce), 1/2 cup***   180
    (Minute Microwave Single/Family Size), 1/2 cup . . .   160
    (Mueller's Chef's Series), 1/2 cup   160
    broccoli *(Lipton* Noodles & Sauce), 1/4 pkg. dry . . .   130
    broccoli *(Lipton* Noodles & Sauce), 1/2 cup**   200
    mushroom *(Noodle Roni)*, 1 serving   160
fettuccini *(Noodle Roni)*, 1 serving   300
garlic and butter *(Mueller's Chef's Series)*, 1/2 cup . . .   170
garlic butter *(Noodle Roni)*, 1 serving   300
herb butter *(Noodle Roni)*, 1 serving   160
Parmesan:
    (Lipton Noodles & Sauce), 1/4 pkg. dry   140
    (Lipton Noodles & Sauce), 1/2 cup**   210
    (Minute Microwave Family Size), 1/2 cup   170
    (Minute Microwave Single Size), 1/2 cup   160
    (Noodle Roni Parmesano), 1 serving   240
pesto *(Noodle Roni)*, 1 serving   220
Romanoff *(Noodle Roni)*, 1 serving   240
sour cream and chives:
    (Lipton Noodles & Sauce), 1/4 pkg. dry   150
    (Lipton Noodles & Sauce), 1/2 cup***   200
    (Mueller's Chef's Series), 1/2 cup   190
Stroganoff:
    (Lipton Noodles & Sauce), 1/4 pkg. dry   130
    (Lipton Noodles & Sauce), 1/2 cup**   200
    (Mueller's Chef's Series), 1/2 cup   190
    (Noodle Roni), 1 serving   350

    * *Prepared according to package directions, except as noted*
   ** *Prepared with whole milk and butter*
  *** *Prepared with 2 tbsp. butter*

PASTA DISHES, CANNED, 7.5 ounces, except as noted
See also "Entrees, Canned & Packaged," "Macaroni Dishes, Canned," and "Noodle Dishes, Canned"

	calories
garden medley *(Lipton Hearty Ones)*, 11 oz.	323
Italiano *(Lipton Hearty Ones)*, 11 oz.	328
rings, in sauce *(Buitoni)*	150
rings or twists, and meatballs, in sauce *(Buitoni)*	210
twists, in sauce *(Buitoni)*	150

PASTA DISHES, FROZEN
See also "Dinners, Frozen" and "Entrees, Frozen"

	calories
Alfredo, w/broccoli *(The Budget Gourmet* Side Dish), 5.5 oz.	200
creamy cheddar *(Green Giant Pasta Accents)*, ½ cup	100
Dijon *(Green Giant* Garden Gourmet), 1 pkg.	260
garden herb *(Green Giant Pasta Accents)*, ½ cup	80
garlic seasoning *(Green Giant Pasta Accents)*, ½ cup	110
Florentine *(Green Giant* Garden Gourmet), 1 pkg.	230
marinara *(Green Giant* One Serving), 5.5 oz.	180
Parmesan, w/sweet peas *(Green Giant* One Serving), 5.5 oz.	170
primavera *(Green Giant Pasta Accents)*, ½ cup	110
and vegetables, in creamy Stroganoff sauce *(Birds Eye Custom Cuisine)*, 4.6 oz.	120
and vegetables, w/white cheese sauce *(Birds Eye Custom Cuisine)*, 4.6 oz.	150
ziti, in marinara sauce *(The Budget Gourmet* Side Dish), 6.25 oz.	220

> **PASTA DISHES, MIXES***, 1/2 cup, except as noted
> *See also "Entrees, Mixes," "Macaroni Dishes,*
> *Mixes," and "Noodle Dishes, Mixes"*

	calories
Alfredo *(McCormick/Schilling Pasta Prima)*, 1 pkg. dry	169
Alfredo *(McCormick/Schilling Pasta Prima)*	253
bacon vinaigrette *(Country Recipe Pasta Salad)*	140
broccoli:	
cheddar, w/fusilli *(Lipton Pasta & Sauce)*, 1/4 pkg. dry	140
cheddar, w/fusilli *(Lipton Pasta & Sauce)***	200
creamy *(Lipton Pasta Salad)*, 1/4 pkg. dry	120
creamy *(Lipton Pasta Salad)*	200
buttermilk, country *(Mueller's Salad Bar)*	250
carbonara Alfredo *(Lipton Pasta & Sauce)*	140
cheese:	
cheddar *(Minute Microwave Single/Family Size)*	160
cheddar, tangy *(Hain Pasta & Sauce)*, 1/4 pkg.	180
supreme *(Lipton Pasta & Sauce)*	139
Parmesan, creamy *(Hain Pasta & Sauce)*, 1/4 pkg.	150
chicken broccoli *(Lipton Pasta & Sauce)*	129
cucumber, creamy *(Mueller's Salad Bar)*	250
Dijon, creamy *(Country Recipe Pasta Salad)*	190
garlic, creamy:	
(Lipton Pasta & Sauce), 1/4 pkg. dry	140
(Lipton Pasta & Sauce)**	210
herb:	
garlic *(McCormick/Schilling Pasta Prima)*, 1 pkg. dry	65
garlic *(McCormick/Schilling Pasta Prima)*, 1/2 cup	326
Italian *(Fantastic Pasta Salad)*	167
Italian *(Hain Pasta & Sauce)*, 1/5 pkg.	110
herb tomato:	
(Lipton Pasta & Sauce), 1/4 pkg. dry	130
(Lipton Pasta & Sauce)***	180
homestyle *(Mueller's Salad Bar)*	250
Italian:	
creamy *(Country Recipe Pasta Salad)*	160
creamy *(Mueller's Salad Bar)*	290

robust *(Lipton* Pasta Salad), 1/4 pkg. dry   130
robust *(Lipton* Pasta Salad)****   190
zesty *(Mueller's* Salad Bar)   140
marinara *(McCormick/Schilling Pasta Prima)*, 1 pkg.
   dry   74
mushroom, creamy:
   (Lipton Pasta & Sauce), 1/4 pkg. dry   140
   (Lipton Pasta & Sauce)**   210
mushroom and chicken flavors *(Lipton* Pasta & Sauce)   124
Oriental, w/fusilli *(Lipton* Pasta & Sauce)   130
Oriental, spicy *(Fantastic* Pasta Salad)   175
pasta salad *(McCormick/Schilling Pasta Prima)*, 1 pkg.
   dry   78
pasta salad *(McCormick/Schilling Pasta Prima)*, 1/2 cup   390
pesto *(McCormick/Schilling Pasta Prima)*, 1 pkg. dry .   37
pesto *(McCormick/Schilling Pasta Prima)*   193
primavera *(Hain* Pasta & Sauce), 1/4 pkg.   140
ranch *(Country Recipe* Pasta Salad)   140
Swiss, creamy *(Hain* Pasta & Sauce), 1/5 pkg.   170

   * Prepared according to package directions, except as noted
   ** Prepared with whole milk and butter
  *** Prepared with butter
**** Prepared with 2 tablespoons oil

SIDE DISHES, MIXES*, 1/2 cup, except as noted
*See also "Macaroni Dishes, Mixes," "Noodle Dishes,
Mixes," "Pasta Dishes, Mixes," and "Vegetables,
Dried & Mixes"*

                                          calories
bean:
   Cajun, and sauce *(Lipton)*, 1/4 pkg. dry   130
   Cajun, and sauce *(Lipton)*   160
   chicken, and sauce *(Lipton)*, 1/4 pkg. dry   120
   chicken, and sauce *(Lipton)*   150
chicken, meatless style *(Hain* 3-Grain Side Dish)   100
couscous:
   (Near East), 1 1/4 oz. dry   120
   (Fantastic Foods)   122

Side Dishes, Mixes*, couscous, continued

whole wheat *(Fantastic Foods)* 111
couscous pilaf:
    (Casbah), 1 oz. dry or ¹/₂ cup cooked 100
    savory *(Quick Pilaf)* 124
herb *(Hain 3-Grain Side Dish)* 80
hush puppy, all varieties *(Golden Dipt)*, 1¹/₄ oz. 120
lentil pilaf *(Casbah)*, 1 oz. dry or ¹/₂ cup cooked 100
polenta *(Fantastic Polenta)* 106
tabbouleh:
    (Fantastic Foods) 161
    (Near East) 170
    salad *(Casbah)*, 1 oz. dry 126
three grain pilaf, w/herbs *(Quick Pilaf)* 142
wheat pilaf *(Casbah)*, 1 oz. dry or ¹/₂ cup cooked 100

* *Prepared according to package directions, except as noted*

RICE, PLAIN,* ¹/₂ cup cooked, except as noted
See also "Rice Dishes, Mixes"

	calories
basmati:	
(Fantastic Foods)	103
brown *(Fantastic Foods)*	102
brown, long *(Arrowhead Mills)*, 2 oz. dry	200
white, long grain *(Texmati)*	82
brown:	
long grain *(Carolina)*	110
long grain *(Mahatma)*	110
long grain *(River)*	110
long grain *(S&W)*, 3.5 oz.	119
long grain *(Uncle Ben's* Whole Grain), ²/₃ cup	130
long grain, quick *(S&W)*, 3.5 oz.	110
long, medium, or short grain *(Arrowhead Mills)*,	
2 oz. dry	200
precooked *(Uncle Ben's)*, ¹/₂ cup	90
white, long grain:	
(Carolina/Mahatma/River)	100
(Uncle Ben's Natural Whole Grain), ²/₃ cup	130

(Water Maid) 100
basmati, *see "basmati," page 186*
parboiled *(Uncle Ben's Converted)*, 2/3 cup 120
precooked *(Carolina/Mahatma* Instant Enriched) .. 110
precooked *(Minute Rice/Minute Rice* Premium) ... 120
precooked *(Minute Rice* Boil in Bag) 90
precooked *(S&W)*, 3.5 oz. 106
precooked *(Success* Boil-In-Bag Enriched) 100
precooked *(Uncle Ben's* Boil-In-Bag) 90
precooked *(Uncle Ben's Rice In An Instant)*, 2/3 cup 120
wild, cooked *(Fantastic Foods)* 83

* *Prepared according to package directions, without added ingredients, except as noted*

RICE DISHES, CANNED

	calories
fried *(La Choy)*, 3/4 cup	180
Spanish:	
(Featherweight), 7.5 oz.	140
(Heinz), 7.25 oz.	150
(Old El Paso), 1/2 cup	70
(Van Camp's), 1 cup	150

RICE DISHES, FROZEN
See also "Vegetable Dishes, Frozen"

	calories
and broccoli:	
au gratin *(Birds Eye For One)*, 5.75 oz.	180
in cheese sauce *(Green Giant* One Serving), 5.5 oz. .	180
in flavored cheese sauce *(Green Giant Rice Originals)*, 1/2 cup	120
country style *(Birds Eye* International Recipes), 3.3 oz.	90
French style *(Birds Eye* International Recipes), 3.3 oz.	110
fried, w/chicken *(Chun King)*, 8 oz.	260
fried, w/pork *(Chun King)*, 8 oz.	270

Rice Dishes, Frozen, continued

Italian blend white rice and spinach, in cheese sauce *(Green Giant Rice Originals)*, 1/2 cup	140
medley *(Green Giant Rice Originals)*, 1/2 cup	100
Oriental, and vegetables *(The Budget Gourmet* Side Dish), 5.75 oz.	210
peas and mushrooms, w/sauce *(Green Giant* One Serving), 5.5 oz.	130
pilaf *(Green Giant Rice Originals)*, 1/2 cup	110
pilaf, w/green beans *(The Budget Gourmet* Side Dish), 5.5 oz.	240
Spanish style *(Birds Eye* International Recipes), 3.3 oz.	110
white and wild rice *(Green Giant Rice Originals)*, 1/2 cup	130
wild, sherry *(Green Giant* Microwave Garden Gourmet), 1 pkg.	210

RICE DISHES, MIXES*, 1/2 cup, except as noted
See also "Rice, Plain"

---

	calories
Alfredo *(Country Inn)***	140
almondine *(Hain* 3-Grain Side Dish)	130
asparagus:	
au gratin *(Country Inn)***	130
w/hollandaise sauce *(Lipton* Rice & Sauce), 1/4 pkg. dry	120
w/hollandaise sauce *(Lipton* Rice & Sauce)***	170
au gratin, herbed *(Country Inn)***	140
au gratin herb *(Success)*	100
beef flavor:	
(Golden Grain/Rice-A-Roni), 1.33 oz. dry	135
(Golden Grain/Rice-A-Roni)	170
(Lipton Rice & Sauce), 1/4 pkg. dry	120
(Lipton Rice & Sauce)	150
(Mahatma)	100
(Minute Microwave Family Size)	160
(Minute Microwave Single Size)	150
(Success)	100
and vermicelli *(Make-it-easy)*, 1.3 oz. dry	130

broccoli:
   almondine *(Country Inn)*** 130
   au gratin *(Country Inn)*** 130
   au gratin *(Golden Grain/Rice-A-Roni Savory*
      Classics), 1.12 oz. dry 129
   au gratin *(Golden Grain/Rice-A-Roni Savory Classics)* 180
   stir-fry *(Suzi Wan* Dinner Recipe), 7.5 oz. 370
brown and wild:
   (Success) 120
   (Uncle Ben's) 130
   *(Uncle Ben's)**** 150
   mushroom recipe *(Uncle Ben's)* 130
   Spanish style or vegetable herb *(Arrowhead Mills*
      Quick Brown Rice), 2 oz. dry 150
   wild rice and herb *(Arrowhead Mills* Quick Brown
      Rice), 2 oz. dry 140
Cajun *(Lipton* Rice & Sauce), 1/4 pkg. dry 120
Cajun *(Lipton* Rice & Sauce) 150
cauliflower au gratin:
   *(Country Inn)*** 130
   (Golden Grain/Rice-A-Roni Savory Classics), 1/2 oz.
      dry 141
   (Golden Grain/Rice-A-Roni Savory Classics) 170
cheddar:
   and broccoli *(Minute* Microwave Single/Family Size) 160
   zesty *(Golden Grain/Rice-A-Roni Savory Classics),*
      1.3 oz. dry 151
   zesty *(Golden Grain/Rice-A-Roni Savory Classics)* .. 180
chicken and chicken flavor:
   (Golden Grain/Rice-A-Roni), 1.33 oz. dry 136
   (Golden Grain/Rice-A-Roni) 170
   (Lipton Rice & Sauce), 1/4 pkg. dry 130
   (Lipton Rice & Sauce) 150
   (Mahatma) 100
   (Minute Microwave Family Size) 160
   (Minute Microwave Single Size) 150
   (Success) 110
   and broccoli *(Suzi Wan)*** 120
   creamy, and mushroom *(Country Inn)*** 140
   drumstick *(Minute)* 150
   homestyle, and vegetables *(Country Inn)*** 140

Rice Dishes, Mixes*, chicken and chicken flavor, continued

honey lemon *(Suzi Wan* Dinner Recipe), 7.5 oz. . . .	370
and mushroom *(Golden Grain/Rice-A-Roni),* 1.25 oz. dry	129
and mushroom *(Golden Grain/Rice-A-Roni)*	180
royale *(Country Inn)***	120
stock *(Country Inn)***	130
and vegetables *(Golden Grain/Rice-A-Roni),* 1.2 oz. dry	124
and vegetables *(Golden Grain/Rice-A-Roni)*	150
and vegetables *(Suzi Wan)***	120
and vermicelli *(Make-it-easy),* 1.3 oz. dry	130
Florentine:	
(Country Inn)**	140
chicken *(Golden Grain/Rice-A-Roni Savory Classics),* 1.12 oz. dry.	108
chicken *(Golden Grain/Rice-A-Roni Savory Classics)*	130
fried:	
(Minute)	160
w/almonds *(Golden Grain/Rice-A-Roni),* 1.04 oz. dry	106
w/almonds *(Golden Grain/Rice-A-Roni)*	140
green bean almondine:	
(Golden Grain/Rice-A-Roni Savory Classics), 1.25 oz. dry	152
(Golden Grain/Rice-A-Roni Savory Classics)	210
casserole *(Country Inn)***	120
herb au gratin, *see "au gratin," page 188*	
herb and butter:	
(Golden Grain/Rice-A-Roni), 1.04 oz. dry	105
(Golden Grain/Rice-A-Roni)	140
(Lipton Rice & Sauce)	150
long grain and wild:	
(Lipton Rice & Sauce Original), ¼ pkg. dry	120
(Lipton Rice & Sauce Original)	150
(Mahatma)	100
(Minute)	150
(Near East)	130
(Uncle Ben's Original/Fast Cooking)	100
(Uncle Ben's Original)***	120
(Uncle Ben's Fast Cooking)***	130
chicken stock sauce *(Uncle Ben's)*	140

chicken stock sauce *(Uncle Ben's)**** 160
mushrooms and herbs *(Lipton* Rice & Sauce),
   1/4 pkg. dry 120
mushrooms and herbs *(Lipton* Rice & Sauce) 150
Mexican *(Old El Paso)* 140
mushroom:
  (Lipton Rice & Sauce), 1/4 pkg. dry 120
  (Lipton Rice & Sauce) 150
  creamy, and wild rice *(Country Inn)*** 140
Oriental *(Hain* 3-Grain Goodness) 120
Parmesan, creamy, and herbs *(Golden Grain/Rice-A-
Roni Savory Classics)*, 1.22 oz. dry 145
Parmesan, creamy, and herbs *(Golden Grain/Rice-A-
Roni Savory Classics)* 170
pilaf:
  (Casbah), 1 oz. dry or 1/2 cup cooked 90
  (Golden Grain/Rice-A-Roni), 1.45 oz. dry 147
  (Golden Grain/Rice-A-Roni) 190
  (Lipton Rice & Sauce), 1/4 pkg. dry 120
  (Lipton Rice & Sauce)*** 170
  (Near East) 140
  (Success) 120
  beef flavored *(Near East)* 140
  brown, w/miso *(Quick Pilaf)* 145
  chicken flavored *(Near East)* 140
  French style *(Minute* Microwave Family Size) 130
  French style *(Minute* Microwave Single Size) 120
  garden *(Golden Grain/Rice-A-Roni Savory Classics)*,
   1.12 oz. dry 113
  garden *(Golden Grain/Rice-A-Roni Savory Classics)* . 140
  lentil *(Near East)* 170
  nutted *(Casbah)*, 1 oz. dry or 1/2 cup cooked 160
  Spanish, brown *(Quick Pilaf)* 136
  vegetable *(Country Inn)*** 120
  wheat *(Near East)* 150
rib roast *(Minute)* 150
risotto:
  (Golden Grain/Rice-A-Roni), 1.5 oz. dry 157
  (Golden Grain/Rice-A-Roni) 200
  chicken and cheese *(Country Inn)*** 120

Rice Dishes, Mixes*, continued

Spanish:

(Golden Grain/Rice-A-Roni), 1.07 oz. dry	107
(Golden Grain/Rice-A-Roni)	150
(Lipton Rice & Sauce), ¼ pkg. dry	120
(Lipton Rice & Sauce)	140
(Mahatma)	100
(Near East)	170
pilaf *(Casbah)*, 1 oz. dry or ½ cup cooked	90

Stroganoff *(Golden Grain/Rice-A-Roni)*, 1.35 oz. dry . .	150
Stroganoff *(Golden Grain/Rice-A-Roni)*	190
sweet and sour *(Suzi Wan)***	130
sweet and sour *(Suzi Wan* Dinner Recipe), 7.5 oz. . . .	340
teriyaki *(Suzi Wan)***	120
teriyaki *(Suzi Wan* Dinner Recipe), 7.5 oz.	360
three-flavor *(Suzi Wan)***	120
vegetable medley *(Country Inn)***	140

w/vegetables, broccoli, and cheddar:

(Lipton Rice & Sauce), ¼ pkg. dry	130
(Lipton Rice & Sauce)***	180

vegetables, spring, and cheese *(Golden Grain/Rice-A-Roni Savory Classics)*, 1.22 oz. dry	141
vegetables, spring, and cheese *(Golden Grain/Rice-A-Roni Savory Classics)*	170

wild, *see "long grain and wild," page 190*

yellow:

(Golden Grain/Rice-A-Roni), 2 oz. dry	196
(Golden Grain/Rice-A-Roni)	250
(Mahatma/Success)	100

  * *Prepared according to package directions, except as noted*
 ** *Prepared without butter*
*** *Prepared with butter*

Chapter 14

PIZZA AND SANDWICHES

PIZZA, FROZEN
See also "Pizza, French Bread"

---

	calories
Canadian bacon:	
(*Jeno's* Crisp'n Tasty), 1/2 pie	250
(*Tombstone*), 1/4 pie	340
(*Totino's Party* Pizza), 1/2 pie	290
(*Celeste* Suprema), 1/4 pie	381
(*Celeste* Suprema Pizza For One), 1 pie	678
cheese:	
(*Celentano* 9-Slice Pizza), 2.7 oz.	150
(*Celentano* Thick Crust), 4.3 oz.	290
(*Celeste*), 1/4 pie	317
(*Celeste* Pizza For One), 1 pie	497
(*Jeno's* Crisp'n Tasty), 1/2 pie	270
(*Jeno's* 4-Pack), 1 pie	160
(*Pillsbury* Microwave), 1/2 pie	240
(*Stouffer's*), 1/2 of 81/2-oz. pkg.	320
(*Stouffer's* Extra Cheese), 1/2 of 91/4-oz. pkg.	370
(*Tombstone*), 1/4 pie	330
(*Totino's Party* Pizza), 1/2 pizza	280
(*Totino's Party* Pizza, Family Size), 1/3 pie	310
(*Totino's* Small Microwave), 3.9-oz. pie	250
(*Weight Watchers*), 5.86-oz. pkg.	300
snack tray (*Jeno's* Snacks), 4 pies or 1/3 pkg.	130
three cheese (*Tombstone* Double Top), 1/4 pie	490

Pizza, Frozen, cheese, continued

three cheese *(Tombstone* Microwave), 7.7-oz. pkg. . . .   520
two cheese *(Tombstone* Thin Crust), 1/4 pie   330

cheese combination:

and hamburger *(Tombstone),* 1/4 pie   360
and hamburger *(Tombstone* Italian Thin Crust),
   1/4 pie   320
and pepperoni *(Tombstone),* 1/4 pie   380
and pepperoni *(Tombstone* Microwave), 7.5-oz. pkg.   530
and pepperoni *(Tombstone* Thin Crust), 1/4 pie   330
and sausage *(Tombstone),* 1/4 pie   350
and sausage, Italian *(Tombstone* Thin Crust), 1/4 pie   330
sausage and mushroom *(Tombstone),* 1/4 pie   360

combination:

(Jeno's 4-Pack), 1 pie   180
(Pillsbury Microwave), 1/2 pie   310
(Totino's Party Pizza), 1/2 pie   340
(Totino's Party Pizza, Family Size), 1/3 pie   380
(Totino's Small Microwave), 4.2-oz. pie   290
(Weight Watchers Deluxe), 7.15-oz. pkg.   330

deluxe:

(Celeste), 1/4 pie   378
(Celeste Pizza For One), 1 pie   582
(Stouffer's), 1/2 of 10-oz. pkg.   370

hamburger:

(Jeno's Crisp'n Tasty), 1/2 pie   290
(Jeno's 4-Pack), 1 pie   180
(Totino's Party Pizza), 1/2 pie   320

pepperoni:

(Celeste), 1/4 pie   368
(Celeste Pizza For One), 1 pie   546
(Jeno's Crisp'n Tasty), 1/2 pie   280
(Jeno's 4-Pack), 1 pie   170
(Pillsbury Microwave), 1/2 pie   300
(Stouffer's), 1/2 of 8 3/4-oz. pkg.   350
(Tombstone Real Deluxe), 1/4 pie   380
(Totino's Party Pizza), 1/2 pie   330
(Totino's Party Pizza, Family Size), 1/3 pie   360
(Totino's Small Microwave), 4 oz.   270
(Weight Watchers), 6.1-oz. pkg.   320
double cheese *(Tombstone* Double Top), 1/4 pie   560

double cheese *(Tombstone Double Top Deluxe)*,
    1/4 pie   550
snack tray *(Jeno's Snacks)*, 4 pies or 1/3 pkg.   140
pocket sandwich, *see "Sandwiches, Frozen, pizza*
    pocket," page 197
sausage:
    (Celeste), 1/4 pie   376
    (Celeste Pizza For One), 1 pie   571
    (Jeno's Crisp'n Tasty), 1/2 pie   300
    (Jeno's 4-Pack), 1 pie   180
    (Pillsbury Microwave), 1/2 pie   280
    (Stouffers), 1/2 of 9³/₈-oz. pkg.   360
    (Tombstone Deluxe), 1/4 pie   350
    (Tombstone Deluxe Microwave), 8.7-oz. pkg.   520
    (Totino's Party Pizza), 1/2 pie   340
    (Totino's Party Pizza, Family Size), 1/3 pie   370
    (Totino's Small Microwave), 4.2 oz.   280
    (Weight Watchers), 6.26-oz. pkg.   320
    Italian *(Tombstone Microwave)*, 8-oz. pkg.   550
    smoked, w/pepperoni seasoning *(Tombstone)*, 1/4 pie   350
    snack tray *(Jeno's Snacks)*, 4 pies or 1/3 pkg.   140
sausage combination:
    (Tombstone), 1/4 pie   370
    and mushroom *(Celeste Pizza For One)*, 1 pie   592
    and pepperoni *(Jeno's Crisp'n Tasty)*, 1/2 pie   300
    and pepperoni *(Stouffer's)*, 1/2 of 9³/₈-oz. pkg. . . .   380
    and pepperoni *(Tombstone Double Top)*, 1/4 pie   540
    and pepperoni *(Tombstone Microwave)*, 8-oz. pkg. . .   560
(Tombstone Thin Crust Supreme), 1/4 pie   340
vegetable:
    (Celeste), 1/4 pie   310
    (Celeste Pizza For One), 1 pie   490

PIZZA, FRENCH BREAD, FROZEN

	calories
Canadian style bacon *(Stouffer's)*, 1/2 pkg.	360
cheese:	
(Banquet Zap), 4.5 oz.	310
(Lean Cuisine), 5¹/₈-oz. pkg.	310

Pizza, French Bread, Frozen, cheese, continued

    (Lean Cuisine Extra Cheese), 5.5-oz. pkg.   350
    (Pillsbury Microwave), 1 piece   370
    (Stouffer's), 1/2 pkg.   340
    (Stouffer's Double Cheese), 1/2 pkg.   410
deluxe:
    (Banquet Zap), 4.8 oz.   330
    (Lean Cuisine), 61/8-oz. pkg.   350
    (Stouffer's), 1/2 pkg.   430
    (Weight Watchers), 6.12-oz. pkg.   330
hamburger *(Stouffer's)*, 1/2 pkg.   410
pepperoni:
    (Banquet Zap), 4.5 oz.   350
    (Lean Cuisine), 5.25-oz. pkg.   340
    (Pillsbury Microwave), 1 piece   430
    (Stouffer's), 1/2 pkg.   410
    (Weight Watchers), 5.25-oz. pkg.   320
pepperoni and mushroom *(Stouffer's)*, 1/2 pkg.   430
sausage:
    (Lean Cuisine), 6-oz. pkg.   350
    (Pillsbury Microwave), 1 piece   410
    (Stouffer's), 1/2 pkg.   420
sausage combination:
    and mushroom *(Stouffer's)*, 1/2 pkg.   410
    and pepperoni *(Pillsbury* Microwave), 1 piece   450
    and pepperoni *(Stouffer's)*, 1/2 pkg.   450
vegetable deluxe *(Stouffer's)*, 1/2 pkg.   420

SANDWICHES, FROZEN
See also "Breakfast Sandwiches, Frozen"

	calories
beef pocket, and broccoli *(Lean Pockets)*, 1 pkg.	250
beef pocket, 'n cheddar *(Hot Pockets)*, 5 oz.	370
cheeseburger *(MicroMagic)*, 4.75 oz.	450
chicken:	
(MicroMagic), 4.5 oz.	390
barbecue *(Tyson* Microwave), 4 oz.	230
breast *(Tyson* Microwave), 3.5 oz.	275
mini *(Tyson* Microwave), 3.5 oz.	230

chicken pocket:
   (Lean Pockets Supreme), 1 pkg.   280
   'n cheddar *(Hot Pockets)*, 5 oz.   310
   Oriental *(Lean Pockets)*, 1 pkg.   250
   Parmesan *(Lean Pockets)*, 1 pkg.   270
ham and cheese pocket *(Hot Pockets)*, 5 oz.   360
hamburger *(MicroMagic)*, 4 oz.   350
pizza pocket:
   (Lean Pockets Pizza Deluxe), 1 pkg.   280
   pepperoni *(Hot Pockets)*, 5 oz.   380
   sausage *(Hot Pockets)*, 5 oz.   360
turkey pocket, w/ham and cheese *(Hot Pockets)*, 5 oz.   320

Chapter 15

FATS, OILS,
AND SALAD DRESSINGS

FATS AND OILS

	calories
butter, 1 tsp., except as noted:	
(Land O'Lakes)	35
(Darigold Lightly Salted)	25
(Hotel Bar/Kellers)	35
whipped *(Breakstone's),* 1 tbsp.	70
whipped *(Land O'Lakes)*	25
fat, imitation *(Rokeach Neutral Nyafat)*	99
margarine, 1 tbsp., except as noted:	
(Country Morning Stick), 1 tsp.	35
(Country Morning Tub), 1 tsp.	30
(Country Morning Light Stick or tub), 1 tsp.	20
(Diet *Mazola)*	50
(Hain Safflower)	100
(Land O'Lakes Stick or Tub), 1 tsp.	35
(Mazola)	100
(Nucoa)	100
(Nucoa Heart Beat)	25
(Nucoa Heart Beat Unsalted)	24
(Parkay)	100
(Weight Watchers)	60
(Weight Watchers Corn Oil)	50
(Weight Watchers Unsalted)	50
soft *(Chiffon* Cup)	90
soft *(Chiffon* Stick)	100
soft (Diet *Parkay)*	50
soft *(Nucoa)*	90

soft *(Parkay)* 100
soft, safflower *(Hain)* 100
spread *(Kraft* "Touch of Butter" Bowl) 50
spread *(Kraft* "Touch of Butter" Stick) 60
spread *(Land O'Lakes* Tub), 1 tsp. 25
spread *(Mazola* Corn Oil Light) 50
spread *(Parkay* Corn Oil Light) 70
spread *(Parkay* 50% Vegetable Oil) 60
spread *(Weight Watchers* Light) 50
spread, w/sweet cream *(Land O'Lakes* Stick), 1 tsp. 30
spread, w/sweet cream *(Land O'Lakes* Tub), 1 tsp. . 25
squeeze *(Parkay)* 100
whipped *(Chiffon)* 70
whipped *(Miracle* Brand Cup) 60
whipped *(Miracle* Brand Stick) 70
whipped *(Parkay* Cup or Stick) 60
oils, 1 tbsp., except as noted:
all varieties *(Crisco)* 120
all varieties *(Hain)* 120
all varieties *(Wesson)* 120
canola *(Nucoa Heart Beat)* 120
corn *(Mazola)* 120
corn spray *(Mazola* No Stick), 2.5-second spray ... 6
olive *(Amore* Pure or Extra Virgin) 120
olive *(Bertolli)* 120
peanut *(Planters)* 120
vegetable spray, regular or butter flavor *(Weight
   Watchers* Cooking Spray), 1-second spray 2
shortening, vegetable, plain or butter flavor *(Crisco)*,
   1 tbsp. 110

SALAD DRESSINGS, READY-TO-SERVE,
one tablespoon, except as noted
See also "Salad Dressings, Mixes"

calories
all varieties, except cucumber, French, or Italian *(Kraft*
   Reduced Calorie) 30
bacon and buttermilk *(Kraft)* 80

Salad Dressings, Ready-to-Serve, continued
bacon and tomato:
    (Estee) 8
    (Kraft) 70
blue cheese:
    (Estee) 8
    (Featherweight Neu Bleu) 4
    (Roka Brand) 60
    (Roka Brand Reduced Calorie) 16
    (S&W Nutradiet) 25
    chunky *(Kraft)* 60
    chunky *(Wish-Bone)* 75
    chunky *(Wish-Bone* Lite) 40
buttermilk:
    (Hain Old Fashioned) 70
    creamy *(Kraft)* 80
Caesar:
    (Lawry's Classic), 1 oz. 130
    (Weight Watchers) 4
    (Wish-Bone) 77
    creamy *(Hain* Regular/Low Salt) 60
    golden *(Kraft)* 70
Chinese vinegar, w/sesame and ginger *(Lawry's*
    Classic), 1 oz. 145
coleslaw *(Kraft)* 70
cucumber:
    creamy *(Featherweight)* 4
    creamy *(Kraft)* 70
    creamy *(Kraft* Reduced Calorie) 25
    dill *(Hain)* 80
Dijon:
    creamy *(Estee)* 8
    creamy *(Featherweight)* 20
    mustard *(Great Impressions)* 57
    vinaigrette *(Hain)* 50
    vinaigrette *(Wish-Bone* Classic) 60
    vinaigrette *(Wish-Bone* Lite Classic) 30
dill, creamy *(Nasoya Vegi-Dressing)* 40
French:
    (Catalina) 70
    (Catalina Reduced Calorie) 16

(Estee)	4
(Featherweight)	14
(Kraft)	60
(Kraft Miracle)	70
(Kraft Reduced Calorie)	25
(S&W Nutradiet)	18
(Wish-Bone Deluxe)	60
(Wish-Bone Lite)	31
(Wish-Bone Lite Sweet'N Spicy)	18
(Wish-Bone Sweet'N Spicy)	63
creamy *(Hain)*	60
garlic *(Wish-Bone)*	55
red *(Wish-Bone* Lite)	17
style *(Weight Watchers)*	10
style *(Wish-Bone* Lite)	30
w/green pepper *(Great Impressions)*	64
garlic:	
creamy *(Estee)*	2
creamy *(Kraft)*	50
creamy *(Wish-Bone)*	74
French *(Wish-Bone)*	55
herb *(Nasoya Vegi-Dressing)*	40
and sour cream *(Hain)*	70
herb:	
(Featherweight)	6
garden *(Featherweight)*	25
savory *(Hain* No Salt Added)	90
homestyle *(Dorothy Lynch)*	55
homestyle *(Dorothy Lynch* Reduced Calorie)	30
honey and sesame *(Hain)*	60
Italian:	
(Featherweight)	4
(Hain Traditional)	80
(Hain Traditional No Salt Added)	60
(Kraft Presto)	70
(Nasoya Vegi-Dressing)	40
(Ott's)	80
(Wish-Bone)	46
(Wish-Bone Lite)	7
(Wish-Bone Robusto)	47
blended *(Wish-Bone)*	37

Salad Dressings, Ready-to-Serve, Italian, continued

w/bleu cheese *(Lawry's* Classic), 1 oz.	186
cheese *(Featherweight)*	20
cheese vinaigrette *(Hain)*	55
w/cheese *(Wish-Bone)*	89
creamy *(Hain* Regular/No Salt Added)	80
creamy *(Kraft* Reduced Calorie)	25
creamy *(S&W/Nutradiet)*	10
creamy *(Wish-Bone)*	56
creamy *(Wish-Bone* Lite)	26
creamy or regular *(Estee)*	4
creamy, w/real sour cream *(Kraft)*	50
herbal *(Wish-Bone* Classics)	70
no oil *(Kraft)*	4
no oil *(S&W/Nutradiet)*	2
w/Parmesan cheese *(Lawry's* Classic), 1 oz.	156
style *(Weight Watchers)*	6
zesty *(Kraft)*	70
zesty *(Kraft* Reduced Calorie)	20
mayonnaise:	
(Bama)	100
(Bennett's Real)	110
(Estee)	45
(Featherweight)	30
(Hain Light Low Sodium)	60
(Hain Real No Salt Added/*Hain* Safflower)	110
(Hellmann's/Best Foods)	100
(Hellmann's/Best Foods Light)	50
(Kraft)	100
(Kraft Light)	50
(Rokeach)	100
(Weight Watchers Regular/Low Sodium)	50
soybean *(Featherweight Soyamaise)*	100
mayonnaise, imitation:	
(Nucoa Heart Beat)	40
(Hellmann's Cholesterol Free)	50
(Weight Watchers Cholesterol Free)	50
(Hain Eggless No Salt Added)	110
tofu *(Nasoya Nayonaise)*	40
mayonnaise type *(see also specific brands):*	
(Bama)	50

(Miracle Whip)	70
(Miracle Whip Light)	45
(Spin Blend)	60
cholesterol free *(Spin Blend)*	40
whipped *(Weight Watchers)*	45
oil and vinegar *(Kraft)*	70
olive oil:	
Italian *(Wish-Bone* Classic)	34
vinaigrette *(Wish-Bone)*	28
vinaigrette *(Wish-Bone* Lite)	16
onion and chive *(Wish-Bone* Lite)	37
onion and chives, creamy *(Kraft)*	70
Oriental spice *(Featherweight)*	20
(Ott's Famous)	40
(Ott's Reduced Calorie *Famous)*	26
poppyseed *(Great Impressions)*, 2 tbsp.	131
poppyseed *(Hain* Rancher's)	60
ranch:	
(Wish-Bone)	78
(Wish-Bone Lite)	42
creamy *(Rancher's Choice)*	90
creamy *(Rancher's Choice* Reduced Calorie)	30
creamy *(Weight Watchers)*	25
red wine:	
vinaigrette *(Wish-Bone)*	51
vinegar *(Estee)*	2
vinegar *(Featherweight)*	6
vinegar, w/Cabernet *(Lawry's* Classics), 1 oz.	138
Russian:	
(Featherweight)	6
(Kraft)	60
(S&W/Nutradiet)	25
(Weight Watchers)	50
(Wish-Bone)	46
(Wish-Bone Lite)	22
creamy *(Kraft)*	60
San Francisco, w/Romano *(Lawry's* Classic), 1 oz.	136
sesame garlic *(Nasoya Vegi-Dressing)*	40
sour *(Friendship Sour Treat)*, 1 oz.	36
sour cream, nondairy *(Crowley)*, 1 oz.	40
Swiss cheese vinaigrette *(Hain)*	60

Salad Dressings, Ready-to-Serve, continued

Thousand Island:

(Estee)	8
(Featherweight)	18
(Hain)	50
(Kraft)	60
(S&W/Nutradiet)	25
(Weight Watchers)	50
(Wish-Bone)	63
(Wish-Bone Lite)	36
and bacon *(Kraft)*	60
tomato, zesty *(Featherweight)*	2
tomato vinaigrette *(Weight Watchers)*	8

vinaigrette, *see specific listings*

vinegar and oil:

balsamic vinegar *(Great Impressions)*	67
red wine vinegar *(Great Impressions)*	64
red wine vinegar *(Kraft)*	60
white wine vinegar *(Great Impressions)*	63
vintage, w/sherry wine *(Lawry's* Classic), 1 oz.	110
white wine, w/Chardonnay *(Lawry's* Classic), 1 oz.	153

SALAD DRESSINGS, MIXES*, one tablespoon,
except as noted
See also "Salad Dressings, Ready-to-Serve"

	calories
all varieties, except buttermilk and ranch *(Good Seasons)*	70
bacon *(Lawry's)*, 1 pkg. dry	65
blue cheese *(Hain* No Oil)	14
buttermilk *(Good Seasons* Farm Style)	60
buttermilk *(Hain* No Oil)	12
Caesar *(Hain* No Oil)	4
Caesar *(Lawry's)*, 1 pkg. dry	75
French *(Hain* No Oil)	12
garlic and cheese *(Hain* No Oil)	6
herb *(Hain* No Oil)	2

Italian:

all varieties *(Good Seasons* Lite)	25

   (Good Seasons No Oil)   6
   (Hain No Oil)..........................   4
   (Lawry's), 1 pkg. dry   45
   w/cheese *(Lawry's),* 1 pkg. dry   74
ranch *(Good Seasons)*   60
ranch *(Good Seasons* Lite)   30
Thousand Island *(Hain* No Oil)...............   12

* *Prepared according to package directions, except as noted*

Chapter 16

SAUCES, GRAVIES, CONDIMENTS, AND SEASONINGS

SAUCES
See also "Gravies" and "Condiments & Seasonings"

---

	calories
Alfredo:	
mix *(French's Pasta Toss)*, 2 tsp. dry	25
mix *(Lawry's Pasta Alfredo)*, 1 pkg.	226
refrigerated *(Contadina Fresh)*, 6 oz.	540
barbecue:	
(Enrico's Original), 1 tbsp.	18
(Estee), 1 tbsp.	18
(Heinz Thick & Rich), 1 tbsp.	18
(Hunt Original), 1 tbsp.	20
(Kraft), 2 tbsp.	40
(Kraft Thick'N Spicy Original), 2 tbsp.	50
(Maull's Lite), 1 tbsp.	12
(Ott's), 1 tbsp.	14
Cajun style *(Golden Dipt)*, 1 fl. oz.	90
chunky *(Kraft Thick'N Spicy)*, 2 tbsp.	60
Dijon and honey *(Lawry's)*, 1/4 cup	203
garlic or hickory smoke *(Kraft)*, 2 tbsp.	40
hickory smoke *(Heinz Thick & Rich)*, 1 tbsp.	19
hickory smoke *(Kraft Thick'N Spicy)*, 2 tbsp.	50
hickory smoke, w/onion bits *(Kraft)*, 2 tbsp.	50
honey *(Hain)*, 1 tbsp.	14
w/honey *(Kraft Thick'N Spicy)*, 2 tbsp.	60

hot or hot hickory smoke *(Kraft)*, 2 tbsp.   40
Italian seasonings *(Kraft)*, 2 tbsp.   50
Kansas City style *(Kraft)*, 2 tbsp.   50
Kansas City style *(Kraft* Thick'N Spicy), 2 tbsp. . . .   60
mesquite *(Enrico's)*, 1 tbsp.   18
mesquite smoke *(Kraft)*, 2 tbsp.   40
mild *(French's Cattleman's)*, 1 tbsp.   25
mushroom *(Heinz* Thick & Rich), 1 tbsp.   14
onion bits *(Kraft)*, 2 tbsp.   50
w/orange juice *(Lawry's* California Grill), 1/4 cup . .   34
Oriental *(La Choy)*, 1 tbsp.   16
sloppy Joe w/beef *(Libby's)*, 1/3 cup   110
smoky *(French's Cattleman's)*, 1 tbsp.   25
smoky *(Ott's)*, 1 tbsp.   14
bearnaise *(Great Impressions)*, 2 tbsp.   192
bolognese *(Progresso)*, 1/2 cup   150
bolognese, refrigerated *(Contadina Fresh)*, 7.5 oz.   230
browning sauce *(Gravymaster)*, 1 tsp.   12
cheese *(see also "Welsh rarebit," page 213)*:
    aged *(White House)*, 3.5 oz.   213
    cheddar or nacho *(Lucky Leaf/Musselman's)*, 4 oz. .   220
    four cheese, refrigerated *(Contadina Fresh)*, 6 oz. . . .   470
    jalapeño *(White House)*, 3.5 oz.   193
    nacho *(Kaukauna)*, 1 oz.   80
    nacho, mix *(McCormick/Schilling)*, 1 pkg.   167
    nacho *(White House)*, 3.5 oz.   193
    mix* *(French's)*, 1/4 cup   80
    mix *(McCormick/Schilling)*, 1 pkg.   138
chicken, mix, 1 pkg.:
    cacciatore *(McCormick/Schilling* Sauce Blend)   132
    creole *(McCormick/Schilling* Sauce Blend)   140
    curry *(McCormick/Schilling* Sauce Blend)   152
    Dijon *(McCormick/Schilling* Sauce Blend)   156
    mesquite marinade *(McCormick/Schilling* Sauce
        Blend)   132
    teriyaki *(McCormick/Schilling* Sauce Blend)   172
chili:
    (Featherweight), 1 tbsp.   8
    (Heinz), 1 tbsp.   17
    (S&W Chili Makin's), 1/2 cup   100
    green, mild *(El Molino)*, 2 tbsp.   10

Sauces, chili, continued

hot dog *(Gebhardt)*, 2 tbsp.	20
hot dog *(Wolf* Brand), 1.25 oz. or ⅙ cup	44
tomato *(Del Monte)*, ¼ cup	70

clam:

red, canned *(Buitoni)*, 5 oz.	190
red, canned *(Ferrara)*, 4 oz.	70
red, refrigerated *(Contadina Fresh)*, 7.5 oz.	120
white, canned *(Ferrara)*, 4 oz.	80
white, refrigerated *(Contadina Fresh)*, 6 oz.	290

cocktail *(see also "seafood," page 211):*

(Del Monte), ¼ cup	70
(Estee), 1 tbsp.	10
(Sauceworks), 1 tbsp.	12
(Stokely), 1 tbsp.	18
regular or extra hot *(Golden Dipt)*, 1 tbsp.	20

Creole, Cajun *(Enrico's* Light), 4 oz.	76
diable *(Escoffier)*, 1 tbsp.	20

duck sauce, *see "sweet and sour," page 211*

enchilada:

(La Victoria), 1 cup	80
(Rosarita), 3 oz.	19
green chili *(Old El Paso)*, ¼ cup	18
hot or mild *(Del Monte)*, ½ cup	45
hot *(El Molino)*, 2 tbsp.	16
hot *(Old El Paso)*, ¼ cup	30
hot or mild *(Ortega)*, 1 oz.	12
mild *(Old El Paso)*, ¼ cup	25

fajita *(Tio Sancho* Skillet Sauce), 1 oz.	14
forestiera, refrigerated *(Contadina Fresh)*, 7.5 oz.	270
herb and garlic, w/lemon juice *(Lawry's)*, ¼ cup	36
hollandaise *(Great Impressions)*, 2 tbsp.	192
hollandaise, mix *(McCormick/Schilling)*, 1 pkg.	203

horseradish:

(Great Impressions), 1 tbsp.	74
(Heinz), 1 tbsp.	75
(Sauceworks), 1 tbsp.	50

lemon butter dill *(Golden Dipt* Cooking Sauce), 1 fl. oz.	110
lobster, rock *(Progresso)*, ½ cup	120
mesquite, w/lime juice *(Lawry's)*, ¼ cup	24
mustard, hot *(Sauceworks)*, 1 tbsp.	35

Newberg, w/sherry, canned *(Snow's)*, 1/3 cup   120
orange, Mandarin *(La Choy)*, 1 tbsp.   24
pasta *(see also "tomato," page 212, and specific listings):*
   (Enrico's All Natural Regular/No Salt Added), 4 oz.   60
   (Estee), 4 oz.   60
   (Featherweight), 4 oz.   60
   (Hunt's Traditional), 4 oz.   70
   (Pastorelli Italian Chef), 4 oz.   81
   (Prego), 4 oz.   130
   (Prego No Salt Added), 4 oz.   110
   (Ragú), 4 oz.   80
   (Ragú Chunky Garden Style), 4 oz.   70
   (Ragú Italian), 4 oz.   90
   (Ragú Homestyle), 4 oz.   50
   (Ragú Thick & Hearty), 4 oz.   100
   mix *(Lawry's* Rich & Thick), 1 pkg.   147
   mix *(McCormick/Schilling)*, 1 pkg.   26
   cheese and garlic, mix *(French's Pasta Toss)*, 2 tsp. .   25
   Italian, mix *(French's Pasta Toss)*, 2 tsp.   25
   Italian style, mix* *(French's)*, 5/8 cup   100
   marinara *(Prego)*, 4 oz.   100
   meat flavor *(Hunt's)*, 4 oz.   70
   meat flavor *(Prego)*, 4 oz.   140
   meat flavor *(Weight Watchers)*, 1/3 cup   50
   mushroom flavor *(Enrico's)*, 4 oz.   60
   mushroom flavor *(Featherweight)*, 4 oz.   60
   mushroom flavor *(Hunt's)*, 4 oz.   70
   mushroom flavor *(Prego)*, 4 oz.   130
   mushroom flavor *(Weight Watchers)*, 1/3 cup   40
   w/fresh mushrooms *(Enrico's* Pasta Sauce), 4 oz. . .   60
   w/mushrooms, mix *(French's)*, 5/8 cup*   100
   w/mushrooms, mix *(Lawry's)*, 1 pkg.   143
   mushroom and green pepper *(Enrico's* All Natural),
     4 oz.   60
   mushroom and green pepper or onion *(Prego* Extra
     Chunky), 4 oz.   100
   pesto, *see "pesto," page 210*
   Romanoff, mix *(French's Pasta Toss)*, 2 tsp.   30
   sausage and green pepper *(Prego* Extra Chunky),
     4 oz.   160
   Sicilian *(Progresso)*, 1/2 cup   30

Sauces, pasta, continued

tomato, garden, w/mushrooms *(Prego Al Fresco)*, 4 oz.	100
tomato, garden, w/peppers *(Prego Al Fresco)*, 4 oz.	100
tomato and onion *(Prego Extra Chunky)*, 4 oz.	110
pepper sauce, hot *(Gebhardt Louisiana Style)*, 1/2 tsp.	0
pepper sauce, hot *(Tabasco)*, 1/4 tsp.	<1
pesto, mix *(French's Pasta Toss)*, 2 tsp. dry	20
pesto, refrigerated *(Contadina Fresh)*, 2.33 oz.	350

picante *(see also "salsa," below)*:

(Estee), 2 tbsp.	8
(Gebhardt), 1 tbsp.	4
(Old El Paso), 2 tbsp.	8
(Pace), 2 tsp.	3
(Wise), 2 tbsp.	12
mild *(Azteca)*, 1 tbsp.	4

pizza:

(Contadina Pizza Squeeze), 1/4 cup	30
(Contadina Quick & Easy Original), 1/4 cup	30
(Enrico's Homemade Style All Natural), 4 oz.	60
(Pastorelli Italian-Chef), 4 oz.	90
(Ragú Pizza Quick), 3 tbsp.	35
w/Italian cheese *(Contadina)*, 1/4 cup	30
w/pepperoni *(Contadina)*, 1/4 cup	40
plum, tangy *(La Choy)*, 1 oz.	45
primavera, creamy *(Progresso)*, 1/2 cup	190
rib sauce *(Dip n'Joy Saucey Rib)*, 1 oz.	60
Robert sauce *(Escoffier Sauce Robert)*, 1 tbsp.	20

salsa, canned or in jars:

brava *(La Victoria)*, 1 tbsp.	6
burrito *(Del Monte)*, 1/4 cup	20
casera *(La Victoria)*, 1 tbsp.	4
green chili *(La Victoria)*, 1 tbsp.	3
green chili, hot *(Ortega)*, 1 oz.	10
green chili, mild *(Del Monte)*, 1/4 cup	20
green chili, mild or medium *(Ortega)*, 1 oz.	8
green jalapeño *(La Victoria)*, 1 tbsp.	4
hot *(Hain)*, 1/4 cup	22
mild *(Hain)*, 1/4 cup	20
mild or hot *(Enrico's Chunky Style)*, 2 tbsp.	8

mild, medium or hot *(Old El Paso* Thick'n Chunky),
  2 tbsp.   6
omelette *(La Victoria)*, 1 tbsp.   6
picante *(La Victoria)*, 1 tbsp.   4
picante *(Old El Paso)*, 2 tbsp.   10
picante *(Ortega)*, 1 oz.   10
picante, hot *(Del Monte)*, 1/4 cup   20
picante, hot and chunky *(Del Monte)*, 1/4 cup   15
ranchera *(Ortega)*, 1 oz.   12
ranchera or red jalapeño *(La Victoria)*, 1 tbsp.   6
roja, mild *(Del Monte)*, 1/4 cup   20
suprema *(La Victoria)*, 1 tbsp.   4
taco, hot or mild *(Ortega)*, 1 oz.   10
taco, mild *(Rosarita)*, 2 oz.   27
Texas *(Hot Cha Cha)*, 1 oz.   6
thick 'n chunky *(Old El Paso)*, 2 tbsp.   6
Victoria *(La Victoria)*, 1 tbsp.   4
seafood *(see also "cocktail," page 208)*:
  Creole *(Great Impressions)*, 1 tbsp.   21
  dipping *(Great Impressions)*, 1 tbsp.   17
  dipping, Polynesian *(Great Impressions)*, 1 tbsp.   38
sour cream, mix *(McCormick/Schilling)*, 1 pkg.   176
soy:
  (Kikkoman), 1 tbsp.   10
  (Kikkoman Lite), 1 tbsp.   11
  (La Choy/La Choy Lite), 1 tsp. . . . .   <1
steak:
  (A.1.), 1 tbsp.   12
  (Estee), 1 tbsp.   15
  (French's), 1 tbsp.   25
  (Heinz 57), 1 tbsp.   15
  (Lea & Perrins), 1 oz.   40
  (Steak Supreme), 1 tbsp.   20
stir-fry *(Kikkoman)*, 1 tsp.   6
stir-fry *(Lawry's)*, 1/4 cup   120
Stroganoff, mix *(Lawry's)*, 1 pkg.   123
Stroganoff, mix* *(Natural Touch)*, 4 oz.   90
sweet and sour:
  (Kikkoman), 1 tbsp.   18
  (La Choy), 1 tbsp.   30
  (Lawry's), 1/4 cup   549

Sauces, sweet and sour, continued

(Sauceworks), 1 tbsp.	25
duck sauce (La Choy), 1 tbsp.	26
regular, Hawaiian, or hot (Great Impressions), 2 tbsp.	102
Szechwan, hot and spicy (La Choy), 1 oz.	48

taco (see also "salsa," page 210):

(Estee), 2 tbsp.	14
(Lawry's Sauce'n Seasoner), 1/4 cup	40
chunky (Lawry's), 1/4 cup	22
green (La Victoria), 1 tbsp.	4
hot or mild (Del Monte), 1/4 cup	15
hot, medium, or mild (Old El Paso), 2 tbsp.	10
hot or mild (Ortega), 1 oz.	12
mild (Enrico's No Salt Added), 2 tbsp.	14
mild or medium (Heinz), 1 tbsp.	6
red (La Victoria), 1 tbsp.	6
red, mild (El Molino), 2 tbsp.	10
western style (Ortega), 1 oz.	8

tartar, 1 tbsp.:

(Golden Dipt)	70
(Golden Dipt Lite)	50
(Great Impressions)	86
(Hellmann's/Best Foods)	70
(Sauceworks)	70
(Weight Watchers)	35
egg-free (Life All Natural)	38
natural lemon and herb flavor (Sauceworks)	70

teriyaki:

(Kikkoman), 1 tbsp.	15
(Kikkoman Baste & Glaze), 1 tbsp.	27
(La Choy Sauce and Marinade), 1 oz.	30
(La Choy Thick and Rich), 1 oz.	41
barbecue marinade (Lawry's), 1/4 cup	164
ginger marinade (Golden Dipt), 1 fl. oz.	120
w/pineapple juice (Lawry's), 1/4 cup	72

tomato (see also "pasta," page 209):

(Contadina), 1/2 cup	30
(Contadina Thick and Zesty), 1/2 cup	40
(Del Monte Regular/No Salt Added), 1 cup	70
(Health Valley Regular/No Salt Added), 1 cup	70
(Hunt's), 4 oz.	30

(Hunt's No Salt Added/Special), 4 oz.	35
(S&W), 1/2 cup	40
(Stokely), 1/2 cup	30
Italian style *(Contadina),* 1/2 cup	30
marinara *(Buitoni),* 1/2 cup	70
marinara, refrigerated *(Contadina Fresh),* 7.5 oz.	100
w/onions *(Del Monte),* 1 cup	100
plum, w/basil, refrigerated *(Contadina Fresh),* 7.5 oz.	100
Welsh rarebit, canned *(Snow's),* 1/2 cup	170
worcestershire:	
(Lea & Perrins), 1 tsp.	5
regular or smoky *(French's),* 1 tbsp.	10
white wine *(Lea & Perrins),* 1 tsp.	3

* *Prepared according to package directions*

GRAVIES
See also "Condiments & Seasonings," "Sauces," and "Seasoning & Roasting Mixes, Dry"

	calories
au jus:	
(Franco-American), 2 oz.	10
mix* *(French's),* 1/4 cup	10
mix* *(Lawry's),* 1 cup	84
mix* *(McCormick/Schilling),* 1/4 cup	20
beef *(Franco-American),* 2 oz.	25
beef, w/chunky beef *(Hormel Great Beginnings),* 5 oz.	136
brown:	
(Heinz), 2 oz. or 1/4 cup	25
(McCormick/Schilling), 1/3 cup	30
w/onions *(Franco-American),* 2 oz.	25
mix* *(French's),* 1/4 cup	20
mix* *(Lawry's),* 1 cup	94
mix* *(McCormick/Schilling),* 1/4 cup	23
mix* *(McCormick/Schilling* Lite), 1/4 cup	10
mix* *(Pillsbury),* 1/4 cup	15
chicken:	
(Franco-American), 2 oz.	50
(Heinz), 2 oz. or 1/4 cup	35

Gravies, chicken, continued

w/chunky chicken *(Hormel Great Beginnings)*, 5 oz.	147
giblet *(Franco-American)*, 2 oz.	30
mix* *(French's* Gravy for Chicken), 1/4 cup	25
mix* *(Lawry's)*, 1 cup	99
mix* *(McCormick/Schilling)*, 1/4 cup	22
country, mix *(Tone's)*, 1 tsp. dry	12
herb, mix* *(McCormick/Schilling)*, 1/4 cup	20
homestyle, mix* *(French's)*, 1/4 cup	20
homestyle, mix* *(Pillsbury)*, 1/4 cup	15
mushroom:	
(Franco-American), 2 oz.	25
(Heinz), 2 oz. or 1/4 cup	25
mix* *(French's)*, 1/4 cup	20
mix* *(McCormick/Schilling)*, 1/4 cup	19
onion, mix* *(French's)*, 1/4 cup	25
onion, mix* *(McCormick/Schilling)*, 1/4 cup	22
pork:	
(Franco-American), 2 oz.	40
(Heinz), 2 oz. or 1/4 cup	25
w/chunky pork *(Hormel Great Beginnings)*, 5 oz.	140
mix* *(French's)*, 1/4 cup	20
mix* *(McCormick/Schilling)*, 1/4 cup	20
turkey:	
(Franco-American), 2 oz.	30
(Heinz), 2 oz. or 1/4 cup	25
w/chunky turkey *(Hormel Great Beginnings)*, 5 oz.	138
mix* *(Lawry's)*, 1 cup	102
mix* *(McCormick/Schilling)*, 1/4 cup	22

* Prepared according to package directions

CONDIMENTS & SEASONINGS
See also "Sauces," "Gravies," "Pure Herbs & Spices," and "Salad Dressings"

	calories
apple pie spice *(Tone's)*, 1 tsp.	9
bacon bits:	
(Hormel), 1 tbsp.	30

(Libby's Bacon Crumbles), 1 tbsp.	25
(Oscar Mayer), 1/4 oz.	20
imitation *(Bac • Os)*, 2 tsp.	25
barbecue spice *(McCormick/Schilling)*, 1/4 tsp.	< 1
barbecue spice *(Tone's)*, 1 tsp.	9
beef marinade seasoning mix *(Lawry's)*, 1 pkg.	49
beef seasoning mix, ground, w/onions *(French's)*, 1/4 pkg. dry	25
beef stew seasoning mix:	
(French's), 1/6 pkg.	25
(Lawry's), 1 pkg.	131
(McCormick/Schilling), 1 pkg.	130
beef Stroganoff seasoning *(McCormick/Schilling)*, 1 pkg.	125
bitters *(Angostura)*, 1/4 tsp.	4
burrito seasoning mix *(Lawry's)*, 1 pkg.	132
Cajun seasoning *(Tone's)*, 1 tsp.	9
capers *(Crosse & Blackwell)*, 1 tbsp.	6
catsup:	
(Del Monte Regular/No Salt Added), 1/4 cup	60
(Estee), 1 tbsp.	6
(Featherweight), 1 tbsp.	6
(Hain Natural Regular/No Salt Added), 1 tbsp.	16
(Heinz/Heinz Hot), 1 tbsp.	16
(Heinz Lite), 1 tbsp.	8
(Hunt's), 1 tbsp.	16
(Hunt's No Salt Added), 1 tbsp.	20
(Smucker's), 1 tsp.	8
(Stokely), 1 tbsp.	20
(Weight Watchers), 2 tsp.	8
celery salt, *see "salt, flavored," page 217*	
cheese topping, cheddar, w/bacon *(Tone's)*, 1 tsp.	10
chili powder *(Gebhardt)*, 1 tsp.	6
chili powder, hot or mild *(Tone's)*, 1 tsp.	8
chili seasoning mix:	
(Lawry's Seasoning Blends), 1 pkg.	143
(McCormick/Schilling), 1 pkg.	18
(Tio Sancho), 1.23 oz.	109
chutney, Major Grey's *(Crosse & Blackwell)*, 1 tbsp.	53
coconut, cream of *(Coco Lopez)*, 2 tbsp.	120
coconut, cream of *(Holland House)*, 1 fl. oz.	81

216   CONDIMENTS & SEASONINGS

Condiments & Seasonings, continued

curry powder *(Tone's)*, 1 tsp.	6
dill seasoning *(McCormick/Schilling Parsley Patch* It's a Dilly)*, 1 tsp.	11
enchilada seasoning mix *(Lawry's)*, 1 pkg.	152
fajita seasoning blend *(Lawry's)*, 1 pkg.	63
garlic bread spread *(Lawry's)*, ½ tbsp.	47
garlic powder, *see "Pure Herbs & Spices, garlic powder," page 220*	
garlic salt, *see "salt, flavored," page 218*	
garlic seasoning:	
(McCormick/Schilling Season All)*, ¼ tsp.	2
(McCormick/Schilling Parsley Patch), 1 tsp.	13
garlic spread concentrate *(Lawry's)*, 1 tbsp.	15
guacamole seasoning blend *(Lawry's)*, 1 pkg.	60
gumbo file powder *(Tone's)*, 1 tsp.	8
hamburger seasoning *(McCormick/Schilling)*, 1 pkg.	130
herbs, seasoning *(Lawry's* Pinch of Herbs)*, 1 tsp.	9
horseradish, prepared:	
(Crowley), 1 oz.	10
(Kraft Regular or Cream Style)*, 1 tbsp.	10
hot, red, or white *(Gold's)*, 1 tsp.	4
Italian seasoning *(McCormick/Schilling)*, ¼ tsp.	1
lemon herb marinade *(Golden Dipt)*, 1 fl. oz.	130
lemon pepper seasoning, 1 tsp.:	
(Lawry's)	6
(McCormick/Schilling Parsley Patch)	13
(McCormick/Schilling Spice Blends)*	7
coarse or fine ground *(Tone's Mr. Pepper)*	12
mayonnaise, *see "Salad Dressings, mayonnaise," page 202*	
meat loaf seasoning:	
(French's), ⅛ pkg.	20
(Lawry's Seasoning Blends)*, 1 pkg.	355
(McCormick/Schilling), 1 pkg.	130
meat marinade, mix *(French's)*, ⅛ pkg.	10
meat marinade, mix *(McCormick/Schilling)*, 1 pkg.	110
meat tenderizer, seasoned or unseasoned *(Tone's)*, 1 tsp.	7
meatball seasoning mix *(French's)*, ¼ pkg.	35
mesquite seasoning *(Tone's)*, 1 tsp.	13
Mexican seasoning *(Tone's)*, 1 tsp.	6

monosodium glutamate *(Tone's)*, 1 tsp.   0
mustard, prepared:
    (Featherweight), 1 tsp.   5
    (Hain Stone Ground), 1 tbsp.   14
    (Kraft Pure), 1 tbsp.   10
    brown, spicy *(Gulden's)*, .25 oz.   8
    Dijon *(French's)*, 1 tsp.   8
    Dijon *(Grey Poupon)*, 1 tbsp.   18
    English *(Life* All Natural), 1 tbsp.   22
    w/horseradish or Medford *(French's)*, 1 tbsp.   16
    horseradish *(Kraft)*.   14
    hot *(Gulden's* Diablo), .25 oz.   8
    jalapeño *(Great Impressions)*, 2 tsp.   7
    mild, creamy *(Gulden's)*, .25 oz.   6
    w/onion *(French's)*, 1 tsp.   8
    spicy *(French's* Bold'n Spicy), 1 tsp.   6
    yellow *(French's)*, 1 tbsp.   10
    yellow *(Heinz)*, 1 tsp.   3
nacho seasoning *(Lawry's* Seasoning Blends), 1 pkg. . . .   141
onion powder, *see "Pure Herbs & Spices, onion*
    powder," page 220
Oriental 5-spice *(Tone)*, 1 tsp.   9
parsley seasoning, all purpose *(McCormick/Schilling*
    Parsley Patch), 1 tsp.   6
pepper, seasoned *(Lawry's)*, 1 tsp.   9
pepper, seasoned, lemon, *see "lemon pepper seasoning,"*
    page 216
pickling spice *(Tone's)*, 1 tsp.   10
pimiento spread *(Price's)*, 1 oz.   80
popcorn seasoning *(McCormick/Schilling Parsley*
    Patch), 1 tsp.   10
pot roast seasoning *(Lawry's* Seasoning Blends), 1 pkg.   122
rice seasoning, Mexican *(Lawry's* Seasoning Blends),
    1 pkg.   94
salad nuggets, *see "Croutons," page 30*
salad seasoning *(McCormick/Schilling* Supreme), 1 tsp.   11
salad topping *(Tone's* American), 1 tsp.   7
salt, regular, kosher, or sea (all brands), 1 tsp.   0
salt, flavored, 1 tsp.:
    butter *(McCormick/Schilling)*   2
    celery *(Tone's)*   6

Condiments & Seasonings, salt, flavored, 1 tsp., continued

garlic *(Lawry's)*	4
garlic *(Morton)*	3
onion *(Tone's)*	1
salt, seasoned, 1 tsp.:	
(Lawry's)	4
(Lawry's Hot n' Spicy)	3
(Lawry's Lite)	8
(McCormick/Schilling)	4
(McCormick/Schilling Salt'n Spice)	3
(Morton)	4
(Morton Nature's Seasons)	3
salt, substitute:	
(Lawry's Salt-Free 17), 1 tsp.	10
(Morton), 1 tsp.	<1
seasoned *(Health Valley Instead of Salt)*, 1 tsp.	11
seasoned *(Lawry's Salt-Free)*, 1 tsp.	3
seasoned *(Morton)*, 1 tsp.	2
sandwich spread:	
(Hellmann's/Best Foods), 1 tbsp.	50
(Kraft), 1 tbsp.	50
meat *(Oscar Mayer* Chub), 1 oz.	67
sesame seasoning, all-purpose *(McCormick/Schilling Parsley Patch)*, 1 tsp.	15
shrimp spice *(Tone's* Craboil), 1 tsp.	10
Sloppy Joe seasoning:	
(Lawry's Seasoning Blends), 1 pkg.	126
mix *(French's)*, 1/8 pkg.	16
mix *(McCormick/Schilling)*, 1 serving	18
sour cream and chive topping *(Tone's)*, 1 tsp.	16
soy sauce, *see "Sauces, soy," page 211*	
spaghetti seasoning *(Tone's)*, 1 tsp.	11
steak seasoning, broiled *(McCormick/Schilling* Spice Blends), 1/4 tsp.	1
taco salad seasoning *(Lawry's* Seasoning Blends), 1 pkg.	124
taco seasoning *(Old El Paso)*, 1 pkg.	100
taco seasoning mix:	
(Lawry's Seasoning Blends), 1 pkg.	118
(McCormick/Schilling), 1 pkg.	103
(Tio Sancho), 1.51 oz.	132
meat *(Ortega)*, 1 oz.	90

taco starter *(Del Monte)*, 8 oz.	140
vinegar:	
all varieties *(Heinz)*, 1 tbsp.	2
cider, distilled *(White House)*, 1 fl. oz. or 2 tbsp.	4
cider or white *(Lucky Leaf/Musselman's)*, 1 fl. oz.	4
white *(Indian Summer)*, 1 cup	30
wine, all varieties *(Regina)*, 1 fl. oz.	4
wine, basil or garlic *(Great Impressions)*, 1 tbsp.	7
wine, hot paprika *(Great Impressions)*, 1 tbsp.	6
wine, raspberry *(Great Impressions)*, 1 tbsp.	7
wine, red *(Great Impressions)*, 1 tbsp.	6
wine, cooking:	
Burgundy or Sauterne *(Regina)*, ¼ cup	2
marsala *(Holland House)*, 1 fl. oz.	9
red *(Holland House)*, 1 fl. oz.	6
sherry *(Holland House)*, 1 fl. oz.	5
sherry *(Regina)*, ¼ cup	20
vermouth or white *(Holland House)*, 1 fl. oz.	2
worcestershire sauce, *see "Sauces, worcestershire," page 213*	

PURE HERBS AND SPICES, one teaspoon
See also "Condiments & Seasonings"

---

	calories
allspice, ground *(Spice Islands)*	6
anise seed *(Tone's)*	7
basil, dried, ground *(Spice Islands)*	3
bay leaf, dried *(Tone's)*	2
caraway seed *(Spice Islands)*	8
cardamom, ground *(Tone's)*	6
cardamom seed *(Spice Islands)*	6
celery seed *(Spice Islands)*	11
chives, freeze-dried *(Tone's)*	<1
cinnamon, ground *(Spice Islands)*	6
cloves, ground *(Spice Islands)*	7
coriander leaf, dried *(Tone's)*	2
coriander seed *(Spice Islands)*	6
cumin seed *(Spice Islands)*	7
dill seed *(Spice Islands)*	9

Pure Herbs and Spices, continued

dill weed, dried *(Tone's)*	3
fennel seed *(Spice Islands)*	8
garlic powder *(Spice Islands)*	5
ginger, ground *(Spice Islands)*	6
mace, ground *(Spice Islands)*	10
marjoram, dried *(Spice Islands)*	4
mustard powder *(Spice Islands)*	9
nutmeg, ground *(Spice Islands)*	11
onion powder *(Spice Islands)*	8
oregano, dried *(Spice Islands)*	6
oregano, ground *(Tone's)*	5
paprika *(Spice Islands)*	7
parsley flakes *(Spice Islands)*	4
pepper, ground:	
black or white *(Spice Islands)*	9
coarse or fine grind *(Tone's Mr. Pepper)*	8
red, chili, or cayenne *(Spice Islands)*	9
poppy seed *(Spice Islands)*	13
rosemary, dried *(Spice Islands)*	5
sage, ground *(Spice Islands)*	4
salt, *see "Condiments & Seasonings, salt," page 217*	
savory, ground *(Spice Islands)*	5
sesame seed *(Spice Islands)*	9
tarragon, ground *(Spice Islands)*	5
thyme, ground *(Spice Islands)*	5
turmeric, ground *(Spice Islands)*	7

Chapter 17

PUDDINGS, CUSTARDS, AND GELATINS

PUDDINGS, READY-TO-SERVE
See also "Puddings, Frozen," "Custards, Puddings & Pie Fillings, Mix," and "Gelatin & Gelatin Desserts"

	calories
all flavors:	
(Estee), 1/2 cup	70
(Featherweight), 1/2 cup	100
(Hunt's Snack Pack Lite), 4 oz.	100
(Jell-O Light Pudding Snacks), 4 oz.	100
(Swiss Miss Lite), 4 oz.	100
except chocolate *(Del Monte* Pudding Cup), 5 oz.	180
butterscotch *(Crowley)*, 4.5 oz.	150
butterscotch *(White House)*, 3.5 oz.	113
butterscotch-chocolate-vanilla swirl *(Jell-O* Pudding Snacks), 4 oz.	180
chocolate:	
(Crowley), 4.5 oz.	190
(Del Monte Pudding Cup), 5 oz.	190
(Hunt's Snack Pack), 4.25 oz.	160
(Jell-O Pudding Snacks), 5.5 oz.	230
(Jell-O Pudding Snacks), 4 oz.	170
(Swiss Miss), 4 oz.	180
(White House), 3.5 oz.	120
fudge *(Del Monte* Pudding Cup), 5 oz.	190
fudge or milk *(Jell-O* Pudding Snacks), 4 oz.	170
chocolate-caramel swirl *(Jell-O* Pudding Snacks), 4 oz.	170

Puddings, Ready-to-Serve, continued

chocolate fudge-milk chocolate swirl *(Jell-O* Pudding
    Snacks), 4 oz. 170
chocolate-vanilla swirl *(Jell-O* Pudding Snacks), 5.5 oz. 240
chocolate-vanilla swirl *(Jell-O* Pudding Snacks), 4 oz. . 170
lemon *(White House),* 3.5 oz. 152
rice *(Crowley),* 4.5 oz. 125
rice *(White House),* 3.5 oz. 111
tapioca:
    (Crowley), 4.5 oz. 135
    (Hunt's Snack Pack), 4.25 oz. 160
    (Jell-O Pudding Snacks), 4 oz. 170
    (Swiss Miss), 4 oz. 150
    (White House), 3.5 oz. 131
vanilla:
    (Crowley), 4.5 oz. 140
    (Featherweight), 1/2 cup 100
    (Hunt's Snack Pack), 4.25 oz. 170
    (Jell-O Pudding Snacks), 5.5 oz. 250
    (Jell-O Pudding Snacks), 4 oz. 180
    (Swiss Miss), 4 oz. 160
    (White House), 3.5 oz. 111
vanilla-chocolate swirl *(Jell-O* Pudding Snacks), 4 oz. . 180

PUDDINGS, FROZEN
See also "Puddings, Ready-to-Serve"

---

                                  calories

bars, all flavors *(Jell-O Pudding Pops),* 1 bar 80
butterscotch *(Rich's),* 3 oz. 130
chocolate:
    (Rich's), 3 oz. 140
    mousse *(Weight Watchers),* 1/2 pkg. or 2.5 oz. 170
praline pecan mousse *(Weight Watchers),* 1/2 pkg. 190
vanilla *(Rich's),* 3 oz. 130

CUSTARDS, PUDDINGS & PIE FILLINGS, MIX*,
1/2 cup, except as noted
See also "Puddings, Ready-to-Serve," "Puddings, Frozen," "Gelatin & Gelatin Desserts," and "Pie Fillings, Canned"

---

	calories
all flavors *(Salada Danish Dessert)*	130
banana *(Jell-O Instant Sugar Free)***	80
banana cream:	
(Jell-O Instant)	160
(Jell-O Microwave)	150
(Royal)	160
(Royal Instant)	180
butter almond, toasted *(Royal Instant)*	170
butter pecan *(Jell-O Instant)*	170
butterscotch:	
(D-Zerta)***	70
(Jell-O/Jell-O Microwave)	170
(Jell-O Instant)	160
(Jell-O Instant Sugar Free)**	90
(Royal)	160
(Royal Instant)	180
(Royal Instant Sugar Free)**	100
cheesecake mousse *(Weight Watchers)****	60
chocolate:	
all varieties *(Jell-O)*	160
all varieties *(Jell-O Instant)*	180
(D-Zerta)***	60
(Jell-O Instant Sugar Free)**	90
(Jell-O Microwave)	170
(Jell-O Sugar Free)**	90
(Royal)	180
(Royal Instant)	190
(Royal Instant Sugar Free)**	110
(Weight Watchers Instant)***	90
chocolate chip *(Royal Instant)*	190
dark'n sweet *(Royal)*	180
dark'n sweet *(Royal Instant)*	190
fudge *(Jell-O Instant Sugar Free)***	100

Custards, Puddings & Pie Fillings, Mix*, chocolate, continued
milk *(Jell-O* Microwave) 160
chocolate mint *(Royal* Instant) 190
chocolate mousse:
   (Jell-O Rich & Luscious) 150
   (Weight Watchers)*** 60
   fudge *(Jell-O Rich & Luscious)* 140
   white, almond *(Weight Watchers)**** 60
coconut, toasted *(Royal* Instant) 170
coconut cream *(Jell-O* Instant) 180
custard *(Royal)* 150
custard, egg, golden *(Jell-O Americana)* 160
flan *(Jell-O)* 150
flan, w/caramel sauce *(Royal)* 150
fudge, see "chocolate," page 223
lemon:
   (Jell-O Instant) 170
   (Royal) 160
   (Royal Instant) 180
lime, key *(Royal)* 160
pistachio:
   (Jell-O Instant) 170
   (Jell-O Instant Sugar Free)** 90
   nut *(Royal* Instant) 170
raspberry mousse *(Weight Watchers)**** 60
rennet custard:
   all flavors *(Junket),* ³⁄₈ oz. dry 40
   all flavors *(Junket)* 120
   all flavors *(Junket)**** 90
rice *(Jell-O Americana)* 170
tapioca, vanilla *(Jell-O Americana)* 160
tapioca, vanilla *(Royal)* 160
vanilla:
   (D-Zerta)*** 70
   (Jell-O/Jell-O Microwave) 160
   (Jell-O Instant) 170
   (Jell-O Instant Sugar Free)** 90
   (Jell-O Sugar Free)** 80
   (Royal) 160
   (Royal Instant) 180
   (Royal Instant Sugar Free)** 100

French *(Jell-O)* 170
French *(Jell-O* Instant) 160

* *Prepared according to package directions, with whole milk, except as noted*
** *Prepared with 2% lowfat milk*
*** *Prepared with skim milk*

GELATIN & GELATIN DESSERTS, 1/2 cup, except as noted

	calories
gelatin, unflavored *(Knox)*, 1 pkt.	25
gelatin bar, frozen, all flavors *(Jell-O Gelatin Pops)*, 1 bar	35
gelatin dessert, all flavors:	
(Estee)	8
mix* *(D-Zerta)*	8
mix* *(Jell-O)*	80
mix* *(Featherweight)*	10
mix* *(Royal)*	80
mix* *(Royal* Sugar Free)	6
gelatin drink mix, orange flavor *(Knox)*, 1 envelope ..	39

* *Prepared according to package directions*

Chapter 18

CAKES, COOKIES, PIES, AND PASTRIES

DESSERT CAKES
See also "Dessert Cakes, Frozen," "Dessert Cakes, Mixes," and "Snack Cakes & Pastries"

	calories
(Awrey's Best Wishes), 1/4 of 6" cake	150
(Awrey's Four-in-One Occasion), 1.3-oz. piece	150
apple streusel *(Awrey's),* 2" × 2" piece	160
banana, iced *(Awrey's),* 2" × 2" piece	140
black forest torte *(Awrey's),* 1/14 cake	350
carrot supreme, iced *(Awrey's),* 2" × 2" piece	210
carrot, three-layer, iced *(Awrey's),* 1/12 cake	390
chocolate:	
(Awrey's), .8-oz. piece	70
(Awrey's Happy Birthday), 1.4-oz. piece	150
double, iced *(Awrey's),* 2" × 2" piece	130
double, two-layer *(Awrey's),* 1/12 cake	250
double, three-layer *(Awrey's),* 1/12 cake	310
double, torte *(Awrey's),* 1/14 cake	340
German, iced *(Awrey's),* 2" × 2" piece	160
German, three-layer *(Awrey's),* 1/12 cake	350
milk, yellow, two-layer *(Awrey's),* 1/12 cake	290
white iced, two-layer *(Awrey's),* 1/12 cake	270
coconut, yellow, three-layer *(Awrey's),* 1/12 cake	350
coconut butter cream *(Awrey's),* 2" × 2" piece	160
coffee, caramel nut *(Awrey's),* 1/12 cake	140
coffee, long John *(Awrey's),* 1/12 cake	160

devil's food, white iced *(Awrey's)*, 2″ × 2″ piece   150
lemon, three-layer *(Awrey's)*, 1/12 cake   320
lemon, yellow, two-layer *(Awrey's)*, 1/12 cake   290
Neapolitan, torte *(Awrey's)*, 1/14 cake   380
orange, frosty, iced *(Awrey's)*, 2″ × 2″ piece   150
orange, three-layer *(Awrey's)*, 1/12 cake   320
peanut butter, torte *(Awrey's)*, 1/14 cake   380
pistachio, torte *(Awrey's)*, 1/14 cake   370
pound *(Drake's)*, 1/10 cake or 1.1 oz.   110
pound, golden *(Awrey's)*, 1/14 loaf   130
raisin spice, iced *(Awrey's)*, 2″ × 2″ piece   160
raspberry nut *(Awrey's)*, 1/16 cake   310
sponge *(Awrey's)*, 2″ × 2″ piece   80
strawberry supreme, torte *(Awrey's)*, 1/14 cake   270
walnut, torte *(Awrey's)*, 1/14 cake   320
yellow *(Awrey's)*, .9-oz. piece   80
yellow, white iced *(Awrey's)*, 2″ × 2″ piece   150

DESSERT CAKES, FROZEN*
*See also "Snack Cakes, Pastries & Pies, Frozen &
Refrigerated"*

---

                                                        calories
apple danish *(Sara Lee Free & Light)*, 1/8 cake   130
banana, single layer, iced *(Sara Lee)*, 1/8 cake   170
black forest, two-layer *(Sara Lee)*, 1/8 cake   190
Boston cream *(Pepperidge Farm* Supreme), 2⅞ oz. . . .   290
Boston cream pie *(Weight Watchers)*, 1/2 pkg. or 3 oz. .   160
carrot:
   (Weight Watchers), 1/2 pkg. or 3 oz.   170
   iced *(Pepperidge Farm* Old Fashioned), 1.5 oz.   150
   single layer, iced *(Sara Lee)*, 1/8 cake   250
cheesecake:
   (Weight Watchers), 1/2 pkg. or 3.9 oz.   210
   brownie *(Weight Watchers)*, 1/2 pkg. or 3.5 oz.   200
   cherry cream *(Sara Lee Original)*, 1/6 cake   243
   cream *(Sara Lee Original)*, 1/6 cake   230
   French *(Sara Lee Classics)*, 1/8 cake   250
   strawberry *(Weight Watchers)*, 1/2 pkg. or 3.9 oz. . . .   180
   strawberry, French *(Sara Lee Classics)*, 1/8 cake . . .   240

Dessert Cakes, Frozen*, cheesecake, continued

strawberry cream *(Sara Lee* Original), 1/6 cake 222
cheesecake, nondairy, all flavors *(Tofutti Better than Cheesecake)*, 1/10 cake or 2 oz. 160
chocolate:
    (Pepperidge Farm Supreme), 27/8 oz. 300
    (Sara Lee Free & Light), 1/8 cake 110
    (Weight Watchers), 1/2 pkg. or 2.5 oz. 180
    double, three layer *(Sara Lee)*, 1/8 cake 220
    fudge layer *(Pepperidge Farm)*, 15/8 oz. 180
    fudge stripe layer *(Pepperidge Farm)*, 15/8 oz. 170
    German *(Weight Watchers)*, 1/2 pkg. or 2.5 oz. 200
    German, layer *(Pepperidge Farm)*, 15/8 oz. 180
    mousse *(Sara Lee* Classics), 1/8 cake 260
coconut layer *(Pepperidge Farm)*, 15/8 oz. 180
coffee, all butter:
    cheese *(Sara Lee)*, 1/8 cake 210
    pecan *(Sara Lee)*, 1/8 cake 160
    streusel *(Sara Lee)*, 1/8 cake 160
devil's food layer *(Pepperidge Farm)*, 15/8 oz. 180
golden layer *(Pepperidge Farm)*, 15/8 oz. 180
lemon coconut *(Pepperidge Farm* Supreme), 3 oz. 280
lemon cream *(Pepperidge Farm* Supreme), 15/8 oz. 170
peach melba *(Pepperidge Farm* Supreme), 31/8 oz. 270
pineapple cream *(Pepperidge Farm* Supreme), 2 oz. 190
pound:
    (Pepperidge Farm Cholesterol Free), 1 oz. 110
    (Sara Lee Free & Light), 1/10 cake 70
    all butter *(Sara Lee* Family Size Original), 1/15 cake . 130
    all butter *(Sara Lee* Original), 1/10 cake 130
    butter *(Pepperidge Farm* Old Fashioned), 1 oz. 130
strawberry:
    cream *(Pepperidge Farm* Supreme), 2 oz. 190
    shortcake *(Sara Lee)*, 1/8 cake 190
    stripe layer *(Pepperidge Farm)*, 1.5 oz. 160
vanilla layer *(Pepperidge Farm)*, 15/8 oz. 190

> **DESSERT CAKES, MIXES***, 1/12 of whole cake,
> except as noted
> *See also "Snack Cakes, Mixes"*

                                                 calories

angel food:
- *(Betty Crocker* Traditional), 1/12 mix, dry 130
- *(Duncan Hines)* 140
- all flavors *(Betty Crocker)*, 1/12 mix, dry 150

apple:
- cinnamon *(Betty Crocker SuperMoist)* 250
- streusel *(Betty Crocker MicroRave)*, 1/6 cake 240
- streusel *(Betty Crocker MicroRave)*, 1/6 cake** 210

banana *(Pillsbury Plus)* 250
black forest cherry *(Pillsbury Bundt)*, 1/16 cake 240
black forest mousse *(Duncan Hines Tiarra)* 260
Boston cream *(Betty Crocker* Classic), 1/8 cake 270
Boston cream *(Pillsbury Bundt)*, 1/16 cake 270

butter:
- brickle *(Betty Crocker SuperMoist)* 250
- chocolate *(Betty Crocker SuperMoist)* 270
- pecan *(Betty Crocker SuperMoist)* 250
- recipe *(Pillsbury Plus)* 260
- recipe, golden *(Duncan Hines)* 270
- yellow *(Betty Crocker SuperMoist)* 260

carrot:
- *(Betty Crocker SuperMoist)* 250
- *(Dromedary)* 232
- *(Estee)*, 1/10 cake 100
- 'n spice *(Pillsbury Plus)* 260

cheesecake, 1/8 cake:
- lemon *(Jell-O No Bake)* 270
- lite *(Royal No-Bake)* 210
- plain or New York style *(Jell-O No Bake)* 280
- real *(Royal No-Bake)* 280

cherries and cream *(Duncan Hines Tiarra)* 250
cherry chip *(Betty Crocker SuperMoist)* 190

chocolate:
- *(Estee)*, 1/10 cake 100
- *(Pillsbury* Microwave), 1/8 cake 210
- dark *(Pillsbury Plus)* 250

Dessert Cakes, Mixes*, chocolate, continued

devil's food, *see "devil's food," below*

double supreme *(Pillsbury* Microwave), ⅛ cake 330

fudge *(Betty Crocker SuperMoist)* 260

fudge *(Duncan Hines* Butter Recipe) 270

fudge *(Pillsbury Bundt Tunnel of Fudge* Microwave),
   ⅛ cake 290

fudge *(Pillsbury Bundt Tunnel of Fudge)*, 1/16 cake . 260

fudge, dark Dutch *(Duncan Hines)* 280

fudge marble *(Duncan Hines)* 260

fudge marble *(Pillsbury Plus)* 270

fudge, w/vanilla frosting *(Betty Crocker MicroRave)*,
   ⅙ cake 310

German *(Betty Crocker SuperMoist)* 260

German *(Pillsbury Plus)* 250

German, w/coconut pecan frosting *(Betty Crocker*
   MicroRave), ⅙ cake 320

milk *(Betty Crocker SuperMoist)* 260

mousse *(Duncan Hines Tiarra)* 270

mousse, Amaretto *(Duncan Hines Tiarra)* 270

pudding *(Betty Crocker* Classic), ⅙ cake 230

Swiss *(Duncan Hines)* 280

w/chocolate frosting *(Pillsbury* Microwave), ⅛ cake 300

w/vanilla frosting *(Pillsbury* Microwave), ⅛ cake .. 300

chocolate chip:

  (Betty Crocker SuperMoist) 280

  (Pillsbury Plus) 270

  chocolate *(Betty Crocker SuperMoist)* 260

chocolate macaroon *(Pillsbury Bundt)*, 1/16 cake 240

cinnamon:

  (Streusel Swirl), 1/16 cake 260

  (Streusel Swirl Microwave), ⅛ cake 240

  pecan *(Betty Crocker MicroRave)*, ⅙ cake 290

coffee *(Aunt Jemima* Easy), 1 serving 156

coffee, apple cinnamon *(Pillsbury)*, ⅛ cake 240

devil's food:

  (Betty Crocker SuperMoist) 260

  (Duncan Hines) 280

  (Pillsbury Plus) 270

  w/chocolate frosting *(Betty Crocker MicroRave)*,
    ⅙ cake 310

fudge, *see "chocolate," page 230*
gingerbread *(Dromedary)*, 2" × 2" square 100
lemon:
  (Betty Crocker SuperMoist) 260
  (Duncan Hines Supreme) 260
  (Estee), 1/10 cake 100
  (Pillsbury Bundt Tunnel of Lemon), 1/16 cake 270
  (Pillsbury Microwave), 1/8 cake 220
  (Pillsbury Plus) 250
  (Streusel Swirl), 1/16 cake 270
  chiffon *(Betty Crocker Classic)* 200
  double supreme *(Pillsbury Microwave)*, 1/8 cake.... 300
  w/lemon frosting *(Betty Crocker MicroRave)*,
    1/6 cake.................... 300
  w/lemon frosting *(Pillsbury Microwave)*, 1/8 cake .. 300
  pudding *(Betty Crocker Classic)*, 1/6 cake 230
marble *(Betty Crocker SuperMoist)* 250
pineapple:
  (Duncan Hines Supreme) 260
  cream *(Pillsbury Bundt)*, 1/16 cake 260
  upsidedown *(Betty Crocker Classic)*, 1/9 cake 250
pound:
  (Dromedary), 1/2" slice 150
  (Estee), 1/10 cake 100
  (Martha White), 1/10 cake 120
  golden *(Betty Crocker Classic)* 200
rainbow chip *(Betty Crocker SuperMoist)* 250
sour cream, chocolate *(Betty Crocker SuperMoist)* 260
sour cream, white *(Betty Crocker SuperMoist)* 180
spice *(Betty Crocker SuperMoist)* 260
spice *(Duncan Hines)* 260
strawberry *(Duncan Hines Supreme)* 260
strawberry *(Pillsbury Plus)* 260
vanilla:
  French *(Duncan Hines)* 260
  golden *(Betty Crocker SuperMoist)* 280
  golden, w/rainbow chip frosting *(Betty Crocker
    MicroRave)*, 1/6 cake 320
white:
  (Betty Crocker SuperMoist) 240
  (Duncan Hines)................ 250

Dessert Cakes, Mixes*, white, continued

(Estee), 1/10 cake	100
(Pillsbury Plus)	240

yellow:

(Betty Crocker SuperMoist)	260
(Duncan Hines)	260
(Pillsbury Microwave), 1/8 cake	220
(Pillsbury Plus)	260
w/chocolate frosting *(Betty Crocker MicroRave),* 1/6 cake	300
w/chocolate frosting *(Pillsbury* Microwave), 1/8 cake	300

* *Prepared according to basic package directions*

> **DESSERT PIES, FROZEN,** 1/6 of whole pie, except as noted
> *See also "Dessert Pies, Mixes," and "Snack Cakes, Pastries & Pies, Frozen & Refrigerated"*

calories

apple:

(Banquet Family Size)	250
(Mrs. Smith's "Pie In Minutes"), 1/8 of 8" pie	210
(Sara Lee Homestyle), 1/10 of 9" pie	280
(Sara Lee Homestyle High), 1/10 of 10" pie	400
(Weight Watchers), 1/2 pkg. or 3.5 oz.	200
Dutch *(Sara Lee* Homestyle), 1/10 of 9" pie	300
streusel *(Sara Lee* Free & Light), 1/8 pie	170
banana cream *(Banquet)*	180
banana cream *(Pet-Ritz)*	170
blackberry or blueberry *(Banquet* Family Size)	270
blueberry *(Mrs. Smith's "Pie In Minutes"),* 1/8 of 8" pie	220
blueberry *(Sara Lee* Homestyle), 1/10 of 9"pie	300

Boston cream, *see "Dessert Cakes, Frozen, Boston cream," page 227*

cherry:

(Banquet Family Size)	250
(Mrs. Smith's "Pie In Minutes"), 1/8 of 8" pie	220
(Sara Lee Homestyle), 1/10 of 9" pie	270
streusel *(Sara Lee* Free & Light), 1/10 pie	160

chocolate cream or coconut cream *(Banquet)*	190
chocolate cream or coconut cream *(Pet-Ritz)*	190
chocolate mocha *(Weight Watchers)*, 2.75 oz.	160
egg custard *(Pet-Ritz)*	200
lemon:	
cream *(Banquet)*	170
cream *(Pet-Ritz)*	190
meringue *(Mrs. Smith's)*, 1/8 of 8" pie	210
mince *(Sara Lee Homestyle)*, 1/10 of 9" pie	300
mincemeat *(Banquet Family Size)*	260
Neapolitan cream *(Pet-Ritz)*	180
peach:	
(Banquet Family Size)	245
(Mrs. Smith's "Pie In Minutes"), 1/8 of 8" pie	210
(Sara Lee Homestyle), 1/10 of 9" pie	280
pecan *(Mrs. Smith's "Pie In Minutes")*, 1/8 of 8" pie ..	330
pecan *(Sara Lee Homestyle)*, 1/10 of 9" pie	400
pumpkin:	
(Banquet Family Size)	200
(Mrs. Smith's "Pie In Minutes"), 1/8 of 8" pie	190
(Sara Lee Homestyle), 1/10 of 9" pie	240
raspberry *(Sara Lee Homestyle)*, 1/10 of 9" pie	280
strawberry cream *(Banquet)*	170
strawberry cream *(Pet-Ritz)*	170
sweet potato *(Pet-Ritz)*	150

DESSERT PIES, MIXES*, 1/8 of pie, except as noted
See also "Dessert Pies, Frozen"

	calories
banana cream *(Jell-O No Bake)*	240
chocolate:	
mint *(Royal No-Bake)*	260
mousse *(Jell-O No Bake)*	260
mousse *(Royal No-Bake)*	230
coconut cream *(Jell-O No Bake)*	260
lemon meringue *(Royal No-Bake)*	310

Dessert Pies, Mixes*, continued

pumpkin *(Jell-O* No Bake)	250
pumpkin *(Libby's)*, 1/6 pie	390

* *Prepared according to package directions*

SNACK CAKES & PASTRIES, one piece, except as noted
See also "Snack Cakes, Pastries & Pies, Frozen & Refrigerated," "Snack Cakes, Mixes," and "Snack Pies"

---

calories

apple:
bar, baked *(Sunbelt)*	130
delight *(Little Debbie)*	140
spice *(Little Debbie)*	270

banana:
(Hostess Suzy Q's)	240
(Tastykake Banana Treat)	138
slices *(Little Debbie)*	340
twins *(Little Debbie)*	250

brownie *(see also "Cookies, brownie," page 242)*:
Dutch chocolate *(Awrey's Cake)*, 1/16 cake	340
fudge *(Little Debbie)*, 2-oz. piece	240
fudge nut *(Awrey's Sheet Cake)*, 1.25-oz. piece	150
fudge nut, iced *(Awrey's Sheet Cake)*, 2.5-oz. piece . .	300
fudge walnut *(Tastykake)*, 3-oz. piece	373
butterscotch *(Tastykake Krimpets)*	118
caramel peanut filled, chocolate coated *(Little Debbie Peanut Cluster)*	230
cherry cordial *(Little Debbie)*	170

chocolate:
(Hostess Choco Bliss)	200
(Hostess Choco-Diles)	240
(Hostess Ding Dongs)	170
(Hostess Ho Hos)	120
(Hostess Suzy Q's)	250
(Little Debbie), 3 oz.	390
(Little Debbie Choco-Cake), 2.7 oz.	330

(Little Debbie Choco-Jel), 1.16 oz.	150
(Little Debbie Holiday Cake)*, 2.4 oz.	310
(Tastykake Creamie)	174
(Tastykake Juniors)	364
(Tastykake Kandy Kakes)	99
(Tastykake Tempty)	94
cream filled *(Drake's Devil Dog)*	160
cream filled *(Drake's Ring Ding)*	180
devil's food, *see "devil's food," page 236*	
fudge crispy *(Little Debbie)*, 2.08 oz.	260
fudge round *(Little Debbie)*, 2.75 oz.	330
mint, cream filled *(Drake's Ring Ding)*	190
roll, cream filled *(Drake's Yodel)*	150
roll, Swiss, cream filled *(Drake's)*	170
slices *(Little Debbie)*, 3 oz.	320
chocolate chip *(Little Debbie)*, 2.4 oz.	320
coconut:	
(Tastykake Juniors)	317
covered *(Hostess Sno Balls)*	150
crunch *(Little Debbie)*, 2 oz.	320
round *(Little Debbie)*, 1.13 oz.	150
coffee:	
(Drake's Jr.)	140
(Drake's Small)	220
(Little Debbie), 2.1 oz.	250
(Tastykake Koffee Kake Juniors)	·317
cinnamon crumb *(Drake's)*	150
cream filled *(Tastykake* Koffee Kake)	143
crumb cake *(Hostess)*	120
cupcakes:	
butter cream, cream filled *(Tastykake)*	125
chocolate *(Hostess)*	180
chocolate *(Tastykake)*	113
chocolate, cream filled *(Drake's Ring Ding)*	100
chocolate, cream filled *(Tastykake)*	130
chocolate creme *(Tastykake* Kreme Kup)	104
golden, cream filled *(Drake's Sunny Doodle)*	100
orange *(Hostess)*	160
danish:	
apple filled *(Awrey's* Round), 4.5 oz.	390
apple filled *(Awrey's* Square), 3 oz.	220

Snack Cakes & Pastries, danish, continued

cheese filled *(Awrey's* Round), 4.5 oz.	420
cheese filled *(Awrey's* Square), 2.5 oz.	210
cinnamon-raisin filled *(Awrey's* Square), 3 oz.	290
cinnamon-walnut *(Awrey's* Round), 2.75 oz.	300
raspberry filled *(Awrey's* Square), 3 oz.	260
strawberry filled *(Awrey's* Round), 4.5 oz.	400
date nut pastry *(Awrey's)*	230
dessert cup *(Little Debbie)*, .79 oz.	80
devil's food *(Little Debbie Devil Cremes)*, 2.5 oz.	300
devil's food *(Little Debbie Devil Squares)*, 2.2 oz.	270

donuts:

all varieties *(Hostess* Family Pack)	120
plain *(Tastykake* Assorted)	172
chocolate coated *(Tastykake* Choco-Dipped)	181
cinnamon *(Tastykake* Assorted)	201
cinnamon *(Hostess Donette Gems)*	60
coated, mini *(Tastykake)*	81
frosted *(Hostess)*, 1.5 oz.	190
frosted *(Hostess Donette Gems)*	80
fudge iced *(Tastykake* Premium)	350
glazed *(Hostess* Old Fashioned)	250
honey wheat *(Tastykake* Premium)	342
honey wheat, mini *(Tastykake)*	65
(Hostess Old Fashioned)	170
orange glazed *(Tastykake* Premium)	357
powdered sugar *(Hostess Donette Gems)*	60
powdered sugar *(Tastykake,* 12/pkg.)	123
powdered sugar *(Tastykake,* Assorted)	195
powdered sugar, mini *(Tastykake,* 6/pkg.)	58
stick *(Little Debbie)*	230
sugared *(Awrey's)*	610
(Drake's Funny Bone)	150
(Drake's Zoinks)	130
fancy *(Little Debbie)*, 2.6 oz.	340
fig *(Little Debbie Figaroos)*, 1.5 oz.	160
golden cremes *(Little Debbie)*, 1.4 oz.	150
honey, glazed *(Hostess)*	370
honey, iced *(Hostess)*	410
(Hostess Lil' Angels)	90
(Hostess O's)	220

(Hostess Tiger Tail)	240
(Hostess Twinkies)	150
jelly *(Tastykake Krimpets)*, 1 oz.	96
jelly roll *(Little Debbie)*, 2.2 oz.	250
lemon stix *(Little Debbie)*, 1.5 oz.	220
(Little Debbie Caravella), 1.2 oz.	200
(Little Debbie Doodle Dandies), 2.5 oz.	320
(Little Debbie Star Crunch), 1.08 oz.	150
marshmallow supreme *(Little Debbie)*, 1.25 oz.	150
peanut butter:	
(Tastykake Kandy Kakes), .7 oz.	103
bar *(Little Debbie)*, 2.5 oz.	370
and jelly sandwich *(Little Debbie)*, 1.13 oz.	150
pecan twins *(Little Debbie)*, 2 oz.	220
pumpkin delights *(Little Debbie)*, 1.1 oz.	140
Swiss roll *(Little Debbie)*, 2.17 oz.	270
vanilla:	
(Little Debbie), 3 oz.	390
(Tastykake Creamie), 1.5 oz.	182
cream filled *(Tastykake Krimpets)*, 1.1 oz.	139

SNACK PIES, one piece
*See also "Dessert Pies, Frozen" and "Snack Cakes,
Pastries & Pies, Frozen & Refrigerated"*

---

	calories
apple:	
(Drake's)	210
(Hostess)	430
(Tastykake), 4 oz.	345
Dutch *(Little Debbie)*, 2.17 oz.	230
French *(Tastykake)*, 4.2 oz.	399
blackberry *(Hostess)*	420
blueberry:	
(Hostess)	420
(Tastykake), 4 oz.	359
apple *(Drake's)*	210
cherry:	
(Hostess)	460
(Tastykake), 4 oz.	368

Snack Pies, cherry, continued
apple *(Drake's)* 220
chocolate pudding *(Tastykake)*, 4.2 oz. 443
coconut creme *(Tastykake)*, 4 oz. 432
lemon:
  (Drake's) 210
  (Hostess) 440
  (Tastykake), 4 oz. 361
marshmallow:
  banana *(Little Debbie)*, 3 oz. 360
  banana or chocolate *(Little Debbie)*, 1.4 oz. 170
  chocolate *(Little Debbie)*, 3 oz. 370
oatmeal creme *(Little Debbie)*, 1.33 oz. 160
peach *(Hostess)* 420
peach *(Tastykake)*, 4 oz. 343
pecan *(Little Debbie)*, 1.83 oz. 170
pineapple *(Tastykake)*, 4 oz. 362
pumpkin *(Tastykake)*, 4 oz. 356
raisin creme *(Little Debbie)*, 1.17 oz. 140
strawberry *(Hostess)* 410
strawberry *(Tastykake)*, 3.7 oz. 373
(Tastykake Tasty Klair), 4 oz. 436
vanilla pudding *(Tastykake)*, 4.2 oz. 437

**SNACK CAKES, PASTRIES & PIES, FROZEN &
REFRIGERATED,** one piece or serving
*See also "Snack Cakes & Pastries," "Snack Pies,"
and "Miscellaneous Desserts"*

	calories
apple crisp *(Weight Watchers)*, 3.5 oz.	190
apple crisp cake *(Sara Lee Lights)*	150
black forest cake *(Sara Lee Lights)*	170
brownie:	
chocolate *(Weight Watchers)*, 1/3 pkg.	100
chocolate chip, double *(Nestlé Toll House Ready to Bake)*, 1.4 oz.	150
hot fudge *(Pepperidge Farm Newport)*, 1 ramikin	400

carrot cake:
   (Pepperidge Farm Classic), 2¼ oz.   260
   (Sara Lee Deluxe)   180
   (Sara Lee Lights)   170
cheesecake:
   classic *(Sara Lee)*   200
   French *(Sara Lee* Lights)   150
   strawberry *(Pepperidge Farm* Manhattan), 1 ramikin   300
   strawberry, French *(Sara Lee* Lights)   150
chocolate cake:
   double *(Pepperidge Farm* Classic), 2¼ oz.   250
   double *(Sara Lee* Lights)   150
   fudge *(Sara Lee)*   190
   German *(Pepperidge Farm* Classic), 2¼ oz.   250
   mousse *(Pepperidge Farm* Dessert Lights), 2½ oz. . . .   190
   mousse *(Sara Lee),* 3-oz. serving   180
   mousse *(Sara Lee* Lights)   170
cobbler, *see "Miscellaneous Desserts, cobbler," page 241*
coconut cake *(Pepperidge Farm* Classic), 2¼ oz.   230
coffee cake:
   apple cinnamon *(Sara Lee* Individually Wrapped) . .   290
   butter streusel *(Sara Lee* Individually Wrapped) . . .   230
   pecan *(Sara Lee* Individually Wrapped)   280
danish:
   apple *(Pepperidge Farm)*   220
   apple *(Sara Lee* Individual)   120
   caramel, w/nuts, refrigerated *(Pillsbury)*   160
   cheese *(Pepperidge Farm)*   240
   cheese *(Sara Lee* Individual)   130
   cinnamon-raisin *(Pepperidge Farm)*   250
   cinnamon-raisin *(Sara Lee* Individual)   150
   cinnamon-raisin, w/icing, refrigerated *(Pillsbury)* . . .   150
   orange, w/icing, refrigerated *(Pillsbury)*   150
   raspberry *(Pepperidge Farm)*   220
donuts, glazed *(Rich's Ever Fresh)*   141
donuts, jelly *(Rich's Ever Fresh)*   213
fudge cake, golden *(Pepperidge Farm* Classic), 2½ oz. . .   260
lemon cake supreme *(Pepperidge Farm* Dessert Lights),
   2¾ oz.   170
lemon cream cake *(Sara Lee* Lights)   180
lemon coconut cake *(Pepperidge Farm* Classic), 2½ oz.   220

Snack Cakes, Pastries & Pies, continued

pies:

    apple berry *(Pepperidge Farm* Bennington), 1 ramikin   280

    Mississippi mud *(Pepperidge Farm)*, 1 ramikin 410

pound cake, all butter *(Sara Lee)* 200

shortcake, strawberry *(Pepperidge Farm* Dessert

    Lights), 3 oz. 170

turnover, *see "Miscellaneous Desserts, turnover," page*

    242

vanilla fudge swirl cake *(Pepperidge Farm* Classic),

    2¼ oz. 250

SNACK CAKES, MIXES*, one piece
See also "Dessert Cakes, Mixes"

                                            calories

brownie:

    (Duncan Hines Gourmet Truffle) 280

    (Duncan Hines Gourmet Turtle) 240

    caramel fudge chunk *(Pillsbury)* 170

    caramel swirl *(Betty Crocker)* 120

    chocolate, German *(Betty Crocker)* 160

    chocolate, milk or fudge *(Duncan Hines)* 160

    chocolate chip *(Betty Crocker)* 140

    frosted *(Betty Crocker)* 160

    frosted *(Betty Crocker MicroRave)* 180

    fudge *(Betty Crocker)* 150

    fudge *(Betty Crocker* Family Size) 140

    fudge *(Betty Crocker* Supreme) 120

    fudge *(Betty Crocker MicroRave)* 150

    fudge *(Pillsbury* Microwave) 190

    fudge *(Robin Hood/Gold Medal* Pouch Mix) 100

    fudge, chewy *(Duncan Hines)* 130

    fudge, deluxe *(Pillsbury/Pillsbury* Family Size) . . . 150

    fudge, deluxe, w/walnuts *(Pillsbury)* 150

    fudge, double *(Pillsbury)* 160

    fudge, peanut butter *(Duncan Hines)* 150

    fudge, triple, chunky *(Pillsbury)* 170

    rocky road, fudge *(Pillsbury)* 170

    walnut *(Betty Crocker)* 140

    walnut *(Betty Crocker MicroRave)* 160

white, Vienna *(Duncan Hines)* 240
date bar *(Betty Crocker* Classic) 60

* *Prepared according to package directions*

> **MISCELLANEOUS DESSERTS,** one piece or serving
> *See also "Snack Cakes, Pastries, & Pies, Frozen &
> Refrigerated"*

	calories
apple crisp, frozen *(Pepperidge Farm* Berkshire)	250
apple dumpling, frozen *(Pepperidge Farm)*	260
apple 'n spice bake or cherries supreme, frozen *(Pepperidge Farm* Dessert Lights)	170
cobbler, apple, deep dish *(Awrey's),* 1/8 pie	320
cobbler, blueberry, deep dish *(Awrey's),* 1/8 pie	310
cobbler, frozen:	
apple *(Pet-Ritz),* 1/6 pkg. or 4.33 oz.	290
apple *(Stilwell),* 4 oz.	200
blackberry *(Pet-Ritz),* 1/6 pkg. or 4.33 oz.	250
blackberry *(Stilwell),* 4 oz.	280
blueberry *(Pet-Ritz),* 1/6 pkg. or 4.33 oz.	370
cherry *(Pet-Ritz),* 1/6 pkg. or 4.33 oz.	280
cherry *(Stilwell),* 4 oz.	250
peach *(Pet-Ritz),* 1/6 pkg. or 4.33 oz.	260
peach *(Stilwell),* 4 oz.	270
strawberry *(Pet-Ritz),* 1/6 pkg. or 4.33 oz.	290
cream puff, Bavarian, frozen *(Rich's)*	150
danish twist, apple *(Sara Lee),* 1/8 pkg.	190
danish twist, cheese or raspberry *(Sara Lee),* 1/8 pkg. . .	200
dulcita, apple, frozen *(Hormel),* 4 oz.	290
dulcita, cherry, frozen *(Hormel),* 4 oz.	300
eclair, chocolate, frozen *(Rich's)*	210
fruit square, apple or blueberry, frozen *(Pepperidge Farm)*	220
fruit square, cherry, frozen *(Pepperidge Farm)*	230
parfait, peach, frozen *(Pepperidge Farm* Dessert Lights)	150
raspberry-vanilla swirl, frozen *(Pepperidge Farm* Dessert Lights)	160

Miscellaneous Desserts, continued

strawberry yogurt dessert, frozen *(Sara Lee Free &
   Light)*, ¹/10 pkg.   120
turnover:
   all flavors except apple, frozen *(Pepperidge Farm)* . .   310
   apple, frozen *(Pepperidge Farm)*   300
   apple or cherry, refrigerated *(Pillsbury)*   170

COOKIES, one piece, except as noted
See also "Cookies, Frozen, Mixes & Refrigerator"

---

                                                          calories
almond:
   (Stella D'oro Breakfast Treats)   101
   (Stella D'oro Chinese Dessert)   169
   supreme *(Pepperidge Farm* Special Collection)   70
   toast *(Stella D'oro* Mandel)   58
almond-date *(Health Valley Fruit Jumbos)*   70
amaranth *(Health Valley Amaranth Cookies)*   90
animal crackers *(Barnum's)*   12
animal crackers *(Keebler)*   14
anise:
   (Stella D'oro Anisette Sponge)   51
   (Stella D'oro Anisette Toast)   46
   (Stella D'oro Anisette Toast Jumbo)   109
apple:
   bar *(Apple Newtons)*   70
   bar, Dutch *(Stella D'oro)*   112
   filled *(Baker's Own)*   70
   pastry, dietetic *(Stella D'oro)*   86
apple n' raisin *(Archway)*   120
apricot-almond *(Health Valley Fancy Fruit Chunks)* . . .   45
apricot-raspberry *(Pepperidge Farm* Fruit Cookies) . . .   50
apricot-raspberry *(Pepperidge Farm* Zurich)   60
arrowroot biscuit *(National)*   20
blueberry filled *(Baker's Own)*   70
brownie:
   chocolate nut *(Pepperidge Farm* Old Fashioned) . . .   55
   cream sandwich *(Pepperidge Farm* Capri)   80
   walnut *(Pepperidge Farm* Beacon Hill)   120

butter flavor:
  (Pepperidge Farm Chessmen) 45
  chocolate coated *(Keebler* Baby Bear), 3 pieces 70
  chocolate coated *(Keebler E.L. Fudge)* 40
caramel patties *(FFV)* 75
(Carr's Hob-Nobs) 72
(Carr's Muesli) 84
chocolate:
  (Stella D'oro Castelets) 64
  (Stella D'oro Margherite) 72
  creme wafer *(Featherweight)* 20
  fudge *(Estee)* 30
  fudge *(Stella D'oro* Swiss) 68
  fudge bar *(Tastykake)*, 1.8 oz. 240
  fudge mint *(Keebler* Grasshopper) 35
  middles *(Nabisco)* 80
  snaps *(Nabisco)*, 4 pieces or .5 oz. 70
  wafer *(Nabisco* Famous Wafers), .5 oz. 70
chocolate chip:
  (Almost Home Real Chocolate Chip) 60
  (Archway) 50
  (Chips Ahoy! Pure Chocolate Chip) 50
  (Drake's) 70
  (Duncan Hines) 55
  (Featherweight) 45
  (Grandma's Big Cookies) 185
  (Keebler Chips Deluxe) 80
  (Keebler Soft Batch) 80
  (Pepperidge Farm Old Fashioned) 50
  (Tastykake Soft'n Chewy) 188
  bar *(Tastykake)* 211
  w/candy coated chocolate *(Keebler* Rainbow Chips
    Deluxe) 80
  chewy *(Chips Ahoy!)* 60
  chocolate *(Drake's)* 65
  chocolate *(Tastykake* Soft'n Chewy) 199
  chocolate chunk *(Chips Ahoy!* Selections) 90
  w/chocolate middle *(Keebler Magic Middles)* 80
  chunk *(Pepperidge Farm* Nantucket) 120
  chunk pecan *(Chips Ahoy!* Selections) 100
  chunk pecan *(Pepperidge Farm* Chesapeake) 120

244   COOKIES

Cookies, chocolate chip, continued

chunk pecan *(Pepperidge Farm Special Collection)*	70
chunky *(Chips Ahoy! Selections)*	90
double *(Featherweight)*	45
fudge *(Almost Home)*	70
fudge *(Grandma's Big Cookies)*	175
milk *(Duncan Hines)*	55
milk macadamia *(Pepperidge Farm Sausalito)*	120
milk macadamia *(Pepperidge Farm Special Collection)*	70
mint *(Keebler Soft Batch)*	80
snaps *(Nabisco)*, 3 pieces	70
striped *(Chips Ahoy!)*	90
toffee *(Pepperidge Farm Old Fashioned)*	50
walnut *(Keebler Soft Batch)*	80

chocolate sandwich:

(Estee)	50
(Little Debbie), 1.8 oz.	250
(Oreo)	50
(Oreo Big Stuf)	250
(Oreo Double Stuf)	70
fudge *(Keebler Chocolate Creme Sandwich)*	80
fudge covered, dark or white *(Oreo)*	110
fudge, w/fudge creme filling *(Keebler E.L. Fudge)*	70
fudge, w/peanut butter creme filling *(Keebler E.L. Fudge)*	50

chocolate filled sandwich:

(Pepperidge Farm Brussels)	55
(Pepperidge Farm Lido)	90
(Pepperidge Farm Milano/Orleans)	60
fudge creme *(Keebler E.L. Fudge)*	60
mint *(Pepperidge Farm Brussels Mint)*	65
mint or orange *(Pepperidge Farm Milano)*	75

chocolate peanut bar *(Ideal)*	90

coconut:

(Drake's)	65
chocolate filled *(Pepperidge Farm Tahiti)*	90
dietetic *(Stella D'oro)*	52
macaroon *(Stella D'oro)*	60
coffee, chocolate praline filled *(Pepperidge Farm Cappucino)*	50

creme sandwich, *see specific listings*
date pecan *(Health Valley Fancy Fruit Chunks)* 45
date pecan *(Pepperidge Farm Kitchen Hearth)* 55
devils food *(FFV Trolley Cakes)* 60
egg biscuit:
   (Stella D'oro) 43
   (Stella D'oro Anginetti) 31
   (Stella D'oro Jumbo) 47
   dietetic *(Stella D'oro)* 43
   dietetic *(Stella D'oro Kitchel)* 8
   Roman *(Stella D'oro)* 137
   sugared *(Stella D'oro)* 75
(FFV Kreem Pilot Bread) 60
(FFV Royal Dainty) 60
(FFV T.C. Rounds) 80
(FFV Tango) 80
fig:
   bar *(Fig Newtons)* 60
   bar *(Keebler)* 60
   bar, vanilla or whole wheat *(FFV)* 70
   pastry, dietetic *(Stella D'oro)* 89
fruit:
   (Health Valley Fruit & Fitness) 40
   slices *(Stella D'oro)* 60
   tropical *(Health Valley Fancy Fruit Chunks)* 40
   tropical *(Health Valley Fruit Jumbos)* 70
fudge, *see "chocolate," page 243*
fudge bar, caramel and peanut *(Heyday)* 110
ginger *(Pepperidge Farm Gingerman)* 35
ginger boys *(FFV)*, 1.25-oz. pkg. 150
gingersnaps:
   (Archway, 80/pkg.) 25
   (Archway, 54/pkg.) 35
   (FFV) 26
   (Nabisco Old Fashioned) 30
graham cracker:
   (Keebler), 4 pieces 70
   (Nabisco) 30
   (Regal) 70
   (Rokeach) 15
   all varieties *(Honey Maid Graham Bites)*, 11 pieces . 60

Cookies, graham cracker, continued

amaranth *(Health Valley Amaranth Graham
    Crackers)*, 7 pieces   110
chocolate *(Keebler Thin Bits)*, 12 pieces   70
chocolate *(Nabisco)*   60
chocolate *(Nabisco Teddy Grahams)*, 11 pieces   60
cinnamon *(Honey Maid)*   30
cinnamon *(Keebler Alpha Grahams)*, 6 pieces   70
cinnamon *(Keebler Cinnamon Crisp)*, 4 pieces   70
cinnamon *(Keebler Thin Bits)*, 12 pieces   70
cinnamon *(Nabisco Teddy Grahams)*, 11 pieces   60
crispy *(Pepperidge Farm Wholesome)*, 4 pieces   70
fudge covered *(Keebler Deluxe)*   45
w/fudge *(Nabisco Cookies'N Fudge)*   45
honey *(Health Valley Fancy)*, 7 pieces   130
honey *(Honey Maid)*   30
honey *(Keebler Honey Grahams)*, 4 pieces   70
honey *(Nabisco Teddy Grahams)*, 11 pieces   60
oat bran *(Health Valley)*, 7 pieces   130
wheat *(Carr's Home Wheat Graham)*   74
hazelnut *(Pepperidge Farm Old Fashioned)*   55
honey, all varieties *(Health Valley Honey Jumbos)*   70
jelly tarts *(FFV)*   60
lemon *(Featherweight)*   45
lemon nut crunch *(Pepperidge Farm Old Fashioned)* . .   55
marshmallow:
    chocolate cake *(Mallomars)*   60
    chocolate cake *(Pinwheels)*   130
    fudge cake *(Nabisco Puffs)*   90
    fudge cake *(Nabisco Twirls)*   140
mint sandwich *(FFV)*   80
mint sandwich *(Mystic Mint)*   90
molasses:
    (Archway)   100
    (Grandma's Old Time Big Cookies)   160
    (Nabisco Pantry)   80
    crisps *(Pepperidge Farm Old Fashioned)*   35
oat bran:
    animal cookies *(Health Valley)*, 7 pieces   110
    fruit *(Health Valley Oat Bran Fruit Jumbos)*   70
    fruit and nut *(Health Valley)*   55

raisin *(Awrey's)* 100
raisin *(Health Valley Fancy Fruit Chunks)* 45
oatmeal:
  (Archway) 110
  (Archway Ruth's Golden) 120
  (Baker's Bonus) 80
  (Drake's) 60
  (FFV) 26
  (Keebler Old Fashion) 80
  (Little Debbie), 2.75 oz. 340
  apple filled *(Archway)* 90
  apple spice *(Grandma's* Big Cookies) 165
  w/chocolate middle *(Keebler Magic Middles)* 80
  date filled *(Archway)* 100
  iced *(Archway)* 140
  Irish *(Pepperidge Farm* Old Fashioned) 45
  chocolate chunk *(Pepperidge Farm* Dakota) 110
oatmeal raisin:
  (Almost Home) 70
  (Archway) 100
  (Duncan Hines) 55
  (Featherweight) 45
  (Keebler Soft Batch) 70
  (Pepperidge Farm Santa Fe) 100
  (Pepperidge Farm Old Fashioned) 55
  (Tastykake Soft'n Chewy) 207
  bar *(Tastykake)* 224
  raisin bran *(Archway)* 100
peach-apricot:
  bar, vanilla or whole wheat *(FFV)* 70
  pastry *(Stella D'oro)* 93
  pastry, dietetic *(Stella D'oro)* 87
peanut *(Health Valley Fancy Peanut Chunks)* 50
peanut butter:
  (Featherweight) 40
  (Grandma's Big Cookies) 205
  chocolate chip *(Keebler Soft Batch)* 80
  chocolate chunk *(Pepperidge Farm* Cheyenne) 110
  chocolate filled *(Pepperidge Farm* Nassau) 80
  cream filled *(Pitter Patter)* 90
  creme wafer *(Featherweight)* 25

Cookies, peanut butter, continued

nut *(Keebler Soft Batch)* 80
peanut butter sandwich:
  (Estee) 50
  (FFV) 85
  (Nutter Butter) 70
peanut creme patties *(Nutter Butter)* 40
pecan crunch *(Archway)* 60
praline pecan *(FFV)* 40
prune pastry, dietetic *(Stella D'oro)* 95
raisin:
  (Stella D'oro Golden Bars) 109
  bar, iced *(Keebler)* 80
  soft *(Grandma's* Big Cookies) 160
raisin bran *(Pepperidge Farm* Kitchen Hearth) 55
raisin nut *(Health Valley Fruit Jumbos)* 70
raisin oatmeal *(Archway)* 50
raspberry bar *(Raspberry Newtons)* 70
raspberry filled:
  (Baker's Own) 70
  (Pepperidge Farm Chantilly) 80
  (Pepperidge Farm Linzer) 120
  chocolate *(Pepperidge Farm* Chocolate Chantilly) ... 90
sandwich, *see specific listings*
sesame *(Stella D'oro* Regina) 48
sesame, dietetic *(Stella D'oro* Regina) 41
shortbread:
  (Lorna Doone), 3 pieces 70
  (Pepperidge Farm Old Fashioned) 75
  w/chocolate cream center *(Keebler Magic Middles)* . 80
  country *(FFV)* 70
  fudge striped *(Keebler* Fudge Stripes) 50
  fudge striped *(Nabisco Cookies'N Fudge)* 60
  pecan *(Nabisco)* 80
  pecan *(Pecan Sandies)* 80
  pecan *(Pepperidge Farm* Old Fashioned) 70
spice drops *(Stella D'oro* Pfeffernusse) 35
(Stella D'oro Angel Bars) 76
(Stella D'oro Angel Wings) 74
(Stella D'oro Angelica Goodies/Love Cookies) 106
(Stella D'oro Como Delight) 145

(Stella D'oro Holiday Trinkets)	38
(Stella D'oro Royal Nuggets)	2
strawberry:	
(Pepperidge Farm Fruit Cookies)	50
bar *(Strawberry Newtons)*	70
creme wafer *(Featherweight)*	20
sugar:	
(Almost Home Old Fashioned)	70
(Pepperidge Farm Old Fashioned)	50
wafer *(Biscos),* 4 pieces	70
wafer, chocolate *(Tastykake),* 2.2-oz. pkg.	367
wafer, vanilla *(Tastykake),* 2.2-oz. pkg.	366
tea biscuit *(Social Tea)*	20
tofu *(Health Valley The Great Tofu Cookie)*	45
vanilla:	
(Featherweight)	45
(Pepperidge Farm Bordeaux/Pirouettes)	35
(Stella D'oro Castelets/Margherite)	72
chocolate coated *(Pepperidge Farm* Orleans)	30
chocolate laced *(Pepperidge Farm* Pirouettes)	30
chocolate nut coated *(Pepperidge Farm* Geneva)	65
shortbread *(Tastykake)*	57
wafer *(Archway)*	30
wafer *(FFV),* 1 oz.	130
wafer *(Nabisco Nilla* Wafers), .5 oz.	60
wafer, creme *(Featherweight)*	20
wafer, golden *(Keebler)*	20
vanilla creme sandwich:	
(Cameo)	70
(Keebler French Vanilla Creme)	80
(Nabisco Cookie Break)	50
(Nabisco Giggles)	60
wafer *(see also specific listings):*	
brown edged *(Nabisco),* .5 oz.	70
creme, fudge covered *(Keebler Fudge Sticks)*	50
creme filled, assorted *(Estee)*	30
creme filled, chocolate, vanilla *(Estee)*	20
fudge striped *(Nabisco Cookies'N Fudge)*	70
snack, chocolate, strawberry, vanilla *(Estee)*	80
snack, chocolate coated *(Estee)*	130

Cookies, continued

waffle cremes *(Biscos)*	35
wheat free *(Health Valley The Great Wheat Free Cookie)*, 4 pieces	130

COOKIES, FROZEN, MIXES*, & REFRIGERATOR,
two pieces, except as noted

---

	calories
chocolate chip:	
frozen *(Nestlé Toll House Ready to Bake)*	150
mix *(Betty Crocker Big Batch)*	120
mix *(Duncan Hines)*	130
refrigerator *(Pillsbury)*, 1 piece	70
double, frozen *(Nestlé Toll House Ready to Bake)* . .	150
w/nuts, frozen *(Nestlé Toll House Ready to Bake)* . .	160
oatmeal raisin:	
frozen *(Nestlé Toll House Ready to Bake)*	130
mix *(Duncan Hines)*	130
refrigerator *(Pillsbury)*, 1 piece	60
peanut butter, mix *(Duncan Hines)*	140
peanut butter, refrigerator *(Pillsbury)*, 1 piece	70
sugar, refrigerator *(Pillsbury)*, 1 piece	70
sugar, golden, mix *(Duncan Hines)*	130

* *Prepared according to package directions*

CAKE FROSTINGS, READY-TO-SPREAD, 1/12 of
container, except as noted

---

	calories
Amaretto almond *(Betty Crocker Creamy Deluxe)*	160
butter pecan *(Betty Crocker Creamy Deluxe)*	170
caramel pecan *(Pillsbury Frosting Supreme)*	160
cherry *(Betty Crocker Creamy Deluxe)*	160
chocolate:	
(Pillsbury Frost It Hot), 1/8 cake	50
all varieties *(Betty Crocker Creamy Deluxe)*	160
all varieties *(Duncan Hines)*	160

w/dinosaurs *(Betty Crocker Creamy Deluxe* Party) .	160
double Dutch *(Pillsbury Frosting Supreme)*	140
fudge *(Pillsbury),* 1/8 cake	110
fudge *(Pillsbury Frosting Supreme)*	150
fudge *(Pillsbury* Funfetti)	140
milk, mint, or mocha *(Pillsbury Frosting Supreme)* . .	150
chocolate chip:	
(Betty Crocker Creamy Deluxe)	170
(Pillsbury Frosting Supreme)	150
double *(Betty Crocker Creamy Deluxe)*	170
chocolate, candy coated *(Betty Crocker Creamy Deluxe* Party)	160
chocolate coconut almond *(Betty Crocker Creamy Deluxe)*	160
coconut almond *(Pillsbury)*	160
coconut almond *(Pillsbury Frosting Supreme)*	150
coconut pecan:	
(Betty Crocker Creamy Deluxe)	160
(Pillsbury)	150
(Pillsbury Frosting Supreme)	160
cream cheese *(Betty Crocker Creamy Deluxe)*	160
cream cheese *(Pillsbury Frosting Supreme)*	160
decorator, all flavors, except chocolate *(Pillsbury),* 1 tbsp.	70
decorator, chocolate *(Pillsbury),* 1 tbsp.	60
fudge, *see "chocolate," page 250*	
lemon *(Betty Crocker Creamy Deluxe)*	170
lemon *(Pillsbury Frosting Supreme)*	160
rainbow chip *(Betty Crocker Creamy Deluxe)*	170
rocky road *(Betty Crocker Creamy Deluxe)*	150
sour cream:	
chocolate or white *(Betty Crocker Creamy Deluxe)* .	160
vanilla *(Pillsbury Frosting Supreme)*	160
strawberry *(Pillsbury Frosting Supreme)*	160
vanilla:	
(Betty Crocker Creamy Deluxe)	160
(Duncan Hines)	160
(Pillsbury), 1/8 cake	120
(Pillsbury Frosting Supreme)	160
(Pillsbury Funfetti, pink and white)	150

Cake Frostings, Ready-To-Spread, continued
white, fluffy *(Pillsbury)* 60
white, fluffy *(Pillsbury* Frost It Hot), 1/8 cake 50

PIE FILLINGS, CANNED
*See also "Custards, Puddings, & Pie Fillings, Mixes"
and "Pies, Mixes"*

---

calories

apple:
   (Comstock), 3.5 oz. 120
   (Comstock Lite), 3.5 oz. 80
   (Lucky Leaf/Musselman's Plus), 4 oz. 121
   (White House), 3.5 oz. 121
   all varieties *(Lucky Leaf/Musselman's)*, 4 oz. 120
apricot *(Comstock)*, 3.5 oz. 110
apricot *(Lucky Leaf/Musselman's)*, 4 oz. 150
banana *(Comstock)*, 3.5 oz. 110
blackberry *(Lucky Leaf/Musselman's)*, 4 oz. 120
blackberry *(Lucky Leaf/Musselman's* Plus), 4 oz. 121
blueberry:
   (Comstock), 3.5 oz. 110
   (Comstock Lite), 3.5 oz. 75
   (Lucky Leaf/Musselman's Plus), 4 oz. 145
   (White House), 3.5 oz. 118
   cultivated *(Lucky Leaf/Musselman's)*, 4 oz. 120
boysenberry *(Lucky Leaf/Musselman's)*, 4 oz. 120
cherry:
   (Comstock), 3.5 oz. 110
   (Comstock Lite), 3.5 oz. 75
   (Lucky Leaf/Musselman's), 4 oz. 120
   (Lucky Leaf/Musselman's Plus), 4 oz. 108
   (White House), 3.5 oz. 141
chocolate *(Comstock)*, 3.5 oz. 130
coconut *(Comstock)*, 3.5 oz. 120
gooseberry *(Lucky Leaf/Musselman's)*, 4 oz. 180
lemon:
   (Comstock), 3.5 oz. 140
   (Lucky Leaf/Musselman's), 4 oz. 200
   French *(Lucky Leaf/Musselman's)*, 4 oz. 180

mincemeat:
  (Borden None Such), 1/3 cup 200
  (Comstock), 3.5 oz. 150
  (Lucky Leaf/Musselman's), 4 oz. 190
  w/brandy *(S&W* Old Fashioned), 4 oz. 234
  w/brandy and rum *(Borden None Such)*, 1/3 cup . . . 220
  condensed *(Borden None Such)*, 1/4 pkg. 220
peach:
  (Comstock), 3.5 oz. 110
  (Lucky Leaf/Musselman's), 4 oz. 150
  (Lucky Leaf/Musselman's Plus), 4 oz. 113
  (White House), 3.5 oz. 117
pineapple *(Comstock)*, 3.5 oz. 100
pineapple *(Lucky Leaf/Musselman's)*, 4 oz. 110
pumpkin:
  (Comstock), 3.5 oz. 100
  (Lucky Leaf/Musselman's), 4 oz. 170
  (Stokely), 1/2 cup 170
  pie mix *(Libby's)*, 1 cup 260
raisin *(Comstock)*, 3.5 oz. 120
raisin *(Lucky Leaf/Musselman's)*, 4 oz. 130
raspberry *(Lucky Leaf/Musselman's)*, 4 oz. 190
strawberry:
  (Comstock), 3.5 oz. 100
  (Lucky Leaf/Musselman's), 4 oz. 120
  (Lucky Leaf/Musselman's Plus), 4 oz. 138
strawberry-rhubarb *(Lucky Leaf/Musselman's)*, 4 oz. . 120
vanilla creme *(Lucky Leaf/Musselman's)*, 4 oz. 150

PASTRY & PIE CRUSTS
See also "Shells & Wrappers"

                       calories
pastry pocket, refrigerated *(Pillsbury)*, 1 piece 240
pie crust shell, frozen or refrigerated:
  (Mrs. Smith's, 8"), 1/8 shell 80
  (Mrs. Smith's 9"), 1/8 shell 90
  (Mrs. Smith's 95/8"), 1/8 shell 120
  (Pet-Ritz), 1/6 shell 110
  (Pet-Ritz, 95/8"), 1/6 shell 170

Pastry & Pie Crusts, pie crust shell, frozen or refrigerated, continued

(Pillsbury All Ready), 1/8 of 2 crust pie	240
deep dish *(Pet-Ritz)*, 1/6 shell	130
graham cracker *(Pet-Ritz)*, 1/6 shell	110
pie crust shell, mix *(Betty Crocker)*, 1/16 pkg.	120
pie crust shell, mix *(Flako)*, 1 serving*	247
pie crust stick *(Betty Crocker)*, 1/8 stick	120
puff pastry, frozen:	
sheets *(Pepperidge Farm)*, 1/4 sheet	260
shells *(Pepperidge Farm* Patty Shells), 1 shell	210
shells, mini *(Pepperidge Farm)*, 1 shell	50
tart shell, frozen *(Pet-Ritz)*, 1 shell	150

* *Prepared according to package directions*

Chapter 19

NUT BUTTERS, JAMS, AND JELLIES

NUT BUTTERS, two tablespoons, except as noted	
	calories
almond butter, raw *(Hain* Natural)	190
almond butter, blanched, toasted *(Hain)*	220
almond or cashew butter *(Westbrae Natural)*	190
cashew butter *(Hain* Raw/Toasted)	190
peanut butter:	
(Estee), 1 tbsp.	100
(S&W/Nutradiet), 1 tbsp.	93
chunky *(Peter Pan* Crunchy Salt Free)	190
chunky or creamy *(Bama)*	200
chunky or creamy *(Featherweight)*, 1 tbsp.	90
chunky or creamy *(Health Valley* No Salt Added)	180
chunky or creamy *(Jif)*	190
chunky or creamy *(Peter Pan)*	190
chunky or creamy *(Skippy)*	190
chunky or creamy *(Smucker's* Natural/No Salt)	200
creamy *(Peter Pan* Creamy Salt Free)	195
creamy *(Woodstock* Old Fashioned Unsalted)	200
sesame tahini, organic *(Arrowhead Mills)*, 1 oz.	170

JAMS, JELLIES, & PRESERVES	
	calories
butter, apple:	
(Bama), 2 tbsp.	25
(Lucky Leaf/Musselman's), 4 oz.	200

Jams, Jellies, & Preserves, butter, apple, continued

(Smucker's Autumn Harvest/Simply Fruit), 1 tsp. . . .	12
(Tap'n Apple), 1 oz.	45
(White House), 1 oz.	50
natural or cider (Smucker's), 1 tsp.	12
butter, honey (Honey Butter), 1 tbsp. or .5 oz.	50
butter, peach (Smucker's), 1 tsp.	15
fruit spreads, all flavors:	
(Polaner All Fruit Spreadable Fruit), 1 tsp.	14
(Smucker's Simply Fruit), 1 tsp.	16
(Weight Watchers), 2 tsp.	16
low sugar (Smucker's), 1 tsp.	8
jams and preserves:	
all flavors (Polaner), 2 tsp.	35
all flavors (S&W/Nutradiet), 1 tsp.	4
all flavors (Smucker's), 1 tsp.	18
all flavors (Smucker's Slenderella), 1 tsp.	8
all flavors (Welch's), 2 tsp.	35
strawberry (Kraft Reduced Calorie), 1 tsp.	8
strawberry (Smucker's Imitation), 1 tsp.	2
jellies:	
all flavors (Bama), 2 tsp.	30
all flavors (Estee), 1 tsp.	2
all flavors (Featherweight), 1 tsp.	4
all flavors (Kraft), 1 tsp.	17
all flavors (Musselman's), 1 oz.	80
all flavors (Polaner), 2 tsp.	35
all flavors (Smucker's), 1 tsp.	18
all flavors (Smucker's Slenderella), 1 tsp.	8
apple (Lucky Leaf/Musselman's), 1 oz.	80
apple-grape or grape (Welch's), 2 tsp.	35
grape (Kraft Reduced Calorie), 1 tsp.	8
grape (Smucker's Imitation), 1 tsp.	2
jalapeño (Great Impressions), 1 tbsp.	58
pepper, green or red (Great Impressions), 1 tbsp. . . .	50
jelly and peanut butter (Bama), 2 tbsp.	150
marmalade, orange (Smucker's), 1 tsp.	18

Chapter 20

SYRUPS, TOPPINGS, AND SWEET BAKING INGREDIENTS

SUGAR
See also "Honey, Molasses, & Syrups"

	calories
brown, packed (all brands), 1 cup	821
cane baton *(Frieda* of California), 1 oz.	21
fruit *(Estee* Fructose), 1 tsp.	12
fruit *(Featherweight* Fructose), 1 pkt. or 1 tsp.	12
granulated (all brands), 1 tbsp.	46
granulated, juice, organic *(Sucanat),* 1 tsp.	12
powdered, unsifted (all brands), 1 tbsp.	31
substitute:	
(Equal), 1 pkt.	4
(Sprinkle Sweet), 1 tsp.	2
(Sweet'n Low), 1 pkt.	4
(Sweet* 10), 1/8 tsp.	0
(Weight Watchers Sweet'ner), 1 pkt.	4
liquid *(Featherweight),* 3 drops	0
liquid table *(S&W/Nutradiet),* 1/8 tsp.	0
saccharin *(Featherweight),* 1/4 grain tablet	0
turbinado *(Hain),* 1 tbsp.	50

HONEY, MOLASSES, & SYRUPS
See also "Sugar," "Dessert Toppings & Syrups," and "Sweet Flavorings & Extracts"

	calories
corn syrup, dark or light *(Karo)*, 1 tbsp.	60
honey, strained or extracted (all brands), 1 tbsp.	60
molasses, dark or light *(Brer Rabbit)*, 1 tbsp.	60
molasses, gold or green *(Grandma's)*, 1 tbsp.	70
pancake syrup:	
(Aunt Jemima ButterLite), 1 fl. oz.	50
(Aunt Jemima Lite), 1 fl. oz.	54
(Aunt Jemima Original), 1 fl. oz.	109
(Estee), 1 tbsp.	4
(Featherweight), 1 tbsp.	16
(Log Cabin Country Kitchen), 1 fl. oz.	100
(Log Cabin Lite), 1 fl. oz.	50
(Log Cabin Pancake and Waffle), 1 fl. oz.	100
(Vermont Maid), 1 tbsp.	50
maple flavored *(S&W)*, 1 tsp.	4

DESSERT TOPPINGS & SYRUPS
See also "Honey, Molasses, & Syrups"

	calories
blueberry *(Estee* Syrup), 1 tbsp.	4
blueberry *(Featherweight* Syrup), 1 tbsp.	16
butterscotch:	
(Kraft), 1 tbsp.	60
caramel flavor *(Smucker's* Special Recipe), 2 tbsp.	160
flavor *(Smucker's)*, 2 tbsp.	140
caramel:	
(Kraft), 1 tbsp.	60
flavored *(Smucker's)*, 2 tbsp.	140
hot *(Smucker's)*, 2 tbsp.	150
chocolate:	
(Estee Syrup), 1 tbsp.	20
(Hershey's Syrup), 1 oz. or 2 tbsp.	80
(Kraft), 1 tbsp.	60
(Smucker's Magic Shell), 2 tbsp.	190

dark, flavored *(Smucker's* Special Recipe), 2 tbsp. ...   130
flavored *(Smucker's* Syrup), 2 tbsp.   130
milk, w/almonds *(Nestlé Candytops),* 1.25 oz.   230
milk, w/crisps *(Nestlé Crunch Candytops),* 1.25 oz. . .   220
white, w/almonds *(Nestlé Candytops),* 1.25 oz.   230
chocolate fudge:
   (Hershey's), 2 tbsp.   100
   (Smucker's), 2 tbsp.   130
   (Smucker's Magic Shell), 2 tbsp.   190
   hot *(Kraft),* 1 tbsp.   70
   hot *(Smucker's),* 2 tbsp.   110
   hot *(Smucker's* Special Recipe), 2 tbsp.   150
   Swiss milk chocolate *(Smucker's),* 2 tbsp.   140
chocolate nut *(Smucker's Magic Shell),* 2 tbsp.   200
fruit syrup, all flavors *(Smucker's),* 2 tbsp.   100
marshmallow *(Marshmallow Fluff),* 1 heaping tsp. . . .   59
marshmallow creme *(Kraft),* 1 oz.   90
nut *(Planters),* 1 oz.   180
peanut butter-caramel *(Smucker's),* 2 tbsp.   150
pecan, in syrup *(Smucker's),* 2 tbsp.   130
pineapple *(Kraft),* 1 tbsp.   50
pineapple *(Smucker's),* 2 tbsp.   130
strawberry:
   (Kraft), 1 tbsp.   50
   (S&W Syrup), 1 tsp.   4
   (Smucker's), 2 tbsp.   120
walnut, in syrup *(Smucker's),* 2 tbsp.   130
whipped, frozen *(Kraft* Real Cream), ¼ cup   30
whipped, pressurized *(Crowley),* 1 tbsp.   20
whipped, nondairy:
   frozen *(Birds Eye Cool Whip),* 1 tbsp.   12
   frozen *(Birds Eye Cool Whip* Lite), 1 tbsp.   8
   frozen *(Kraft* Whipped Topping), ¼ cup   35
   frozen, extra creamy *(Birds Eye Cool Whip* Dairy
      Recipe), 1 tbsp.   14
   mix* *(D-Zerta),* 1 tbsp.   8
   mix* *(Dream Whip),* 1 tbsp.   10
   mix* *(Featherweight),* 1 tbsp.   4
   pressurized *(Rich's Richwhip),* ¼ oz.   20

Dessert Toppings & Syrups, whipped, nondairy, continued
  prewhipped *(Estee)*, 1 tbsp.   4
  prewhipped *(Rich's Richwhip)*, 1 tbsp.   12

* *Prepared according to package directions*

SWEET FLAVORINGS & EXTRACTS*, one
teaspoon, except as noted
See also "Honey, Molasses, & Syrups"

	calories
almond extract:	
(Virginia Dare)	7
pure *(Durkee)*	13
pure *(Ehlers)*	12
anise extract, pure *(Durkee)*	16
anise extract, pure *(Ehlers)*	26
banana extract, imitation *(Durkee)*	15
banana extract, imitation *(Ehlers)*	20
black walnut flavor *(Durkee)*	4
brandy flavor *(Durkee)*	15
brandy flavor *(Ehlers)*	16
cherry extract, pure *(Burton's)*	9
cherry extract, imitation *(Ehlers)*	16
chocolate flavor *(Durkee)*	7
chocolate flavor *(Ehlers)*	10
coconut flavor *(Durkee)*	8
coconut flavor *(Ehlers)*	17
coffee flavor, pure *(Burton's)*	9
grenadine:	
(Garnier)	17
(Holland House)	15
(Rose's), 1 fl. oz.	65
lemon extract:	
(Virginia Dare)	22
imitation *(Durkee)*	17
pure *(Ehlers)*	30
maple extract, imitation *(Durkee)*	6
maple extract, imitation *(Ehlers)*	9

orange extract:
   (Virginia Dare) 22
   imitation *(Durkee)* 14
   pure *(Ehlers)* 30
orgeat syrup *(Garnier)* 17
peppermint extract, imitation *(Durkee)* 15
peppermint extract, pure *(Ehlers)* 24
pineapple:
   extract, imitation *(Ehlers)* 14
   flavor, imitation *(Durkee)* 6
   flavor, pure *(Burton's)* 12
raspberry extract:
   imitation *(Burton's)* 10
   imitation *(Ehlers)* 14
   pure *(Burton's)* 8
rose extract, pure *(Burton's)* 9
rum:
   extract, imitation *(Burton's)* 11
   flavor, imitation *(Durkee)* 14
   flavor, pure *(Ehlers)* 19
strawberry extract:
   imitation *(Durkee)* 12
   imitation *(Ehlers)* 16
   pure *(Burton's)* 10
vanilla:
   extract, imitation *(Durkee)* 3
   extract, pure *(Virginia Dare)* 10
   extract, pure *(Durkee)* 8
   extract, pure *(Ehlers)* 13
   flavor, imitation *(Durkee)* 3

* Note: If a flavoring that contains alcohol is added to a recipe before cooking, the alcohol (which frequently contributes a major portion of the calories) will be evaporated and the calories reduced.

MISCELLANEOUS SWEET BAKING INGREDIENTS, one ounce, except as noted

	calories
butterscotch chips *(Nestlé* Toll House Morsels)	150

Miscellaneous Sweet Baking Ingredients, continued

chocolate, bars:

semi-sweet *(Hershey's* Premium)	140
semi-sweet *(Nestlé)*	160
semi-sweet or unsweetened *(Baker's)*	140
sweet *(Baker's German)*	140
unsweetened *(Hershey's)*	190
unsweetened *(Nestlé)*	180
white *(Nestlé* Premier), .5 oz.	80
chocolate, pre-melted *(Nestlé Choco Bake)*	190

chocolate chips:

milk *(Baker's)*	140
milk *(Baker's* Big Chip), ¼ cup	240
milk *(Hershey's)*	150
milk or mint *(Nestlé* Toll House Morsels)	150
mint *(Hershey's)*, 1.5 oz. or ¼ cup	230
semi-sweet *(Baker's)*, ¼ cup	200
semi-sweet *(Baker's* Big Chip), ¼ cup	220
semi-sweet *(Nestlé* Toll House Morsels)	150
semi-sweet, regular or mini *(Hershey's)*, ¼ cup	220
vanilla (white), milk *(Hershey's)*, ¼ cup	240

chocolate chunks or pieces:

milk *(Hershey's* Chunks)	160
milk or semi-sweet *(Nestlé Toll House Treasures)*	150
semi-sweet *(Hershey's* Chunks)	140
white *(Nestlé Toll House Premier Treasures)*	160
chocolate shreds *(Tone's)*, 1 tsp.	21
cocoa, *see "Cocoa & Flavored Mixes, Dry, cocoa," page 286*	

coconut, dried:

(Baker's Angel Flake), ⅓ cup	120
canned *(Baker's Angel Flake)*, ⅓ cup	110
shredded *(Baker's* Premium Shred), ⅓ cup	140
toasted *(Baker's Angel Flake)*, ⅓ cup	200
peanut butter baking chips *(Reese's)*, ¼ cup	230

Chapter 21

CANDY AND
CHEWING GUM

CANDY

	calories
almond, candy coated *(Brach's* Jordan Almonds), 1 oz.	120
(Baby Ruth), 1 oz.	130
(Brach's Royals), 1 oz.	100
bridge mix *(Brach's)*, 1 oz.	130
(Butterfinger), 1 oz.	130
butterscotch:	
(Brach's Disks), 1 oz.	110
(Callard & Bowser), 1 oz.	115
(Featherweight), 1 piece	25
candy cane *(Brach's)*, 1 oz.	110
candy cane *(Spangler)*, 1 piece	60
candy corn *(Heide)*, 1 piece	9
candy corn, Indian or three color *(Brach's)*, 1 oz.	100
caramel:	
(Brach's Milk Maid), 1 oz.	110
(Featherweight), 1 piece	30
(Kraft), 1 piece	35
(Sugar Babies Regular/Tidbits), 15/8-oz. pkg.	180
(Sugar Daddy), 13/8-oz. pop	150
chocolate *(Brach's* Milk Maid), 1 oz.	110
chocolate, vanilla *(Estee)*, 1 piece	20
chocolate coated *(Pom Poms)*, 1 oz.	100
chocolate coated, w/cookies *(Twix)*, 2-oz. piece	140
milk chocolate coated *(Rolo)*, 1.93 oz. or 8 pieces	270

Candy, caramel, continued

w/peanut, chocolate coated *(Oh! Henry)*, 2 oz.	280
carob milk bar *(Caroby)*, 4 sections	150
cherry:	
(Heide Jersey Cherries), 1 piece	13
chocolate cream *(Brach's)*, 1 oz.	110
dark or milk chocolate coated *(Brach's)*, 1 oz.	110
chocolate:	
(Brach's I Luv U), 1 oz.	150
(Brach's Jots), 1 oz.	130
almond *(Estee)*, 2 squares	60
almond *(Featherweight)*, 1 section	90
w/almonds *(Hershey's Golden Almond/Solitaires)*,	
1.6 oz. or ½ bar	260
w/almonds, roasted *(Cadbury)*, 1 oz.	150
assorted, wrapped *(Brach's)*, 1 oz.	110
babies *(Heide)*, 1 piece	12
bell, in foil *(Brach's)*, 1 oz.	150
candy coated *(M&M's)*, 1.69 oz.	250
w/caramel *(Caramello)*, 1.6 oz.	220
coconut *(Estee)*, 2 squares	60
cream *(Callard & Bowser)*, 1 oz.	120
crunch *(Estee)*, 2 squares	45
crunch *(Featherweight)*, 1 section	80
dark, deluxe *(Estee)*, 2 squares	60
dark, sweet *(Hershey's Special Dark)*, 1.45 oz.	220
w/fruit and nuts *(Cadbury)*, 1 oz.	150
fruit & nut *(Estee)*, 2 squares	60
w/krisps and honey *(Cadbury)*, 1 oz.	150
milk *(Brach's* Stars), 1 oz.	150
milk *(Cadbury Dairy Milk)*, 1 oz.	150
milk *(Estee)*, 2 squares	60
milk *(Featherweight)*, 1 section	80
milk *(Hershey's)*, 1.55 oz.	240
milk *(Hershey's Kisses)*, 1.46 oz. or 9 pieces	220
milk *(Nabisco* Stars), 1 oz.	160
milk *(Nestlé)*, 1.45 oz.	220
milk, w/almonds *(Hershey's)*, 1.45 oz.	230
milk, w/almonds *(Nestlé)*, 1.45 oz.	230
milk, creamy *(Hershey's Symphony)*, 1.75 oz.	270

milk, creamy, w/almonds and toffee chips *(Hershey's
Symphony)*, 1.75 oz. 280
milk, w/crisps *(Krackel)*, 1.55 oz. 230
milk, w/crisps *(Nestlé Crunch)*, 1.4 oz. 210
milk, w/crisps and nuts *(Nestlé 100 Grand)*, 1.5 oz. . 200
milk, w/fruit and nuts *(Chunky)*, 1.4 oz. 210
milk, w/peanuts *(Brach's* Peanut Clusters), 1 oz. . . . 150
milk, w/peanuts *(Mr. Goodbar)*, 1.75 oz. 290
mint or peanut *(Estee)*, 2 squares 60
w/peanuts, candy coated *(M&M's)*, 1.74 oz. 250
white, w/almonds *(Nestlé Alpine)*, 1.25 oz. 210
chocolate, tofu:
(Barat Passionettes), 1 piece 70
w/almonds *(Barat* Bar), 1 oz. 170
w/almonds and raisins *(Barat* Bar), 1 oz. 160
mints or pastilles *(Barat* Bits), .75 oz. 120
mints, after dinner *(Barat)*, 1 piece 40
peanuts, dipped *(Barat* Bits), .75 oz. 120
raisins, smothered *(Barat* Bits), 1 oz. 120
truffle, w/praline *(Barat* Bar), 1 oz. 170
chocolate chips, *see "Miscellaneous Sweet Baking
Ingredients, chocolate chips," page 262*
cinnamon disks, hearts or Imperial *(Brach's)*, 1 oz. . . . 110
coconut, chocolate coated:
(Mounds), 1.9-oz. piece 260
(Sunbelt Macaroo), 2 oz. 288
dark or milk chocolate *(Bounty)*, 1.05 oz. 150
w/almonds *(Almond Joy)*, 1.76-oz. piece 250
coconut, Neapolitan *(Brach's)*, 1 oz. 120
coffee flavor *(Brach's)*, 1 oz. 120
cough drops *(Beech-Nut)*, 1 piece 10
cough drops *(Halls* Cough Tablets), 1 piece 15
creme center, chocolate coated, 1 piece:
(Spangler Opera Creme Chocolate Drop) 80
caramel, w/nuts *(Spangler* Peanut Cluster) 100
cherry, maple, or vanilla creme, w/nuts *(Spangler*
Peanut Cluster) 110
fudge, w/peanuts or pecans *(Spangler* Cluster) 140
mint, dark chocolate coated *(Spangler Bittersweets)* . 80
eggs, creme *(Cadbury)*, 1.37 oz. 190
eggs, creme *(Cadbury* Mini), 1 oz. 140

Candy, continued

eggs, malted milk, chocolate *(Brach's)*, 1 oz.   130
eggs, pastel *(Brach's* Fiesta), 1 oz.   120
(Estee Estee-ets), 5 pieces   35
filled, assorted *(Brach's)*, 1 oz.   110
fruit flavored:
   all flavors *(Brach's* Fruit Bunch), 1 oz.   90
   all flavors *(Skittles)*, 2.3 oz.   265
   all flavors, chews *(Bonkers!)*, 1 piece   20
   all flavors, chews *(Rascals)*, 1 piece   4
   all flavors, chews *(Starburst)*, 2.07 oz.   240
   all flavors, drops *(Featherweight)*, 1/3 oz.   30
fudge *(Kraft* Fudgies), 1 piece   35
fudge, all varities *(Woodys)*, 1 oz.   120
gum drops, *see "jellied and gummed," below*
halvah *(Fantastic Foods)*, 1.5-oz. bar   232
hard *(see also specific listings):*
   (Estee), 2 pieces   25
   all flavors *(Life Savers)*, 1 piece   8
   fruit flavored drops *(Heide)*, 1 piece   11
   sour balls *(Brach's)*, 1 oz.   110
hearts *(Brach's* Conversation Hearts)   110
(Heath Bits'O Brickle), 3 oz.   448
(Heath Soft'n Crunchy Bar), 2 pieces   190
(Heide Red Hot Dollars), 1 piece   9
holiday mix *(Brach's)*, 1 oz.   110
honey *(Bit-O-Honey)*, 1.7 oz.   200
(Hot Tamales), 1 piece   9
jellied and gummed *(see also specific listings):*
   beans, gummi bears, hearts, mints, spearmint leaves,
     spice, worms *(Brach's)*, 1 oz.   100
   beans *(Just Born Teenee Beanee* Gourmet), 1 piece .   4
   beans, large *(Heide)*, 1 piece   9
   cherry, sour *(Brach's* Jels), 1 oz.   100
   cinnamon *(Brach's* Cinnamon Bears), 1 oz.   80
   eggs *(Brach's/Brach's* Tiny), 1 oz.   100
   eggs *(Just Born* Petite), 1 piece   4
   eggs *(Rodda)*, 1 piece   7
   eggs, speckled *(Brach's)*, 1 oz.   110
   fruit flavored *(Jujyfruits)*, 1 oz. or 11 pieces   100
   gum drops *(Estee)*, 4 pieces   25

gummi bears *(Estee)*, 4 pieces	20
gummi bears *(Heide)*, 1 piece	3
(Heide Fish), 1 piece	21
(Heide Jujubes), 1 piece	3
(Heide Mexican Hats), 1 piece	10
juicy *(Callard & Bowser)*, 1 oz.	90
(Jolly Joes), 1 piece	9
lemon drops *(Brach's)*, 1 oz.	110

licorice:

(Brach's Red Laces/Twists/Twin Twists), 1 oz.	100
(Pearson's Licorice Nip), 1 oz.	120
candy coated *(Good & Fruity/Good & Plenty)*, 1 oz.	106
cherry *(Y&S Bites/Nibs)*, 1 oz.	100
drops *(Diamond)*, 1 piece	14
strawberry *(Y&S Twizzlers)*, 1 oz.	100

lollipop:

all flavors *(Brach's Pops)*, 1 oz.	110
all flavors *(Estee)*, 1 piece	25
all flavors *(Life Savers)*, 1 piece	45
all flavors, except chocolate *(Tootsie Pop)*, 1 oz.	111
chocolate *(Tootsie Pop)*, 1 oz.	110
lozenge *(Listerine* Throat Lozenge), 1 piece	9
malted milk balls, chocolate coated *(Brach's)*, 1 oz. . . .	130
(Mars), 1.76-oz. bar	240

marshmallow *(see also specific listings)*:

(Brach's Perkys Circus Peanuts), 1 oz.	100
(Campfire), 2 large or 24 mini pieces	40
(Funmallows), 1 piece	30
(Kraft Jet-Puffed), 1 piece	25
(Spangler Circus Peanuts), 1 oz. or 4 pieces	110
coconut, toasted *(Just Born)*, 1 piece	30
miniature *(Funmallows/Kraft)*, 10 pieces	18
(Mike & Ikes), 1 piece	9
(Milky Way), 2.15-oz. bar	280
(Milky Way Dark), 1.76 oz.	220

mint *(see also "peppermint" and specific listings)*:

(Brach's Coolers/Kentucky Mint/Starlight), 1 oz. . . .	110
(Brach's Creme de Menthe), 1 oz.	150
(Brach's Jots/Pearls), 1 oz.	120
(Certs Sugar Free), 1 piece	6
(Featherweight Cool Blue) 1 piece	25

Candy, mint, continued

(Mint Meltaway), .33-oz. piece	50
all flavors *(Breath Savers)*, 1 piece	8
assorted *(Brach's* Dessert Mints), 1 oz.	110
butter or party *(Kraft)*, 1 piece	8
clear *(Clorets)*, 1 piece	8
mini *(Certs* Sugar Free), 1 piece	1
parfait *(Brach's)*, 1 oz.	150
pressed *(Clorets)*, 1 piece	6

mint, chocolate coated:

(Junior Mints), 1 oz. or 12 pieces	120
(York Peppermint Pattie), 1.5 oz.	180
dark chocolate *(After Eight)*, 1 piece	35
regular, creme, or thin *(Brach's)*, 1 oz.	110
(Munch), 1.42-oz. bar	220
(Necco Sky Bar), 1.5-oz. bar	196
nonpareils *(Nestlé Sno-Caps)*, 1 oz.	140
nonpareils, dark chocolate *(Brach's)*, 1 oz.	140

nougat:

chocolate coated *(Charleston Chew!)*, 1 oz.	120
jelly *(Brach's)*, 1 oz.	100
kisses *(Brach's)*, 1 oz.	110
nut *(Brach's* Nut Goodies), 1 oz.	130
orange *(Brach's* Orangettes), 1 oz.	100
orange sticks, chocolate coated *(Brach's)*, 1 oz.	110
ornaments, Christmas *(Brach's)*, 1 oz.	150

peanut:

(Brach's Jots), 1 oz.	140
butter toffee *(Flavor House)*, 1 oz.	150
chocolate coated *(Brach's)*, 1 oz.	150
chocolate coated *(Brach's* Small), 1 oz.	140
chocolate coated *(Goobers)*, 1⅜ oz.	220
chocolate coated *(Nabisco)*, 1 oz.	160
filled *(Brach's)*, 1 oz.	110
French burnt *(Brach's)*, 1 oz.	130
peanut brittle *(Estee)*, ¼ oz.	35
peanut brittle *(Kraft)*, 1 oz.	130

peanut butter:

(PB Max), 1.48 oz.	240
candy coated *(Reese's Pieces)*, 1.85 oz.	260
chocolate coated, w/cookies *(Twix)*, 1.77-oz. bar	130

cup *(Estee)*, 1 piece	40
cup, chocolate coated *(Reese's)*, 1.8 oz.	280
kisses *(Brach's)*, 1 oz.	110
peanut caramel cluster *(Brach's)*, 1 oz.	150
peanut parfait *(Brach's)*, 1 oz.	160
peppermint kisses *(Brach's)*, 1 oz.	100
peppermint swirls *(Featherweight)*, 1 piece	20
popcorn, caramel coated:	
(Estee), 1-oz. bag	140
(Orville Redenbacher), 2.5 cups	240
and peanuts *(Cracker Jack)*, 1 oz.	120
raisins, chocolate coated:	
(Brach's), 1 oz.	130
(Estee), 10 pieces	30
(Nabisco), 1 oz. or 29 pieces	130
(Raisinets), 1 3/8 oz.	180
raspberry, filled *(Brach's)*, 1 oz.	110
ribbon, crimp *(Brach's)*, 1 oz.	110
rock *(Brach's Cut Rock)*, 1 oz.	110
(Snickers), 2.07-oz. bar	280
straws, mint filled *(Brach's)*, 1 oz.	110
taffy, all flavors *(Brach's Salt Water Taffy)*, 1 oz.	100
(3 Musketeers), 2.13-oz. bar	260
toffee:	
(Brach's), 1 oz.	110
(Callard & Bowser), 1 oz.	135
(Kraft), 1 piece	30
(Skor), 1.4 oz.	220
English *(Bits 'O Heath)*, 3 1/2 oz.	520
English *(Heath Bar)*, 2 pieces	180
(Tootsie Roll), 1 oz.	112
wafer, assorted *(Necco)*, 2.02-oz. roll	225
wafer bar, chocolate coated *(Kit Kat)*, 1.63 oz.	250

CHEWING GUM, one piece, except as noted

	calories
(Beech-Nut)	10
(Big Red)	10
(Care*Free)	8

Chewing Gum, continued

(Chewels)	8
(Clorets Stick)	9
(Dentyne)	6
(Dentyne Sugarless)	5
(Doublemint)	10
(Extra)	8
(Freedent)	10
(Freshen-Up)	13
(Juicy Fruit)	10
(Sticklets)	7
(Wrigley's Spearmint)	10
balls *(Brach's Gumdinger)*, 1 oz.	110

bubble:

(Bubble Yum)	25
(Bubble Yum Sugarless)	20
(Bubblicious)	25
(Bubblicious Sugarless)	5
(Care*Free)	10
(Extra)	7
(Hubba Bubba)	23
(Hubba Bubba Original Sugar Free)	14
grape *(Hubba Bubba* Sugar Free)	13

candy coated:

(Beechies)	6
(Chiclets)	6
(Chiclets Tiny), 1 pkg.	8
(Clorets)	6

Chapter 22

ICE CREAM AND
FROZEN CONFECTIONS

ICE CREAM & FROZEN CONFECTIONS
See also "Yogurt, Frozen," and "Baskin-Robbins"

---

	calories
ice, cherry, Italian *(Good Humor)*, 6 fl. oz.	138
ice bars, 1 bar:	
all flavors *(Gold Bond* Twin Pop)	60
all flavors *(Good Humor* Ice Stripes), 1.5 fl. oz.	35
all flavors *(Popsicle* Big Stick), 3.5 fl. oz.	80
all flavors, all natural *(Popsicle)*, 1.75 fl. oz.	40
banana or lime *(Popsicle)*, 1.75 fl. oz.	50
cherry *(Good Humor Calippo)*, 4.5 fl. oz.	138
grape *(Popsicle)*, 2.2 fl. oz.	50
lemon *(Good Humor Calippo)*, 4.5 fl. oz.	112
orange *(Good Humor Calippo)*, 4.5 fl. oz.	111
raspberry, root beer, or strawberry *(Popsicle)*, 1.75 fl. oz.	50
wildberry *(Popsicle)*, 1.75 fl. oz.	40
ice cream, 1/2 cup, except as noted:	
all flavors *(Borden Olde Fashioned Recipe)*	130
butter almond *(Breyers)*	170
butter crunch *(Sealtest)*	150
butter pecan *(Breyers)*	180
butter pecan *(Frusen Glädjé)*	280
butter pecan *(Häagen-Dazs)*	390
butter pecan *(Lady Borden)*	180
butter pecan *(Sealtest)*	160

Ice Cream & Frozen Confections, ice cream, 1/2 cup, continued

cherry vanilla *(Breyers)*	150
caramel nut sundae *(Häagen-Dazs)*	310
chocolate *(Breyers)*	160
chocolate *(Frusen Glädjé)*	240
chocolate *(Häagen-Dazs)*	270
chocolate or triple chocolate stripe *(Sealtest)*	140
chocolate, deep *(Häagen-Dazs)*	290
chocolate, deep, peanut butter *(Häagen-Dazs)*	330
chocolate, Swiss, almond *(Frusen Glädjé)*	270
chocolate chip *(Sealtest)*	150
chocolate-chocolate chip *(Breyers)*	180
chocolate-chocolate chip *(Frusen Glädjé)*	270
chocolate-chocolate chip *(Häagen-Dazs)*	290
chocolate mint *(Breyers)*	170
chocolate chip vanilla *(Frusen Glädjé)*	280
chocolate swirl *(Borden)*	130
coffee *(Breyers)*	150
coffee *(Frusen Glädjé)*	260
coffee *(Häagen-Dazs)*	270
coffee *(Sealtest)*	140
cookies n' cream *(Breyers)*	170
heavenly hash *(Sealtest)*	150
honey vanilla *(Häagen-Dazs)*	250
macadamia brittle *(Häagen-Dazs)*	280
maple walnut *(Sealtest)*	160
mocha chip *(Frusen Glädjé)*	280
peach *(Breyers)*	130
praline and cream *(Frusen Glädjé)*	280
rum raisin *(Häagen-Dazs)*	250
strawberry *(Borden)*	130
strawberry *(Breyers)*	130
strawberry *(Frusen Glädjé)*	230
strawberry *(Häagen-Dazs)*	250
strawberry *(Sealtest)*	130
vanilla *(Breyers)*	150
vanilla *(Eagle* Brand Homestyle)	150
vanilla *(Frusen Glädjé)*	230
vanilla *(Good Humor* Cup), 3 fl. oz.	98
vanilla *(Häagen-Dazs)*	260
vanilla, French vanilla, or vanilla fudge *(Sealtest)* . .	140

vanilla fudge *(Häagen-Dazs)* 270
vanilla fudge twirl *(Breyers)* 160
vanilla Swiss almond *(Frusen Glädjé)* 270
vanilla Swiss almond *(Häagen-Dazs)* 290
vanilla toffee chunk *(Frusen Glädjé)* 270
vanilla-chocolate-strawberry *(Breyers)* 150
vanilla-chocolate-strawberry *(Sealtest)* 140
vanilla-chocolate-strawberry *(Sealtest Cubic Scoops)* . 130
vanilla-orange *(Sealtest Cubic Scoops)* 130
vanilla-raspberry *(Sealtest Cubic Scoops)* 130
vanilla-raspberry swirl *(Frusen Glädjé)* 230
ice cream, substitute and imitation, 1/2 cup, except as
  noted:
all flavors *(Sealtest Free)* 100
all flavors, hard or soft-serve *(Lite-Lite Tofutti)* 90
cappuccino *(Tofutti* Love Drops) 230
chocolate *(Simple Pleasures)*, 4 oz. 140
chocolate *(Tofutti* Love Drops) 230
chocolate, supreme *(Tofutti)* 210
chocolate chip *(Low, Lite'n Luscious)* 100
coffee *(Simple Pleasures)*, 4 oz. 120
Jamoca Swiss almond *(Low, Lite'n Luscious)* 90
peach *(Simple Pleasures)*, 4 oz. 135
pineapple coconut *(Low, Lite'n Luscious)* 90
rum raisin *(Simple Pleasures)*, 4 oz. 130
strawberry *(Low, Lite'n Luscious)* 80
strawberry *(Simple Pleasures)*, 4 oz. 120
vanilla *(Tofutti)* 200
vanilla *(Tofutti* Love Drops) 220
vanilla, chocolate dipped *(Tofutti O's)*, 1 piece 40
vanilla-almond bark *(Tofutti)* 230
wildberry *(Tofutti)* 210
ice cream bars, 1 piece:
(Good Humor Fat Frog), 3 fl. oz. 154
(Good Humor Halo Bar), 2.5 fl. oz. 230
(Heath), 3 fl. oz. 170
(Klondike), 5 fl. oz. 280
(Klondike Krispy), 5 fl. oz. 290
(Klondike Lite), 2.5 fl. oz. 140
almond, toasted *(Good Humor)*, 3 fl. oz. 212
assorted *(Good Humor Whammy)*, 1.6 fl. oz. 95

Ice Cream & Frozen Confections, ice cream bars, 1 piece, continued

caramel almond *(Häagen-Dazs* Crunch)	240
chip candy crunch *(Good Humor)*, 3 fl. oz.	255
chocolate *(Klondike)*, 5 fl. oz.	270
chocolate, w/dark chocolate coating *(Häagen-Dazs)* .	390
chocolate, milk, w/almonds, milk chocolate coated *(Nestlé* Premium), 3.7 fl. oz.	350
chocolate, w/milk chocolate coating *(Nestlé Quik)* . .	210
chocolate eclair *(Good Humor)*, 3 fl. oz.	188
chocolate fudge cake *(Good Humor)*, 6.3 fl. oz.	214
chocolate fudge sundae *(Bakers Fudgetastic)*	220
chocolate fudge sundae, crunchy *(Bakers Fudgetastic)*	230
peanut butter *(Häagen-Dazs* Crunch)	270
strawberry shortcake *(Good Humor)*, 3 fl. oz.	176
vanilla *(Häagen-Dazs* Crunch)	220
vanilla, w/caramel peanut center, milk chocolate coated *(Oh! Henry)*, 3 fl. oz.	320
vanilla, chocolate coated *(Good Humor)*, 3 fl. oz. . . .	198
vanilla, w/dark chocolate coating *(Häagen-Dazs)* . . .	390
vanilla, w/milk chocolate coating *(Häagen-Dazs)* . . .	360
vanilla, w/milk chocolate coating and almonds *(Häagen-Dazs)*	370
vanilla, w/milk chocolate coating and crisps *(Nestlé Crunch)*, 3 fl. oz.	180
vanilla, w/white chocolate coating *(Nestlé Alpine* Premium), 3.7 fl. oz.	350
ice cream bars, substitute and imitation 1 bar:	
(Good Humor Cool Shark), 3 fl. oz.	68
(Good Humor Jumbo Jet Star), 4.5 fl. oz.	85
(Good Humor Milky Pop), 1.5 fl. oz.	45
amaretto-chocolate swirl *(Crystal Light Cool N'Creamy)*	60
chocolate *(Weight Watchers* Treat Bars), 2.75 oz. . . .	100
chocolate dip *(Weight Watchers)*, 1.7 oz.	110
chocolate fudge *(Good Humor)*, 2.5 fl. oz.	127
chocolate fudge, double *(Crystal Light Cool N'Creamy)*	50
chocolate fudge, double *(Weight Watchers)*, 1.75 oz. .	60
chocolate fudge swirl *(Sealtest Free)*	90
chocolate mousse *(Weight Watchers)*, 1.75 oz.	35
chocolate/vanilla *(Crystal Light Cool N'Creamy)* . . .	50

English toffee crunch *(Weight Watchers)*, 1.7 oz. ... 120
orange-vanilla *(Crystal Light Cool N'Creamy)* 30
orange-vanilla *(Weight Watchers* Sugar Free Treat
   Bars), 1.75 oz. 30
strawberry finger *(Good Humor)*, 2.5 fl. oz. 49
vanilla fudge or vanilla strawberry swirl *(Sealtest
   Free)* 80
vanilla sandwich *(Weight Watchers)* 150
ice cream cones or cups:
   filled *(Good Humor* King Cone), 5.5 fl. oz. 290
   boysenberry *(Good Humor* King Cone), 5 fl. oz. ... 340
   vanilla-chocolate cup *(Good Humor* Combo), 6 fl. oz. 201
ice cream mix, all flavors *(Salada)*, 1 cup* 310
ice cream sandwiches, 1 piece:
   chocolate chip cookie *(Good Humor)*, 2.7 fl. oz. ... 204
   chocolate chip cookie *(Good Humor)*, 4 fl. oz. 246
   vanilla *(Good Humor)*, 3 fl. oz. 191
   vanilla *(Good Humor)*, 2.5 fl. oz. 165
   vanilla *(Klondike)*, 5 fl. oz. 230
ice cream and sorbet, *see "sorbet," page 276*
ice milk, 1/2 cup:
   caramel nut *(Light N' Lively)* 120
   chocolate *(Borden)* 100
   chocolate *(Breyers* Light) 120
   chocolate *(Darigold* Lite) 110
   chocolate *(Weight Watchers Grand Collection)* 110
   chocolate chip *(Light N' Lively)* 120
   chocolate chip *(Weight Watchers Grand Collection)* . 120
   chocolate fudge twirl *(Breyers* Light) 130
   chocolate swirl *(Weight Watchers Grand Collection)* . 120
   coffee *(Light N' Lively)* 100
   cookies n' cream *(Light N' Lively)* 110
   heavenly hash *(Breyers* Light) 150
   heavenly hash *(Light N' Lively)* 120
   Neapolitan *(Weight Watchers Grand Collection)* 110
   pecan pralines'n creme *(Weight Watchers Grand
      Collection)* 120
   praline almond *(Breyers* Light) 130
   strawberry *(Borden)* 90
   strawberry *(Breyers* Light) 110
   toffee fudge Parfait *(Breyers* Light) 140

Ice Cream & Frozen Confections, ice milk, 1/2 cup, continued

vanilla *(Borden)*	90
vanilla *(Breyers* Light)	120
vanilla *(Light N' Lively)*	100
vanilla *(Weight Watchers Grand Collection)*	100
vanilla-chocolate almond *(Light N' Lively)*	120
vanilla-chocolate-strawberry *(Breyers* Light)	120
vanilla-chocolate-strawberry *(Light N' Lively)*	100
vanilla-fudge swirl *(Light N' Lively)*	110
vanilla-raspberry Parfait *(Breyers* Light)	130
vanilla-raspberry swirl *(Light N' Lively)*	110
ice milk cone *(Gold Bond* Olde Nut Sundae), 3 fl. oz.	230

sherbet:

all flavors *(Sealtest)*, 1/2 cup	130
orange *(Bordon)*, 1/2 cup	110
orange *(Darigold)*, 1/2 cup	120

sherbet bar, 1 bar:

all flavors *(Creamsicle* Sugar Free), 1.75 fl. oz.	25
all flavors *(Fudgsicle* Fat Free), 1.75 fl. oz.	70
all flavors *(Fudgsicle* Sugar Free), 1.75 fl. oz.	35
chocolate *(Fudgsicle)*, 1.75 oz.	70
chocolate, fudge nut dip *(Fudgsicle* Sugar Free), 2.1 fl. oz.	130

sorbet:

blueberry, key lime or orange, and cream *(Häagen-Dazs)*, 1/2 cup	190
orange, mandarin *(Dole)*, 4 oz.	110
peach or pineapple *(Dole)*, 4 oz.	120
raspberry *(Dole)*, 4 oz.	110
raspberry *(Frusen Glädjé)*, 1/2 cup	140
raspberry, and cream *(Häagen-Dazs)*, 1/2 cup	180
strawberry *(Dole)*, 4 oz.	110

* *Prepared according to package directions*

Chapter 23

NUTS, CHIPS, PRETZELS, AND RELATED SNACKS

NUTS & SEEDS, SHELLED, one ounce, except as noted
See also "Nut Butters"

	calories
almonds:	
(Beer Nuts)	180
(Dole)	170
all varieties *(Planters)*	170
cashews:	
(Beer Nuts)	170
dry-roasted *(Planters* Regular/Unsalted)	160
dry-roasted, whole *(Guys)*	170
honey-roasted *(Planters)*	170
honey-roasted, w/peanuts *(Planters)*	170
oil-roasted *(Flavor House)*	180
oil-roasted *(Planters* Fancy)	170
oil-roasted, halves *(Planters/Planters* Unsalted)	170
macadamia nuts, oil-roasted *(Mauna Loa)*	210
mixed nuts:	
w/peanuts *(Guy's)*	170
dry-roasted *(Planters)*	160
dry-roasted *(Planters* Unsalted)	170
oil-roasted *(Flavor House)*	180
peanuts:	
(Beer Nuts)	180
(Little Debbie), 1.25 oz.	230

Nuts & Seeds, Shelled, peanuts, continued

(Weight Watchers), 1 pouch	100
cocktail, oil-roasted (Planters Regular/Unsalted)	170
dry-roasted (Flavor House Regular/Unsalted)	180
dry-roasted (Frito-Lay's), 1⅛ oz.	190
dry-roasted (Guy's)	170
dry-roasted (Planters)	160
dry-roasted (Planters Unsalted)	170
honey-roasted (Eagle Honey Roast)	170
honey-roasted (Flavor House)	160
honey-roasted (Planters)	170
honey-roasted, dry-roasted (Planters)	160
oil-roasted (Flavor House)	170
oil-roasted (Planters)	170
redskin, oil-roasted (Planters)	170
Spanish (Guy's)	170
Spanish, dry-roasted (Planters)	160
Spanish, oil-roasted (Flavor House)	170
pecans, halves, pieces, or chips (Planters)	190
pistachios, dry-roasted (Planters)	170
pistachios, roasted (Dole)	163
sesame nut mix, dry roasted (Planters)	160
sunflower seed kernels:	
dried (Arrowhead Mills)	160
dry-roasted (Flavor House)	180
walnuts:	
black (Planters)	180
English or Persian (Diamond)	192
English or Persian (Planters)	190

CHIPS, PUFFS, & SIMILAR SNACKS, one ounce, except as noted
See also "Popcorn," "Pretzels," "Crackers," and "Nuts & Seeds, Shelled"

	calories
carrot chips (Hain Regular/No Salt Added)	150
carrot chips, barbecue (Hain)	140
cheddar sticks (Flavor Tree), ¼ cup	129

corn chips:
    (Azteca Unsalted) 140
    (Bachman) 160
    (Dipsy Doodles Rippled Corn Chips) 160
    (Featherweight Low Salt) 170
    (Fritos/Fritos Dip Size) 150
    (Fritos Crisp'n Thin) 160
    (Health Valley Regular/No Salt Added) 160
    (Planters) 160
    (Snyder's) 160
    all varieties *(Wise)* 160
    barbecue flavor *(Bachman* BBQ) 150
    barbecue flavor *(Fritos* Bar-B-Q) 150
    blue *(Arrowhead Mills* Corn Curls Regular/Unsalted) 120
    chili cheese *(Fritos)* 160
    ranch *(Fritos Wild'n Mild)* 150
    tortilla, *see "tortilla chips," page 281*
    yellow corn *(Arrowhead Mills)*, 3/4 oz. 90
corn crisps and puffs:
    (Bugles) 150
    (Chee • tos Puffs/Puffed Balls) 160
    (Cheez Doodles Baked Corn Puffs) 150
    (Cheez Doodles Fried Corn Puffs) 160
    (Featherweight Cheese Curls Low Salt) 150
    (Jax Baked) 140
    (Jax Crunchy) 160
    (Planters Cheez Balls/Curls) 160
    (Wise Cheez Waffies) 140
    cheddar cheese *(Health Valley)* 160
    crunchy *(Chee • tos)* 150
    crunchy *(Chee • tos* Light) 140
    nacho cheese *(Bugles)* 160
onion flavored chips *(Funyuns)* 140
onion flavored rings *(Wise)* 130
pasta snack chip *(Bachman Pastapazazz)* 150
pork rind snack *(Baken • ets)* 160
potato chips and crisps:
    all varieties *(Eagle)* 150
    all varieties *(Health Valley)* 160
    all varieties *(Pringle's)* 170
    all varieties *(Pringle's* Light) 150

Chips, Puffs, & Similar Snacks, potato chips and crisps, continued

all varieties *(Zapp's* Original Kettle/Lite)	150
(Bachman Regular/Unsalted/Ridge/Ruffled)	160
(Bachman Kettle Cooked)	140
(Barrel O'Fun)	150
(Cape Cod/Cape Cod Waves Regular/No Salt)	150
(Cottage Fries No Salt Added)	160
(Featherweight Low Salt)	160
(King Kold Regular/Rip-L)	150
(Lay's Regular/Unsalted).....................	150
(Munchos)	150
(O'Boisies)	150
(Ruffles)	150
(Ruffles Light)	130
(Snacktime Krunchers!)	150
(Wise Plain or Rippled/*Wise Ridgies)*	150
(Wise New York Deli)	160
au gratin or dill *(King Kold)*	150
barbecue *(Bachman)*	150
barbecue *(King Kold* BBQ)	140
barbecue *(Lay's* Bar-B-Q)	150
barbecue *(Ruffles)*	150
barbecue *(Wise/Wise Ridgies)*	150
Cajun *(Ruffles Cajun Spice)*	150
cheddar and sour cream *(Ruffles)*	150
dill and sour cream *(Cape Cod* Regular/No Salt)...	150
hot *(Bachman)*	150
hot *(Wise)*	160
jalapeño *(Snacktime Krunchers!)*	150
mesquite *(Ruffles* Mesquite Grille)	160
mesquite *(Snacktime Krunchers!)*	150
onion-garlic *(King Kold)*	150
onion-garlic *(Wise)*	150
ranch *(Ruffles)*	160
salt and vinegar *(Lay's)*	150
Saratoga style *(Bachman* Kettle Cooked)	140
skins, all flavors *(Tato Skins)*	150
sour cream and onion *(Bachman)*	150
sour cream and onion *(King Kold)*	150
sour cream and onion *(Lay's)*	160
sour cream and onion *(O'Boisies)*	150

sour cream and onion *(Ruffles)* 150
sour cream and onion *(Wise Ridgies)* 160
vinegar *(Bachman)* 150
potato sticks, shoestring, canned *(Allens)* 140
sesame chips *(Flavor Tree)*, 1/4 cup 163
sesame sticks *(Flavor Tree)*, 1/4 cup 133
sesame sticks *(Flavor Tree No Salt)*, 1/4 cup 131
snack chips or mix:
  (Eagle) 140
  (Flavor Tree Party Mix, Regular/No Salt), 1/4 cup . . 163
  (Pepperidge Farm Classic) 140
  (Ralston Chex Traditional) 120
  (Super Snax) 137
  all flavors *(Great Snackers)*, 1 pouch 60
  cheddar or nacho *(Ralston Chex)* 130
  lightly smoked *(Pepperidge Farm)* 150
  sour cream and onion *(Ralston Chex)* 130
  spicy *(Pepperidge Farm)* 140
sour cream and onion sticks *(Flavor Tree)*, 1/4 cup . . . 127
taro snack chips *(Ray's)* 139
tortilla chips:
  all varieties *(Doritos)* 140
  all varieties *(Doritos* Light) 120
  all varieties *(Featherweight* Low Salt) 150
  (Bachman Regular/No Salt) 140
  (Buenitos Tortilla Chips Regular/No Salt Added) . . 150
  (La Famous Regular/No Salt Added) 140
  (Laura Scudder's Restaurant Style Lightly Salted) . . 140
  (Old El Paso Nachips) 150
  (Tostitos) 140
  blue *(Bearitos* Organic) 146
  blue *(Bearitos* Organic No Salt) 137
  crispy *(Old El Paso)* 150
  nacho *(Bachman)* 140
  nacho *(Bravos* Strips) 140
  nacho *(Bravos* Rounds) 150
  nacho *(Laura Scudder's* Triangles) 140
  nacho *(Tio Sancho)*, 1/2 oz. 70
  nacho, jalapeño flavor *(Bravos)* 150
  nacho, jalapeño flavor *(Laura Scudder's* Strips) 150
  nacho, sharp *(Tostitos)* 150

Chips, Puffs, & Similar Snacks, tortilla chips, continued

picante flavor, savory and mild *(Laura Scudder's*
Restaurant Style Strips)   150
ranch *(Eagle)*   140
sesame *(Hain* Regular/No Salt Added)   140
sesame, cheese *(Hain)*   160
taco style *(Hain)*   160
yellow corn *(Bearitos* Organic)   143
yellow corn *(Bearitos* Organic No Salt)   148
wasabi snack chips *(Eden)*   130

POPCORN, popped, except as noted	

	calories
(Bachman), 1/2 oz.	80
(Bachman Lite), 1/2 oz.	50
(Bearitos Organic Lite), 1 oz.	132
(Bearitos Organic No Salt), 1 oz.	108
(Bearitos Organic Traditional), 1 oz.	140
(Bonnie Lee), popped w/out oil and salt, 1 oz.	109
(Bonnie Lee), popped w/oil and salt, 1 oz.	172
(Frito-Lay's), 1/2 oz.	70
(Jiffy Pop Pan Popcorn), 4 cups	130
(Laura Scudder's Tender Baby White Corn), 1/2 oz. . .	80
(Orville Redenbacher Natural), 3 cups	80
(Orville Redenbacher Natural Salt Free), 3 cups	90
(Weight Watchers Lightly Salted), .66-oz. pkg.	80
(Wise Tender Baby White Corn), 1/2 oz.	80
(Wise Tender Eating Baby Popcorn), 1/2 oz.	70
butter flavor:	
(Jiffy Pop Pan Popcorn), 4 cups	130
(Orville Redenbacher Regular/Salt Free), 3 cups . . .	80
(Wise), 1/2 oz.	80
cheese and cheese flavor:	
(Bachman), 1/2 oz.	90
(Bearitos Organic), 1 oz.	137
(Frito-Lay's), 1/2 oz.	80
cheddar *(Orville Redenbacher)*, 3 cups	160
cheddar, white *(Bachman)*, 1/2 oz.	70
cheddar, white *(Cape Cod)*, 1/2 oz.	80

cheddar, white *(Clover Club)*, 1/2 oz.	70
cheddar, white *(Keebler* Deluxe), 1 oz.	140
cheddar, white *(Laura Scudder's)*, 1/2 oz.	70
cheddar, white *(Weight Watchers)*, .66-oz. bag	100
cheddar, white *(Wise)*, 1/2 oz.	70
honey caramel *(Keebler* Pop Deluxe), 1 oz.	120
microwave, 3 cups, except as noted:	
(Featherweight Natural Low Salt)	80
(Weight Watchers), 1 oz. or 1 pkg.	100
butter flavor *(Featherweight* Low Salt)	100
natural or butter flavor *(Jiffy Pop)*, 4 cups	140
natural or butter flavor *(Jolly Time)*	150
natural or butter flavor *(Orville Redenbacher* Lite)	50
natural or butter flavor *(Pillsbury)*	210
natural or butter flavor *(Planters)*	140
natural or butter flavor *(Pop • Secret)*	100
natural or butter flavor *(Pop • Secret* Light)	70
natural or butter flavor *(Pop Weaver's)*, 4 cups	140
natural or butter flavor *(Pops-Rite)*	90
cheddar cheese flavor *(Jolly Time)*	180
cheese flavor *(Pop • Secret)*, 1/3 pkg. unpopped	170
frozen *(Pillsbury* Salt-Free)	170
frozen, original or butter flavor *(Pillsbury)*	210
white:	
(Jolly Time), 4 cups	75
or yellow, air popped *(Pops-Rite)*, 1 oz.	100
or yellow, oil popped *(Pops-Rite)*, 1 oz.	220
yellow *(Jolly Time)*, 4 cups	88

PRETZELS, one ounce, except as noted

	calories
(A & Eagle)	110
(Estee Unsalted), 5 pieces	25
(Featherweight Low Salt), 20 pieces	110
all varieties:	
(Bachman)	110
(Rokeach)	110
(Rold Gold)	110
except Dutch and twists *(Mr. Salty)*	110

Pretzels, continued

beer *(Quinlan)*	110
braids or knots *(Keebler* Butter Pretzels)	110
cheddar flavor *(Combos),* 1.8 oz.	240
Dutch *(Mr. Salty),* 2 pieces	110
logs *(Quinlan)*	103
oat bran *(Quinlan)*	115
rice bran *(Quinlan* No-Salt)	101
sticks *(Quinlan)*	105

thins:

(Quinlan)	104
(Quinlan Ultra Thins)	106
tiny *(Quinlan)*	109
tiny *(Quinlan* No-Salt)	115
twists *(Mr. Salty),* 5 pieces	110

GRANOLA & SNACK BARS, one bar
See also "Breakfast Bars"

---

calories

granola bars:

all varieties, except oat bran-honey graham *(Nature Valley)*	120
w/almonds, chewy *(Sunbelt)*	120
caramel nut *(Quaker Granola Dipps)*	148
chocolate chip *(Quaker Chewy)*	128
chocolate chip *(Quaker Granola Dipps)*	139
chocolate chip, chewy *(Sunbelt)*	150
chocolate chip, chocolate coated *(Hershey's)*	170
chocolate chip, fudge dipped, chewy *(Sunbelt)*	220
w/chocolate chips, chewy *(Sunbelt)*	220
chocolate fudge *(Quaker Granola Dipps)*	160
chocolate graham and marshmallow *(Quaker Chewy)*	126
cocoa creme, chocolate coated *(Hershey's)*	180
Common Sense, raspberry filled *(Kellogg's Smart Start)*	170
cookies and creme, chocolate coated *(Hershey's)*	170
corn flakes, mixed berry filled *(Kellogg's Smart Start)*	170
honey and oats *(Quaker Chewy)*	125
nut and raisin, chunky *(Quaker Chewy)*	131

(Nutri • Grain) blueberry or strawberry *(Kellogg's Smart Start)* 180
oat bran-honey graham *(Nature Valley)* 110
oats and honey, chewy *(Sunbelt)* 130
oats and honey, fudge dipped, chewy *(Sunbelt)* 190
peanut butter *(Quaker Chewy)* 128
peanut butter *(Quaker Granola Dipps)* 170
peanut butter, chocolate coated *(Hershey's)* 180
peanut butter, chocolate coated *(Kudos)* 190
peanut butter chocolate chip *(Quaker Chewy)* 131
peanut butter chocolate chip *(Quaker Granola Dipps)* 174
w/peanuts, fudge dipped, chewy *(Sunbelt)*, 2.25 oz. . 300
raisin bran *(Kellogg's Smart Start)* 160
raisin and cinnamon *(Quaker Chewy)* 128
w/raisins, chewy *(Sunbelt)* 150
w/raisins, fudge dipped, chewy *(Sunbelt)* 200
(Rice Krispies), w/almonds *(Kellogg's Smart Start)* . 130
snack bars:
apple *(Health Valley Apple Bakes)* 100
date *(Health Valley Date Bakes)* 100
fruit *(Health Valley Fruit & Fitness)* 100
oat bran, almond and date *(Health Valley Oat Bran Jumbo Fruit Bars)* 170
oat bran, apricot *(Health Valley Oat Bran Apricot Bakes)* 100
oat bran, fig and nut *(Health Valley Fig & Nut Bakes)* 110
oat bran, fruit and nut *(Health Valley Oat Bran Jumbo Fruit Bars)* 150
oat bran, raisin and cinnamon *(Health Valley Oat Bran Jumbo Fruit Bars)* 140
raisin *(Health Valley Raisin Bakes)* 100
rice bran, almond and date *(Health Valley Rice Bran Jumbo Fruit Bars)* 190

Chapter 24

COCOA, COFFEE, TEA, AND SOFT DRINKS

COCOA & FLAVORED MIXES, DRY
See also "Dessert Toppings & Syrups" and "Flavored Milk Beverages"

---

	calories
all flavors, 1 pouch:	
(Carnation Instant Breakfast)	130
(Carnation Instant Breakfast No Sugar Added)	70
except vanilla *(Pillsbury* Instant Breakfast)	130
chocolate flavor:	
(Hershey's), .8 oz. or 3 tsp.	90
(Nestlé Quik), ¾ oz. or 2½ heaping tsp.	90
(Nestlé Quik Sugar Free), 1 heaping tsp.	18
fudge milkshake *(Weight Watchers)*, 1 pkt.	70
cocoa, powder:	
(Bensdorp), 1 oz.	130
(Hershey's), 1 oz. or ⅓ cup	120
(Hershey's European), 1 oz.	90
(Nestlé), 1.5 oz. or ½ cup	180
cocoa mix:	
(Carnation 70-Calorie), 1 pkt.	70
(Featherweight), .44 oz.	50
(Hills Bros), 2 tbsp.	110
(Hills Bros Sugar Free), 3 tsp.	60
(Swiss Miss Lite), 1 pkt.	70
(Swiss Miss Sugar Free), 1 pkt.	50
all varieties *(Carnation* Sugar Free), 1 pkt.	50
Amaretto creme *(Swiss Miss)*, 1.25 oz.	150
chocolate, double rich, or milk *(Swiss Miss)*, 1 pkt. .	110

chocolate, milk, or rich *(Carnation)*, 1 pkt. 110
chocolate, milk, and marshmallow *(Weight
  Watchers)*, 1 pkt. 60
chocolate creme *(Swiss Miss)*, 1.25 oz. 150
chocolate fudge *(Carnation)*, 1-oz. pkt. 110
w/marshmallows, regular or chocolate *(Carnation)*,
  1 pkt. or 4 heaping tsp. 110
w/mini marshmallows *(Swiss Miss)*, 1 oz. 110
mint *(Featherweight)*, .44 oz. 50
malted milk flavor *(Carnation Original)*, 3 heaping tsp. 90
malted milk flavor, chocolate *(Carnation)*, 3 heaping
  tsp. 80
orange sherbet milkshake *(Weight Watchers)*, 1 pkt. . . . 70
strawberry flavor *(Nestlé Quik)*, ¾ oz. or 2½ heaping
  tsp. 80
vanilla flavor *(Pillsbury Instant Breakfast)*, 1 pouch . . 140

COFFEE*

	calories
plain:	

ground roast *(Chock Full O'Nuts Regular/
  Decaffeinated)*, 6 fl. oz. 2
freeze-dried *(Taster's Choice Original/Colombian/
  Maragor)*, 8 fl. oz. 4
instant *(Kava)*, 1 tsp. powder 2
instant *(Nescafé/Nescafé Decaf)*, 8 fl. oz. 4
instant *(Nescafé Classic/Brava/Silka)*, 8 fl. oz. 4
instant, w/chicory *(Nescafé Mountain Blend/
  Mountain Blend Decaffeinated)*, 8 fl. oz. 6
instant, w/chicory *(Sunrise)*, 8 fl. oz. 6
flavored, 6 fl. oz.:
all flavors, except café Francais *(General Foods
  International Sugar Free)* 30
café Amaretto *(General Foods International)* 50
café Francais *(General Foods International)* 60
café Francais *(General Foods International Sugar
  Free)* 35
café Irish creme *(General Foods International)* 50
café Vienna *(General Foods International)* 60

Coffee*, flavored, 6 fl. oz., continued
  café Vienna *(Hills Bros Cafe Coffees)* 60
  chocolate, double Dutch *(General Foods*
    International) 50
  chocolate mint, Dutch *(General Foods* International) 50
  mocha *(General Foods* International Suisse Mocha) . 50
  mocha *(MJB)* 52
  mocha, banana nut *(MJB* Sugar Free) 39
  mocha, cherry *(MJB)* 53
  mocha, fudge *(MJB* Sugar Free) 39
  mocha mint *(MJB)* 53
  mocha mint *(MJB* Sugar Free) 37
  mocha, Swiss *(Hills Bros* Cafe Coffees) 60
  mocha, Swiss *(Hills Bros* Cafe Coffees Sugar Free) . . 40
  mocha, vanilla *(MJB* Sugar Free) 39
  orange cappuccino *(General Foods* International) . . . 60
  orange capri *(Hills Bros* Cafe Coffees) 60
substitute (cereal grain beverage):
  (Kaffree Roma), 8 fl. oz. 6
  (Pero), 1 serving, powder 4
  (Pionier), 1 serving, powder 6
  regular or coffee flavor *(Postum* Instant), 6 fl. oz. . . 12

* Brewed or prepared according to package directions, except as noted

---

TEA, PLAIN, FLAVORED, & HERBAL*, eight fluid
ounces, except as noted

                                                          calories
plain:
  (Nestea), 6 fl. oz. 0
  caffeine-free *(Celestial Seasonings)* 4
  instant, regular or decaffeinated *(Lipton),* 6 fl. oz. . . . 0
  instant, lemon flavor *(Lipton),* 6 fl. oz. 3
flavored or special blend *(see also "herbal," page 289):*
  all flavors *(Celestial Seasonings* Fruit & Tea) . . . . . . <3
  Amaretto *(Celestial Seasonings Amaretto Nights)* . . . 3
  (Bigelow Chinese Fortune), 5¼ fl. oz. 1
  (Bigelow Constant Comment), 5¼ fl. oz. 1
  (Bigelow English Teatime), 5¼ fl. oz. 1

(Celestial Seasonings Classic English Breakfast) 3
(Celestial Seasonings Morning Thunder) 3
chocolate orange *(Celestial Seasonings Bavarian
    Chocolate Orange)* 7
cinnamon *(Bigelow Cinnamon Stick)*, 5¼ fl. oz. ... 1
cinnamon *(Celestial Seasonings Cinnamon Vienna)* .. 2
darjeeling *(Celestial Seasonings Darjeeling Gardens)* . 3
darjeeling or Earl Grey *(Bigelow)* 5¼ fl. oz. 1
Earl Grey *(Celestial Seasonings Extraordinary Earl
    Grey)* 3
Irish cream *(Celestial Seasonings Irish Cream Mist)* . 3
lemon *(Bigelow Lemon Lift)*, 5¼ fl. oz. 1
mint *(Bigelow Plantation Mint)*, 5¼ fl. oz. 1
mint, Swiss *(Celestial Seasonings)* .... <3
raspberry *(Bigelow Raspberry Royale)*, 5¼ fl. oz. ... 1
raspberry *(Celestial Seasonings* Fruit & Tea) 2
herbal, all varieties (all brands), 6 fl. oz. .... < 10
iced, canned or bottled:
    (Shasta), 12 fl. oz. 124
    w/lemon *(Lipton* Presweetened) 83
    w/lemon *(Lipton* Sugar Free) .... <1
    w/lemon *(Nestea* Sugar Free) 2
    w/lemon *(Nestea* Sugar Sweetened) 70
    w/lemon *(Veryfine)* 80
    w/natural lemon flavor *(Lipton* Aseptic), 8.45 oz. .. 96
    lemon flavored *(Wyler's* Fruit Tea Punch), 12 oz. .. 118
iced, instant or mix:
    (Crystal Light Sugar Free Decaffeinated) 4
    (Lipton Sugar Free Regular/Decaffeinated) 1
    (Nestea 100%) 2
    (Nestea 100% Decaffeinated) 0
    flavored, all flavors *(Nestea* Ice Teasers) 6
    lemon flavor *(Lipton* Regular/Decaffeinated), 6 fl. oz. 55
    lemon flavor *(Nestea)* 6
    lemon flavor *(Nestea* Presweetened) 70
    lemon flavor *(Nestea* Sugar Free) 4
    lemon flavor, *(Nestea* Sugar Free Decaffeinated),
      2 tsp. 6

---

* *Brewed or prepared according to package directions, except as noted*

> **SOFT DRINKS & MIXERS,** six fluid ounces, except as noted
> *See also "Fruit & Fruit-Flavored Drinks" and "Cocktail Mixes, Nonalcoholic"*

	calories
all flavors *(Natural 90* Diet)	2
all flavors *(Schweppes* Royal)	35
berry, red *(Shasta)*	79
berry, wild *(Health Valley)*	71
cherry, black *(Shasta)*	81
cherry cola:	
(Coca-Cola)	76
(Diet Coke)	<1
(Diet Wild Cherry Pepsi)	<1
(Pepsi Wild Cherry)	82
(Shasta)	70
cherry-lime *(Spree)*	79
chocolate *(Yoo-Hoo),* 9 fl. oz.	140
citrus mist *(Shasta)*	85
club soda (all brands)	0
cola:	
(Coca-Cola Regular/Caffeine-free)	77
(Coca-Cola Classic)	72
(Diet Coke Regular/Caffeine-free)	<1
(Diet Pepsi Regular/Caffeine-free)	<1
(Jolt)	85
(Pepsi Regular/Caffeine-free)	80
(Pepsi Light)	<1
(Shasta)	74
(Shasta Free)	76
(Spree)	74
(Tab Regular/Caffeine-free)	<1
cherry, *see "cherry cola," above*	
collins mixer:	
(Canada Dry), 8 fl. oz.	80
(Schweppes)	75
(Shasta)	59
cream *(A&W)*	84
cream *(Shasta* Creme)	77
(Dr. Diablo)	70

(Dr Pepper Regular/Caffeine-free)	75
(Dr Pepper Diet Regular/Caffeine-free)	<2
(Fresca)	2
fruit punch *(Shasta)*	87
ginger ale:	
(Canada Dry), 8 fl. oz.	90
(Canada Dry Golden), 8 fl. oz.	100
(Fanta)	63
(Health Valley)	77
(Shasta)	60
(Spree)	60
plain or raspberry *(Schweppes)*	65
plain or raspberry *(Schweppes* Sugar Free Diet)	2
ginger beer *(Schweppes)*	70
grape:	
(Canada Dry Concord), 8 fl. oz.	130
(Fanta)	86
(Schweppes)	95
(Shasta)	89
grapefruit:	
(Schweppes)	80
(Spree)	77
(Wink), 8 fl. oz.	120
half & half *(Canada Dry),* 8 fl. oz.	110
lemon, bitter *(Schweppes)*	82
lemon sour *(Schweppes)*	79
lemon-lime:	
(Diet Slice)	8
(Schweppes)	72
(Shasta)	73
(Slice)	75
(Spree)	77
lemon-tangerine *(Spree)*	83
lime, Mandarin *(Spree)*	77
(Mello Yello)	87
(Mello Yello Diet)	3
(Mountain Dew)	90
(Mountain Dew Diet)	2
(Mr. Pibb)	71
orange:	
(Diet Slice)	6

Chapter 25

FAST-FOOD CHAINS
AND RESTAURANTS

NOTE: The listings in this section—which are broken down by restaurant rather than by food category—are generally based on one "average" or "standard" serving. The caloric content of a serving may vary slightly according to restaurant location. And, of course, individual orders that result in a change of ingredients or quantity of ingredients will alter the caloric value. Wherever possible, the weight of a serving has been included as a guide.

ARBY'S

	calories
sandwiches:	
beef 'n cheddar, 7 oz.	455
chicken breast, 6.5 oz.	493
ham 'n cheese, 5.5 oz.	292
roast beef, regular, 5.2 oz.	353
roast beef, super, 8.3 oz.	501
roast chicken club, 8.3 oz.	610
turkey deluxe, 7 oz.	375
french fries, 2.5 oz.	246
potato cakes, 3 oz.	204
shake, Jamocha, 11.5 oz.	368

ARTHUR TREACHER'S

	calories
chicken, 2 patties, 4.8 oz.	369
chicken sandwich, 5.5 oz.	413
chips, 4 oz.	276
cod tail shape, bake 'n broil, 5 oz.	245
coleslaw, 3 oz.	123
fish, 2 pieces, 5.2 oz.	355
fish sandwich, 5.5 oz.	440
Krunch Pup, 2-oz. piece	203
Lemon Luvs, 3-oz. piece	276
shrimp, 7 pieces, 4.1 oz.	381

BASKIN-ROBBINS, one regular scoop

	calories
ice, daiquiri	140
ice cream:	
almond fudge	270
chocolate	275
chocolate chip	260
chocolate raspberry truffle	310
pralines'n cream	280
rocky road	300
strawberry	220
vanilla	240
vanilla, French	280
sherbet, rainbow	160
sorbet, red raspberry	140
sugar cone, 1 cone	60
waffle cone, 1 cone	140

BURGER KING

	calories
breakfast bagel sandwich:	
regular	387
w/bacon	438

w/ham	418
w/sausage	731
breakfast *Croissan'wich:*	
regular	304
w/bacon	354
w/ham	335
w/sausage	538
French toast sticks	449
Great Danish	500
scrambled egg platter:	
regular	468
w/bacon	536
w/sausage	702
sandwiches:	
bacon double cheeseburger	510
bacon double cheeseburger deluxe	592
barbeque bacon double cheeseburger	536
BK Broiler chicken	379
cheeseburger	317
chicken Specialty Sandwich	688
double cheeseburger	483
ham and cheese Specialty Sandwich	471
hamburger	275
mushroom Swiss double cheeseburger	473
Whaler fish sandwich	488
Whopper	628
Whopper, w/cheese	711
Whopper Jr.	322
Whopper Jr. w/cheese	364
tenders, chicken, 6 pieces	236
tenders, fish, 6 pieces	267
salad, 1 serving:	
chef salad	180
chicken salad	140
garden salad	90
side salad	20
dressings, 1 pkt.:	
bleu cheese	300
French	280
house	260
Italian, reduced calorie	30

Burger King, dressings, 1 pkt., continued
Thousand Island	240
sauces and condiments:	
bacon bits, 1 pkt.	16
croutons, 1 pkt.	19
ranch dipping sauce, 1 oz.	171
sweet & sour sauce, 1 oz.	45
tartar dipping sauce, 1 oz.	174
side dishes:	
french fries, regular	227
onion rings	274
tater tenders, 2.5 oz.	213
apple pie	305

CARL'S JR.

calories
breakfast:	
bacon, 2 strips, .4 oz.	50
eggs, scrambled, 2.4 oz.	120
English muffin, w/margarine, 2 oz.	180
French toast dips, w/out syrup, 4.7 oz.	480
hash brown nuggets, 3 oz.	170
hot cakes, w/margarine, w/out syrup, 5.5 oz.	360
sausage, 1 patty, .5 oz.	190
Sunrise Sandwich, w/bacon, 4.5 oz.	370
Sunrise Sandwich, w/sausage, 6.1 oz.	500
sandwiches:	
California Roast Beef 'n Swiss, 7.4 oz.	360
Charbroiler BBQ Chicken Sandwich, 6.3 oz.	320
Charbroiler Chicken Club Sandwich, 8.3 oz.	510
Country Fried Steak Sandwich, 7.2 oz.	610
Double Western Bacon Cheeseburger, 7.5 oz.	890
Famous Star Hamburger, 8.1 oz.	590
fish fillet, 7.9 oz.	550
Happy Star hamburger, 3 oz.	220
Old Time Star hamburger, 5.9 oz.	400
Super Star hamburger, 10.6 oz.	770
Western Bacon Cheeseburger, 7.5 oz.	630

potatoes:
    bacon and cheese, 14.1 oz.   650
    broccoli and cheese, 14 oz.   470
    cheese, 14.2 oz.   350
    Fiesta, 15.2 oz.   550
    Lite, 9.8 oz.   250
    sour cream and chive, 10.4 oz.   350
salad-to-go:
    chef, 10.7 oz.   180
    chicken, 10.9 oz.   206
    garden, 4.1 oz.   46
    taco, 14.3 oz.   356
salad dressing, 1 oz.:
    blue cheese   151
    French, reduced calorie   38
    house   110
    Italian   120
    Thousand Island   110
side dishes:
    french fries, regular, 6 oz.   360
    onion rings, 3.2 oz.   310
    zucchini, 4.3 oz.   300
soup, 6.6 oz.:
    Boston clam chowder   140
    broccoli, cream of   140
    chicken noodle, old fashioned   80
    Lumber Jack Mix vegetable   70
bakery products:
    blueberry muffin, 3.5 oz.   256
    bran muffin, 4 oz.   220
    brownie, fudge, 4.5 oz.   597
    chocolate chip cookie, 2.5 oz.   327
    cinnamon roll, 4 oz.   459
    danish (varieties), 4 oz.   519
shakes, regular, 11.6 oz.   353

DAIRY QUEEN

	calories
chicken nuggets, all white, 3.5 oz.	276
chicken nuggets sauce, BBQ, 1 oz.	41
hamburgers:	
single, 5.2 oz.	360
double, 7.4 oz.	530
triple, 10 oz.	710
w/cheese, single, 5.7 oz.	410
w/cheese, double, 8.4 oz.	650
w/cheese, triple, 10 oz.	820
hot dogs:	
3.5 oz.	280
w/cheese, 4 oz.	330
w/chili, 4.5 oz.	320
sandwiches:	
chicken breast fillet, 7.1 oz.	608
chicken breast fillet, w/cheese, 7.6 oz.	661
DQ Hounder, 5.3 oz.	480
DQ Hounder, w/cheese, 5.8 oz.	533
DQ Hounder, w/chili, 7.3 oz.	575
fish fillet, 6.2 oz.	430
fish fillet, w/cheese, 6.7 oz.	483
side dishes:	
french fries, 2.5 oz.	200
french fries, large, 4 oz.	320
lettuce, .5 oz.	2
onion rings, 3 oz.	280
tomato, .5 oz.	4
desserts and shakes:	
Buster Bar, 5.3 oz.	448
Chipper Sandwich, 4 oz.	318
cone, small, 3 oz.	140
cone, regular, 5 oz.	240
cone, large, 7.5 oz.	340
cone, dipped, small, 3.2 oz.	190
cone, dipped, regular, 5.5 oz.	340
cone, dipped, large, 8.3 oz.	510
Dilly Bar, 3 oz.	210
DQ Sandwich, 2.1 oz.	140

float, 14 oz. 410
freeze, 14 oz. 500
Fudge Nut Bar, 5 oz. 406
Heath Blizzard, regular, 14.3 oz. 800
malt, small, 8.5 oz. 438
malt, regular, 14.7 oz. 760
malt, large, 17.2 oz. 889
Mr. Misty, small, 8.7 oz. 190
Mr. Misty, regular, 11.6 oz. 250
Mr. Misty, large, 15.5 oz. 340
Mr. Misty Float, 14.5 oz. 390
Mr. Misty Freeze, 14.5 oz. 500
Mr. Misty Kiss, 3.1 oz. 89
parfait, 10 oz. 430
Peanut Buster Parfait, 10.8 oz. 740
shake, small, 8.5 oz. 409
shake, regular, 14.7 oz. 710
shake, large, 17.2 oz. 813
sundae, small, 3.7 oz. 190
sundae, regular, 6.2 oz. 310
sundae, large, 8.7 oz. 440

DOMINO'S PIZZA, two slices

	calories
cheese	376
deluxe	498
double cheese/pepperoni	545
ham	417
pepperoni	460
sausage/mushroom	430
veggie	498

DRUTHER'S*

	calories
bacon and egg:	
biscuit, 3.1 oz.	258
plate, fried egg, 10 oz.	721

Druther's*, bacon and egg, continued

plate, scrambled egg, 11.1 oz.	742
biscuits and gravy, 8.1 oz.	331

ham and egg:

biscuit, 3.5 oz.	217
plate, fried egg, 10.9 oz.	681
plate, scrambled egg, 12.1 oz.	762

sausage and egg:

biscuit, 3.3 oz.	246
plate, fried egg, 10.6 oz.	741
plate, scrambled egg, 10 oz.	762
1 sausage, 1 biscuit, 1.7 oz.	179
2 sausages, 2 biscuits, 3.4 oz.	358

cheeseburger:

4.7 oz.	380
deluxe quarter, 8.7 oz.	660
double, 6.4 oz.	500
chicken, 8 pieces, 2.6 lbs.	3,664
chicken, 12 pieces, 3.9 lbs.	5,496

chicken dinner:

2-piece, breast and wing, 14 oz.	970
2-piece, leg and thigh, 13.4 oz.	925
3-piece, breast, thigh, and leg, 1.1 lb.	1,281
3-piece, breast, thigh, and wing, 1.1 lb.	1,309

chicken snack:

breast and wing, 14 oz.	970
breast and wing, 7.5 oz.	595
thigh and leg, 13.4 oz.	925
thigh and leg, 7 oz.	549
fish and chips, 11.2 oz.	729
fish dinner, 13.3 oz.	770
fish sandwich, 4.8 oz.	349
hamburger, 4.4 oz.	327

* *Values for all dishes or dinners are complete as served, including accompanying biscuits, potatoes, coleslaw, hush puppies, etc.*

DUNKIN' DONUTS, one piece

	calories
apple filled, w/cinnamon sugar, 2.9 oz.	250
Bavarian filled, w/chocolate frosting, 2.9 oz.	240
blueberry filled, 2.4 oz.	210
buttermilk ring, glazed, 2.6 oz.	290
cake ring, plain, 2.2 oz.	270
cake ring, chocolate, w/glaze, 2.5 oz.	324
coffee roll, glazed, 2.9 oz.	280
cookies:	
chocolate chunk, 1.5 oz.	200
chocolate chunk, w/nuts, 1.5 oz.	210
oatmeal pecan raisin, 1.6 oz.	200
croissant:	
plain, 2.5 oz.	310
almond, 3.7 oz.	420
chocolate, 3.3 oz.	440
cruller, French, w/glaze, 1.3 oz.	140
jelly filled, 2.4 oz.	220
lemon filled, 2.9 oz.	260
muffins:	
apple spice, 3.5 oz.	300
blueberry, 3.6 oz.	280
bran, w/raisins, 3.7 oz.	310
corn, 3.4 oz.	340
cranberry nut, 3.5 oz.	290
oat bran, 3.4 oz.	330
Munchkins, yeast, w/glaze, .4 oz.	43
whole wheat ring, glazed, 2.9 oz.	330
yeast ring, chocolate frosted, 1.9 oz.	200
yeast ring, glazed, 1.9 oz.	200

GODFATHER'S PIZZA

	calories
original cheese:	
mini, 1/4 pie, 2.8 oz.	190
small, 1/6 pie, 3.6 oz.	240
medium, 1/8 pie, 4 oz.	270

Godfather's Pizza, original cheese, continued

   large, 1/10 pie, 4.4 oz. 297

   large, hot slice, 1/8 pie, 5.5 oz. 370

original combo:

   mini, 1/4 pie, 3.8 oz. 240

   small, 1/6 pie, 5.6 oz. 360

   medium, 1/8 pie, 6.2 oz. 400

   large, 1/10 pie, 6.8 oz. 437

   large, hot slice, 1/8 pie, 8.5 oz. 550

thin crust cheese:

   small, 1/6 pie, 2.6 oz. 180

   medium, 1/8 pie, 3 oz. 210

   large, 1/10 pie, 3.4 oz. 228

thin crust combo:

   small, 1/6 pie, 4.3 oz. 270

   medium, 1/8 pie, 4.9 oz. 310

   large, 1/10 pie, 5.4 oz. 336

stuffed cheese:

   small, 1/6 pie, 4.4 oz. 310

   medium, 1/8 pie, 4.8 oz. 350

   large, 1/10 pie, 5.2 oz. 381

stuffed combo:

   small, 1/6 pie, 6.3 oz. 430

   medium, 1/8 pie, 7 oz. 480

   large, 1/10 pie, 7.6 oz. 521

HARDEE'S

                                                 calories

Big Country Breakfast:

   bacon, 7.7 oz. 660

   country ham, 9 oz. 670

   ham, 8.9 oz. 620

   sausage, 9.7 oz. 850

biscuit:

   bacon, 3.3 oz. 360

   bacon and egg, 4.4 oz. 410

   bacon, egg, and cheese, 4.8 oz. 460

   Biscuit 'N' Gravy, 7.8 oz. 440

   Canadian Rise 'N' Shine, 5.7 oz. 470

chicken, 5.1 oz.	430
Cinnamon 'N' Raisin, 2.8 oz.	320
country ham, 3.8 oz.	350
country ham and egg, 4.9 oz.	400
ham, 3.7 oz.	320
ham and egg, 4.9 oz.	370
ham, egg, and cheese, 5.3 oz.	420
Rise 'N' Shine, 2.9 oz.	320
sausage, 4.2 oz.	440
sausage and egg, 5.3 oz.	490
steak, 5.2 oz.	500
steak and egg, 6.3 oz.	550
Hash Rounds, 2.8 oz.	230
margarine/butter blend, .2 oz.	35
pancake syrup, 1.5 oz.	120

pancakes, 3 pieces:

4.8 oz.	280
w/2 bacon strips, 5.3 oz.	350
w/1 sausage patty, 6.2 oz.	430

sandwiches:

Big Deluxe burger, 7.6 oz.	500
Big Roast Beef, 4.7 oz.	300
Big Twin, 6.1 oz.	450
cheeseburger, 4.3 oz.	320
cheeseburger, bacon, 7.7 oz.	610
cheeseburger, quarter pound, 6.4 oz.	500
chicken breast, grilled, 6.8 oz.	310
Chicken Fillet, 6.1 oz.	370
Fisherman's Fillet, 7.3 oz.	500
hamburger, 3.9 oz.	270
hot dog, all beef, 4.2 oz.	300
Hot Ham 'N' Cheese, 5.3 oz.	330
Mushroom 'N' Swiss burger, 6.6 oz.	490
roast beef, regular, 4 oz.	260
Turkey Club, 7.3 oz.	390

salads, side dishes and special items:

Chicken Stix, 9 pieces, 5.3 oz.	310
Chicken Stix, 6 pieces, 3.5 oz.	210
Crispy Curls, 3 oz.	300
fries, big, 5.5 oz.	500
fries, large, 4 oz.	360

Hardee's, salads, side dishes and special items, continued

fries, regular, 2.5 oz.	230
salad, chef, 10.4 oz.	240
salad, chicken 'n' pasta, 14.6 oz.	230
salad, garden, 8.5 oz.	210
salad, side, 4 oz.	20

salad dressings, 2 oz.:

blue cheese	210
French, reduced calorie	130
house	290
Italian	90
Thousand Island	250

sauces and condiments:

barbecue dipping sauce, 1 oz.	30
barbecue sauce, .5-oz. pkt.	14
Big Twin sauce, .5 oz.	50
catsup, .5 oz.	14
catsup, .4-oz. pkt.	12
honey sauce, .5 oz.	45
horseradish, .25-oz. pkt.	25
mayonnaise, .5 oz.	50
mustard, .3-oz. pkt.	6
sweet mustard dipping sauce, 1 oz.	50
sweet 'n' sour dipping sauce, 1 oz.	40
tartar sauce, .7 oz.	90

desserts and shakes:

apple turnover, 3.2 oz.	270
Big Cookie, 1.7 oz.	250
Cool Twist cone, chocolate, 4.2 oz.	200
Cool Twist cone, vanilla or vanilla/chocolate, 4.2 oz.	190
Cool Twist sundae, caramel, 6 oz.	330
Cool Twist sundae, hot fudge, 5.9 oz.	320
Cool Twist sundae, strawberry, 5.9 oz.	260
shake, chocolate, 12 oz.	460
shake, strawberry, 12 oz.	440
shake, vanilla, 12 oz.	400

JACK-IN-THE-BOX

calories

breakfast crescent:
  Canadian, 4.7 oz. 452
  sausage, 5.5 oz. 584
  supreme, 5.1 oz. 547
Breakfast Jack, 4.4 oz. 307
hash browns, 2.2 oz. 116
jelly, grape, .5 oz. 38
pancake platter, 8.1 oz. 612
scrambled egg platter, 8.8 oz. 662
sandwiches:
  bacon cheeseburger, 8.1 oz. 705
  beef fajita pita, 6.2 oz. 333
  cheeseburger, 4 oz. 315
  cheeseburger, double, 5.3 oz. 467
  cheeseburger, ultimate, 10 oz. 942
  chicken fajita pita, 6.7 oz. 292
  chicken fillet, grilled, 7.2 oz. 408
  chicken supreme, 8.1 oz. 575
  fish supreme, 8 oz. 554
  hamburger, 3.4 oz. 267
  Jumbo Jack, 7.8 oz. 584
  Jumbo Jack, w/cheese, 8.5 oz. 677
  Swiss and bacon burger, 6.6 oz. 678
Mexican food:
  guacamole, 1 oz. 55
  salsa, 1 oz. 8
  taco, 2.9 oz. 191
  taco, super, 4.8 oz. 288
salads:
  chef, 14 oz. 295
  Mexican chicken, 14.6 oz. 442
  side, 4 oz. 51
  taco, 14.2 oz. 503
finger foods:
  chicken strips, 4 pieces, 4.4 oz. 349
  chicken strips, 6 pieces, 6.6 oz. 523
  egg rolls, 3 pieces, 6 oz. 405
  egg rolls, 5 pieces, 10 oz. 675

Jack-In-The-Box, finger foods, continued

shrimp, 10 pieces, 3 oz.	270
shrimp, 15 pieces, 4.4 oz.	404
taquitos, 5 pieces, 5 oz.	363
taquitos, 7 pieces, 7 oz.	508

side dishes:

fries, small, 2.4 oz.	221
fries, regular, 3.9 oz.	353
fries, jumbo, 4.8 oz.	442
onion rings, 3.8 oz.	382

dressings and sauces:

BBQ sauce, 1 oz.	44
bleu cheese dressing, 2.5 oz.	262
buttermilk dressing, 2.5 oz.	362
mayo-mustard sauce, .7 oz.	124
mayo-onion sauce, .7 oz.	143
French dressing, reduced calorie, 2.5 oz.	176
seafood cocktail sauce, 1 oz.	32
sweet and sour sauce, 1 oz.	40
Thousand Island dressing, 2.5 oz.	312

desserts and shakes:

apple turnover, 4.2 oz.	410
cheesecake, 3.5 oz.	309
shake, chocolate, 11.4 oz.	330
shake, strawberry, 11.6 oz.	320
shake, vanilla, 11.2 oz.	320

KENTUCKY FRIED CHICKEN

	calories
chicken, *Original Recipe:*	
breast, center, 4.1 oz.	283
breast, side, 3.2 oz.	267
drumstick, 2 oz.	146
thigh, 3.7 oz.	294
wing, 1.9 oz.	178
chicken, *Extra Tasty Crispy:*	
breast, center, 4.8 oz.	342
breast, side, 3.9 oz.	343
drumstick, 2.4 oz.	204

thigh, 4.2 oz.	406
wing, 2.3 oz.	254
chicken, *Kentucky Nuggets*, .6-oz. piece	46

Kentucky Nuggets sauces:
barbeque, 1 oz.	35
honey, .5 oz.	49
mustard, 1 oz.	36
sweet and sour, 1 oz.	58

chicken, *Lite N' Crispy:*
breast, center	220
breast, side	204
drumstick	121
thigh	246
hot wings, six pieces	376

side dishes:
buttermilk biscuit, 2.3 oz.	235
Chicken Littles sandwich, 1.7 oz.	169
coleslaw, 3.2 oz.	119
Colonel's chicken sandwich, 5.9 oz.	482
corn-on-the-cob, 5 oz.	176
french fries, regular, 2.7 oz.	244
mashed potatoes and gravy, 3.5 oz.	71

LITTLE CAESARS

	calories

Little Caesars Meals:
cheese pizza and tossed salad	600
pizza w/green peppers, onions, mushrooms, and tossed salad	640

pizza, single slice:
cheese, 2.2 oz.	170
pepperoni, green peppers, onions, mushrooms, 2.7 oz.	190

sandwiches:
ham and cheese	520
Italian sub	590
tuna melt	700
vegetarian	620

Little Caesars, continued

salads, w/low-calorie dressing:

antipasto salad, 12 oz.	170
Greek salad, 11 oz.	140
tossed salad, 11 oz.	8

McDONALD'S

	calories
biscuit:	
w/bacon, egg, and cheese, 5.5 oz.	440
w/biscuit spread, 2.6 oz.	260
w/sausage, 4.3 oz.	440
w/sausage and egg, 6.3 oz.	520
danish:	
apple, 4.1 oz.	390
cinnamon raisin, 3.9 oz.	440
iced cheese, 3.9 oz.	390
raspberry, 4.1 oz.	410
eggs, scrambled, 3.5 oz.	140
hash brown potatoes, 1.9 oz.	130
hotcakes, w/butter and syrup, 6.2 oz.	410
muffins:	
apple bran, 3 oz.	190
Egg McMuffin, 4.9 oz.	290
English, w/butter, 2.1 oz.	170
English, w/out butter	140
Sausage McMuffin, 4.1 oz.	370
Sausage McMuffin w/egg, 5.9 oz.	440
sausage, pork, 1.7 oz.	180
sandwiches and chicken:	
Big Mac, 7.6 oz.	560
cheeseburger, 4.1 oz.	310
Chicken McNuggets, 4 oz.	290
Filet-O-Fish, 5 oz.	440
hamburger, 3.6 oz.	260
McChicken, 6.7 oz.	490
McD.L.T., 8.3 oz.	580
McLean Deluxe, 7.3 oz.	320
McLean Deluxe, w/cheese, 7.7 oz.	370

Quarter Pounder, 5.9 oz. 410
Quarter Pounder, w/cheese, 6.8 oz. 520
Chicken *McNuggets* sauces:
    barbeque, 1 oz. 50
    honey, 1.5 oz. 45
    hot mustard, 1 oz. 70
    sweet and sour, 1 oz. 60
french fries:
    small, 2.4 oz. 220
    medium, 3.4 oz. 320
    large, 4.3 oz. 400
salads:
    chef, 10 oz. 230
    chunky chicken, 8.8 oz. 140
    garden, 7.5 oz. 110
    side salad, 4.1 oz. 60
dressings and condiments:
    bacon bits, .1 oz. 16
    bleu cheese dressing, 1/5 pkt. 70
    croutons, .4 oz. 50
    French dressing, red, reduced calorie, 1/4 pkt. 40
    peppercorn dressing, 1/5 pkt. 80
    Thousand Island dressing, 1/5 pkt. 78
    vinaigrette dressing, lite, 1/4 pkt. 15
desserts and shakes:
    apple pie, 2.9 oz. 260
    cookies, chocolaty chip, 2.3 oz. 330
    cookies, *McDonaldland,* 2.3 oz. 290
    milk shake, lowfat, chocolate or strawberry, 10.3 oz. 320
    milk shake, lowfat, vanilla, 10.3 oz. 290
    yogurt, frozen, cone, vanilla, 3 oz. 100
    yogurt frozen, sundae, hot caramel, 6.1 oz. 270
    yogurt frozen, sundae, hot fudge, 6 oz. 240
    yogurt, frozen, sundae, strawberry, 6 oz. 210

PIZZA HUT

calories

hand-tossed, 2 slices of medium pie:
    cheese, 7.8 oz. 518

Pizza Hut, hand-tossed, 2 slices of medium pie, continued

pepperoni, 6.9 oz.	500
supreme, 8.4 oz.	540
super supreme, 8.6 oz.	463

pan pizza, 2 slices of medium pie:

cheese, 7.2 oz.	492
pepperoni, 7.4 oz.	540
supreme, 9 oz.	589
super supreme, 9.1 oz.	563

Personal Pan Pizza, 1 whole pie:

pepperoni, 9 oz.	675
supreme, 9.3 oz.	647

Thin 'n Crispy, 2 slices of medium pie:

cheese, 5.2 oz.	398
pepperoni, 5.1 oz.	413
supreme, 7.1 oz.	459
super supreme, 7.2 oz.	463

PONDEROSA

	calories
chicken breast, 5.5 oz.	98
chicken wings, 2 pieces	213

fish, baked:

bake 'r broil, 5.2 oz.	230
baked scrod, 7 oz.	120

fish, broiled:

halibut, 6 oz.	170
roughy, 5 oz.	138
salmon, 6 oz.	192
swordfish, 5.9 oz.	271
trout, 5 oz.	228
fish, fried, 3.2 oz.	190
fish nuggets, 1 piece	31
hot dog, 1.6 oz.	144
shrimp, fried, 7 pieces	231
shrimp, mini, 6 pieces	47

steak, precooked weight:

chopped, 4 oz.	225
chopped, 5.3 oz.	296

Kansas City Strip, 5 oz.	138
New York Strip, choice, 8 oz.	314
New York Strip, choice, 10 oz.	384
porterhouse, choice, 16 oz.	640
ribeye, choice, 6 oz.	282
ribeye, non-graded, 5 oz.	219
sirloin, choice, 7 oz.	241
sirloin tips, choice, 5 oz.	473
T-bone, choice, 10 oz.	444
T-bone, non-graded, 8 oz.	178
teriyaki, 5 oz.	174
steak kabobs, meat only, 3 oz. precooked	153
steak sandwich, 4 oz.	408
side dishes, sauces and condiments:	
BBQ sauce, 1 tbsp.	25
beans, baked, 4 oz.	170
beans, green, 3.5 oz.	20
cauliflower, breaded, 4 oz.	115
carrots, 3.5 oz.	31
cheese, herb, garlic spread, 1 tbsp.	100
cheese sauce, 2 oz.	52
corn, 3.5 oz.	90
gravy, brown or turkey, 2 oz.	25
macaroni and cheese, 1 oz.	17
margarine, liquid, 1 tbsp.	100
margarine, whipped, 1 tbsp.	34
okra, breaded, 4 oz.	124
onion rings, breaded, 4 oz.	213
peas, 3.5 oz.	67
potatoes, baked, 7.2 oz.	145
potatoes, french fried, 3 oz.	120
potatoes, mashed, 4 oz.	62
potato wedges, 3.5 oz.	130
rice pilaf, 4 oz.	160
rolls, dinner, 1 piece	184
rolls, sourdough, 1 piece	110
salad oil, 1 tbsp.	120
shells, pasta, 2 oz.	78
shortening, liquid, 1 oz.	249
sour cream, 1 tbsp.	26
spaghetti, 2 oz.	78

Ponderosa, side dishes, sauces and condiments, continued

spaghetti sauce, 4 oz.	110
stuffing, 4 oz.	230
sweet and sour sauce, 1 oz.	37
tortilla chips, 1 oz.	150
winter mix, 3.5 oz.	25
zucchini, breaded, 4 oz.	102

desserts:

banana pudding, 1 oz.	52
ice milk, chocolate, 3.5 oz.	152
ice milk, vanilla, 3.5 oz.	150
mousse, chocolate, 1 oz.	78
mousse, strawberry, 1 oz.	74
sprinkles, chocolate or rainbow, .18 oz.	24
strawberry glaze, 1 oz.	37

toppings:

caramel, 1 oz.	100
chocolate, 1 oz.	89
strawberry, 1 oz.	71
whipped, 1 oz.	80
wafer, vanilla, 2 cookies	35

QUINCY'S

	calories
catfish filets, 2 pieces, 6.9 oz.	309
chicken breast, grilled, 5 oz.	145
chicken strips, 4 pieces, 4.5 oz.	318
hamburger, 1/4 lb., 6.7 oz.	403
hamburger, 1/4 lb., w/cheese, 7.2 oz.	451
shrimp, 7 pieces, 3.9 oz.	248

steak:

chopped, 5.8 oz.	466
chopped, luncheon, 4 oz.	350
country style, w/mushroom sauce, 6 oz.	288
filet, 5.6 oz.	331
ribeye, 7.3 oz.	665
sirloin, 5.9 oz.	649
sirloin, large, 7.7 oz.	852
sirloin, petite, 4 oz.	446

```
  sirloin club, 4.8 oz. . . . . . . . . . . . . . . . . . . . . .        283
  sirloin tips, 4 oz. . . . . . . . . . . . . . . . . . . . . . .        236
  T-Bone, 7.8 oz. . . . . . . . . . . . . . . . . . . . . . .        1,045
side dishes:
  beans, green, 4.3 oz. . . . . . . . . . . . . . . . . . . .         40
  coleslaw, 2.1 oz. . . . . . . . . . . . . . . . . . . . . . .         60
  cornbread, 1.9 oz. . . . . . . . . . . . . . . . . . . . . .        178
  margarine, 1 oz. . . . . . . . . . . . . . . . . . . . . . .        204
  mushroom sauce, 3 oz. . . . . . . . . . . . . . . . . . .         27
  peppers and onions, 4 oz. . . . . . . . . . . . . . . . .         80
  potato, baked, w/out butter, 8.8 oz. . . . . . . . . . . .        181
  steak fries, 5.5 oz. . . . . . . . . . . . . . . . . . . . . .        426
soups:
  broccoli, cream of, 9.2 oz. . . . . . . . . . . . . . . . .        193
  chili, w/beans, 9.2 oz. . . . . . . . . . . . . . . . . . . .        346
  clam chowder, 9.2 oz. . . . . . . . . . . . . . . . . . . .        198
  vegetable beef, 8.6 oz. . . . . . . . . . . . . . . . . . .         78
```

RAX

calories

```
sandwiches:
  BBC (beef, bacon and cheddar), 8 oz. . . . . . . . . . . .        720
  BBQ, 5.7 oz. . . . . . . . . . . . . . . . . . . . . . . . . .        420
  fish, 7 oz. . . . . . . . . . . . . . . . . . . . . . . . . . . .        460
  ham and Swiss, 7.9 oz. . . . . . . . . . . . . . . . . . .        430
  Philly beef and cheese, 8.25 oz. . . . . . . . . . . . . .        480
  roast beef, large, 8 oz. . . . . . . . . . . . . . . . . . .        570
  roast beef, regular, 5.25 oz. . . . . . . . . . . . . . . .        320
  roast beef, small (Uncle Al), 3.1 oz. . . . . . . . . . . .        260
  turkey bacon club, 9 oz. . . . . . . . . . . . . . . . . . .        670
sandwich condiments and ingredients:
  American cheese slices, .5 oz. . . . . . . . . . . . . . . .         60
  bacon, .5-oz. slice . . . . . . . . . . . . . . . . . . . . . .         80
  BBC sauce, .75 oz. . . . . . . . . . . . . . . . . . . . . .        140
  BBQ sauce, regular or smoky, 1 oz. . . . . . . . . . . .         40
  BBQ meat topping, 3.25 oz. . . . . . . . . . . . . . . . .        140
  bun, hoagie, 6", 3 oz. . . . . . . . . . . . . . . . . . . .        280
  bun, kaiser, 4", 2.25 oz. . . . . . . . . . . . . . . . . . .        180
  bun, small, 1.7 oz. . . . . . . . . . . . . . . . . . . . . . .        180
```

Rax, sandwich condiments and ingredients, continued

catsup, 1 tbsp.	6
fish, 3.5 oz.	230
ham, 2.5 oz.	70
horseradish sauce, .75 oz.	10
lettuce, shredded, ¼ cup	2
mayonnaise, .75 oz.	150
Philly vegetables, 2 oz.	30
pickle, 2.3-oz. spear	8
roast beef, 2.8 oz.	140
Swiss cheese slices, .5 oz.	30
tartar sauce, .5 oz.	50
tomatoes, .5-oz. slice	2
turkey, 2.5 oz.	80
french fries, large, 4.5 oz.	390
french fries, regular, 3 oz.	260
potatoes:	
plain, 8.8 oz.	270
plain, w/margarine, 9.3 oz.	370
BBQ, w/cheese (2 oz.), 14.3 oz.	730
cheese (3 oz.) and bacon, 12.8 oz.	780
cheese (3 oz.) and broccoli, 13.8 oz.	760
chili and cheese (2 oz.), 14.3 oz.	700
potato topping ingredients:	
bacon bits, .5 oz.	40
BBQ meat sauce, 2.5 oz.	110
broccoli, 1.5 oz.	16
cheese sauce, 3 oz.	370
chili, 3 oz.	80
liquid margarine, 1 tbsp.	100
onion, diced, .5 oz.	10
sour topping, 3.5 oz.	130
drive-thru salad, w/out dressing:	
chef salad, 12.5 oz.	230
garden salad, 10.5 oz.	160
dressings, 1 tbsp.:	
blue cheese	50
blue cheese "lite"	35
French	60
French "lite"	40
Italian	50

Italian "lite" 30
oil 130
poppy seed 60
ranch 45
Thousand Island 70
Thousand Island "lite" 40
vinegar 2

Mexican bar:
  banana pepper rings, 1 tbsp. 2
  cheese sauce, 3.5 oz. 420
  cheese sauce, nacho, 3.5 oz. 470
  green onions, 1/4 cup 10
  jalapeño peppers, 1 oz. 6
  olives, 3.5 oz. 110
  refried beans, 3 oz. 120
  sour topping, 3.5 oz. 130
  Spanish rice, 3.5 oz. 90
  spicy meat sauce, 3.5 oz. 80
  taco sauce, 3.5 oz. 30
  taco shells, 1 piece 40
  tomatoes, 1 oz. 6
  tortilla, 1 piece 110
  tortilla chips, 1 oz. 140

pasta bar:
  Alfredo sauce, 3.5 oz. 80
  chicken noodle soup, 3.5 oz. 40
  creme of broccoli soup, 3.5 oz. 50
  Parmesan cheese substitute, 1 oz. 80
  pasta shells, 3.5 oz. 170
  pasta/vegetable blend, 3.5 oz. 100
  rainbow rotini, 3.5 oz. 180
  spaghetti, 3.5 oz. 140
  spaghetti sauce, 3.5 oz. 80
  spaghetti sauce, w/meat, 3.5 oz. 150

desserts:
  chocolate chip cookie, 1 piece 130
  milkshake*, chocolate or strawberry 560
  milkshake*, vanilla 500

Rax, desserts, continued
   whipped topping, 1 dollop   50
hot cocoa mix, 6 fl. oz. 110

* *Without whipped topping*

ROY ROGERS

	calories
breakfast pastry:	
apple swirls	328
cheese swirls	383
cinnamon roll	376
crescent roll	287
crescent sandwich:	
regular	408
w/bacon	446
w/ham	456
w/sausage	564
egg and biscuit platter:	
regular	557
w/bacon	607
w/ham	605
w/sausage	713
pancake platter w/syrup and butter:	
regular	386
w/bacon	436
w/ham	434
w/sausage	542
chicken, fried:	
breast	412
breast and wing	604
leg (drumstick)	140
leg and thigh	436
nuggets, 6 pieces	288
thigh	296
wing	192
sandwiches:	
bacon cheeseburger	552
bar burger	573

cheeseburger	525
cheeseburger, small	275
Express burger	561
Express bacon cheeseburger	641
Express cheeseburger	613
fish sandwich	514
hamburger	472
hamburger, small	222
roast beef, regular	350
roast beef, w/cheese	403
roast beef, large	373
roast beef, large, w/cheese	427

side dishes:

biscuit	231
coleslaw	110
fries, 4 oz.	320
fries, small, 3 oz.	238
fries, large, 5.5 oz.	440

salad dressings, 2 tbsp.:

bacon 'n tomato	136
blue cheese	150
Italian, lo-cal	70
Ranch	155
Thousand Island	160

desserts and shakes:

shake, chocolate	358
shake, strawberry	315
shake, vanilla	306
sundae, caramel	293
sundae, hot fudge	337
sundae, strawberry	216
Vitari, 1 oz.	30

7-ELEVEN

	calories
Big Bite (2-oz. beef weiner), 3.4 oz.	287
Big Bite, super (4-oz. beef weiner), 5.4 oz.	460
burritos:	
bean and cheese, 10 oz.	616

7-Eleven, burritos, continued

beef and bean, 5 oz.	308
beef and bean, green chili, 10 oz.	617
beef and bean, red chili, 5 oz.	308
beef and bean, red hot, 5 oz.	310
beef and bean, red hot, 10 oz.	620
beef and bean, red hot, premium, 5.2 oz.	359
beef, bean and cheese, 5.2 oz.	395
beef and potato, 5.2 oz.	394
chicken and rice, premium, 5 oz.	244
chicken, breast of, 4.8 oz.	405
chimichanga, beef, 5 oz.	363
enchilada, beef and cheese, 6.5 oz.	369
fajitas, 5 oz.	311
sandito, ham and cheese, 5 oz.	347
sandito, pizza, 5 oz.	345
tacos, soft, twin, 5.9 oz.	399
Deli-Shoppe microwave products:	
bacon cheeseburger, 6 oz.	558
bagel and cream cheese, 4 oz.	338
char sandwich, large, 8.4 oz.	713
fish sandwich, w/cheese, 5.2 oz.	433
sausage, red hot, large, 9.3 oz.	845
turkey, wedge, 3.4 oz.	193

SHAKEY'S

	calories
chicken, fried (3 pieces), and potatoes	947
chicken, fried (5 pieces), and potatoes	1,700
Hot Ham and Cheese	550
pizza, *Homestyle Pan Crust,* 1/10 of 12" pie:	
cheese only	303
onion, green pepper, black olives, mushrooms	320
pepperoni	343
sausage, mushroom	343
sausage, pepperoni	374
Shakey's Special	384
pizza, thick crust, 1/10 of 12" pie:	
cheese only	170

green pepper, black olives, mushrooms   162
pepperoni   185
sausage, mushrooms   179
sausage, pepperoni   177
Shakey's Special   208
pizza, thin crust, 1/10 of 12″ pie:
cheese only   133
onion, green pepper, black olives, mushrooms   125
pepperoni   148
sausage, mushrooms   141
sausage, pepperoni   166
Shakey's Special   171
potatoes, 15 pieces   950
Shakey's Super Hot Hero   810
spaghetti, w/meat sauce and garlic bread   940

SKIPPER'S

calories

thick cut cod:
3 piece, fries   665
4 piece, fries   759
5 piece, fries   853
famous fish fillets:
1 fish, fries   558
2 fish, fries   733
3 fish, fries   908
seafood combos:
jumbo shrimp, 1 fish, fries   720
original shrimp, 1 fish, fries   728
clam strips, 1 fish, fries   868
oysters, 1 fish, fries   885
seafood baskets:
jumbo shrimp, fries   707
original shrimp, fries   723
clam strips, fries   1,003
oysters, fries   1,038
Skipper's Platter, fries   1,038
chicken tenderloin strips:
5 piece, fries   793

Skipper's, chicken tenderloin strips, continued

   3 piece, 1 fish, fries 805

   3 piece, original shrimp, fries 800

salads & lite catch:

   2 fish, small green salad 409

   3 chicken, small green salad 305

   1 fish, 2 chicken, small green salad 399

   small green salad 59

   shrimp and seafood salad 167

Create A Catch:

   fish sandwich 524

   double fish sandwich 698

   chicken sandwich 606

   chicken strip 82

   fish fillet 175

   fries 383

   clam chowder cup 100

   clam chowder pint 200

   coleslaw, 5 oz. 289

condiments, 1 tbsp.:

   barbeque sauce 25

   cocktail sauce 20

   tartar sauce 65

salad dressing, 1 pouch:

   premium blue cheese 222

   gourmet Italian 140

   lo-cal Italian 17

   ranch house 188

   1000 Island 160

root beer float 302

TACO BELL

                                                         calories

burrito:

   bean, red sauce, 7.3 oz. 447

   beef, red sauce, 7.3 oz. 493

   chicken, 6 oz. 334

   combination, red sauce, 7 oz. 407

   Supreme, red sauce, 9 oz. 503

cinnamon twist, 1.2 oz.   171
Enchirito, red sauce, 7.5 oz.   382
Meximelt, 3.7 oz.   266
Meximelt, chicken, 3.8 oz.   257
nachos:
   3.7 oz.   346
   BellGrande, 10.1 oz.   649
   Supreme, 5.1 oz.   367
pintos 'N cheese, red sauce, 4.5 oz.   190
pizza, Mexican, 7.9 oz.   575
taco:
   2.75 oz.   183
   Bellgrande, 5.7 oz.   335
   chicken, 3 oz.   171
   soft, 3.25 oz.   225
   soft, chicken, 3.8 oz.   213
   soft, steak, 3.5 oz.   218
   soft, *Supreme,* 4.4 oz.   272
   Supreme, 3.25 oz.   230
taco salad, 21 oz.   905
taco salad, w/out shell, 18.3 oz.   484
tostada, red sauce, 5.5 oz.   243
tostada, chicken, red sauce, 5.8 oz.   264
side orders and condiments:
   green sauce, 1 oz.   4
   guacamole, .7 oz.   34
   jalapeño peppers, 3.5 oz.   20
   nacho cheese, 2 oz.   103
   Pico De Gallo, .7 oz.   6
   ranch dressing, 2.6 oz.   236
   red sauce, 1 oz.   10
   salsa, .35 oz.   18
   sour cream, .7 oz.   46
   taco sauce, 1 pkt.   2
   taco sauce, hot, 1 pkt.   3

TACO JOHN'S

	calories
apple grande, 3 oz.	257
beans, refried, 9.5 oz.	331
burrito:	
bean, 5 oz.	249
beef, 5 oz.	355
combo, 5 oz.	302
smothered, w/green chili, 12.3 oz.	405
smothered, w/Texas chili, 12.3 oz.	518
super, 8.3 oz.	434
chili, Texas, 9.5 oz.	430
chimi, 12 oz.	487
churro, 1.2 oz.	122
enchilada, 7 oz.	379
nachos, 4 oz.	407
nachos, super, 11.25 oz.	657
Potato Ole Large, 6 oz.	414
taco:	
Bravo, super, 8 oz.	485
burger, 6 oz.	332
regular, 4.3 oz.	228
soft shell, 5 oz.	276
taco salad, super, 12.3 oz.	450
tostada, 4.3 oz.	228

WENDY'S

	calories
sandwiches:	
bacon cheeseburger, Jr., 5.5 oz.	430
Big Classic, 9.2 oz.	570
cheeseburger, Kid's Meal, 4.1 oz.	300
cheeseburger, Jr., 4.4 oz.	310
chicken club, 7.2 oz.	506
chicken sandwich, 6.9 oz.	440
chicken sandwich, grilled, 6.2 oz.	340
fish fillet sandwich, 6 oz.	460
hamburger, patty, 1/4 lb.	180

hamburger, Jr., 3.9 oz.	260
hamburger, Kid's Meal, 3.7 oz.	260
hamburger, plain, single, 4.4 oz.	340
hamburger, single, w/everything, 7.4 oz.	420
steak sandwich, country fried, 5.1 oz.	440
Swiss Deluxe, Jr., 5.8 oz.	360
chicken breast fillet, 3.5 oz.	220
chicken fillet, grilled, 2.5 oz.	100
chicken nuggets, crispy, 6 pieces	280
chili, regular, 9 oz.	220
baked potato, hot stuffed:	
plain, 8.8 oz.	250
bacon and cheese, 12.3 oz.	570
broccoli and cheese, 13 oz.	500
cheese, 12.3 oz.	590
chili and cheese, 14.1 oz.	510
sour cream and chives, 11 oz.	460
salads and side dishes:	
chef salad, take out, 9.1 oz.	130
french fries, small, 3.2 oz.	240
garden salad, take out, 8.1 oz.	70
taco salad, 17.3 oz.	530
salad dressings and sauces, 1 tbsp., except as noted:	
bacon and tomato, reduced calorie	45
barbecue nuggets sauce, 1 oz.	50
blue cheese	90
celery seed	70
French	60
French, sweet red	70
Hidden Valley Ranch	50
honey nuggets sauce, .5 oz.	45
Italian Caesar	80
Italian, golden	45
Italian, reduced calorie	25
mustard, sweet, nuggets sauce, 1 oz.	50
sweet and sour nuggets sauce, 1 oz.	45
Thousand Island	70
desserts:	
frosty, dairy, small, 8.6 oz.	340
pudding, butterscotch or chocolate, 1/4 cup	90

WHITE CASTLE

calories

sandwiches:

cheeseburger, 2.3 oz.	200
chicken sandwich, 2.25 oz.	186
fish sandwich, w/out tartar sauce, 2.1 oz.	155
hamburger, 2.1 oz.	161
sausage sandwich, 1.7 oz.	196
sausage and egg sandwich, 3.4 oz.	322

side dishes:

french fries, 3.4 oz.	301
onion chips, 3.3 oz.	329
onion rings, 2.1 oz.	245

condiments:

bun, .9 oz.	74
cheese, .3 oz.	31

Chapter 26

SPIRITS, WINES, LIQUEURS, BEERS, AND RELATED DRINKS

DISTILLED SPIRITS*, one fluid ounce

---

	calories
80 proof	67
84 proof	70
86 proof	72
90 proof	75
94 proof	78
97 proof	81
100 proof	83
104 proof	87

* *Distilled spirits—applejack, bourbon, brandy, gin, rum, tequila, vodka; blended Canadian, Irish and rye whisky; Scotch whisky—are not listed by brand name because their calorie content is determined entirely by the amount of alcohol they contain. The higher the proof (alcoholic content), the more calories in the spirit. Different brands of liquor may not taste the same, but if they are the same proof there is no difference in their caloric content. This applies only to distilled spirits.*

COCKTAIL MIXES, NONALCOHOLIC, one fluid ounce, except as noted
See also "Soft Drinks & Mixers"

---

	calories
Bloody Mary, bottled *(Holland House* Smooth N'Spicy)	3
daiquiri:	
bottled *(Holland House)*	36
instant** *(Bar-Tender's)*, 3½ fl. oz.	177
instant *(Holland House)*, .56 oz. dry	65

Cocktail Mixes, Nonalcoholic, daiquiri, continued

raspberry, bottled *(Holland House)*	30
strawberry, bottled *(Holland House)*	31
mai tai, bottled *(Holland House)*	32
mai tai, instant *(Holland House)*, .56 oz.	64
Manhattan, bottled *(Holland House)*	28
Margarita:	
bottled *(Holland House)*	27
instant *(Holland House)*, .5 oz................	57
strawberry, bottled *(Holland House)*	31
strawberry, instant *(Holland House)*, .56 oz.	66
old fashioned, bottled *(Holland House)*	33
piña colada, bottled *(Holland House)*	33
piña colada, instant *(Holland House)*, .56 oz.	82
sweet and sour, bottled *(Holland House)*	34
Tom Collins, bottled *(Holland House)*	47
Tom Collins, instant *(Holland House)*, .56 oz........	65
whiskey sour:	
bottled* *(Holland House)*	37
instant* *(Bar-Tender's)*, 3½ fl. oz.	177
instant *(Holland House)*, .56 oz. dry	64

** *Prepared according to package directions, with liquor*

TABLE WINES, four fluid ounces
See also "Aperitif & Dessert Wines" and "Wine Coolers"

	calories
Beaujolais, *see "Burgundy, red," page 327*	
Bordeaux, red *(see also "claret," page 328)*:	
(Château La Garde)	108
(Château Olivier)	108
(Château Pontet-Canet, Crus & Fils Frères)	96
Bordeaux rouge *(Chanson Père & Fils)*	108
Bordeaux rouge *(Crus & Fils Frères)*	84
Margaux *(B & G)*	84
Medoc *(Crus & Fils Frères)*	96
St. Emilion *(B & G)*	84
St. Emilion or St. Julien *(Crus & Fils Frères)*	92

APERITIF & DESSERT WINES, two fluid ounces
See also "Table Wines" and "Wine Coolers"

	calories
Asti Spumante *(Gancia)*	84
(DuBonnet Blonde)	76
(DuBonnet Rouge)	95
Madeira:	
(Hiram Walker)	84
(Leacock)	80
(Sandeman & Co.)	84
muscatel *(Gold Seal)*	105
port:	
(Hiram Walker Porto Branco)	92
(Partners Port)	94
all varieties, domestic *(Gold Seal)*	105
ruby *(Hiram Walker)*	92
ruby, domestic *(Italian Swiss Colony* Gold Medal)	86
ruby, domestic *(Taylor)*	100
ruby, imported *(Robertson Bros. & Co.* Black Label)	92
ruby, imported *(Sandeman & Co.)*	92
tawny *(Hiram Walker)*	92
tawny, domestic *(Taylor)*	96
tawny, imported *(Sandeman & Co.)*	92
Sauternes *(B & G)*	64
Sauternes *(Chateau Voigny)*	64
sherry:	
(Hiram Walker Armada Cream)	82
domestic *(Gold Seal* Private Reserve New York State)	93
domestic *(Taylor* New York State)	88
domestic *(Taylor* New York State Cream)	100
imported *(Williams & Humbert* Dry Sack)	80
sherry, dry:	
(Hiram Walker Cocktail)	70
domestic *(Gold Seal* Private Reserve New York State Cocktail)	81
domestic *(Taylor* New York State Pale Dry Cocktail)	76
imported *(Sandeman* Cocktail)	72
vermouth, dry:	
domestic *(Lejon* Extra Dry)	68

Aperitif & Dessert Wines, vermouth, dry, continued

  domestic *(Taylor* Extra Dry)   68
  imported *(C & P* Extra Dry)   74
  imported *(Gancia* Dry)   84
  imported *(Noilly Prat* Extra Dry)   68
vermouth, sweet:
  domestic *(Lejon)*   88
  domestic *(Taylor)*   88
  imported *(C & P)*   94
  imported *(Gancia* Bianco)   88
  imported *(Gancia* Rosso)   102
  imported *(Noilly Prat)*   86
white tokay *(Taylor)*   96

WINE COOLERS, 12 fluid ounces
See also "Table Wines" and "Aperitif & Dessert Wines"

	calories
(Bartles & Jaymes Premium Original)	195
berry *(Bartles & Jaymes* Premium)	214
black cherry *(Bartles & Jaymes* Premium)	210
blush *(Bartles & Jaymes* Premium)	188
citrus *(White Mountain)*	194
cranberry *(White Mountain)*	237
crystal *(White Mountain)*	234
orange *(White Mountain)*	210
peach *(Bartles & Jaymes* Premium)	215
peach *(White Mountain)*	255
raspberry *(White Mountain)*	234
red *(Bartles & Jaymes* Premium)	216
tropical *(Bartles & Jaymes* Premium)	228

LIQUEURS & FLAVORED SPIRITS, one fluid ounce

	calories
Amaretto *(Hiram Walker)*	76
Amaretto and cognac *(Hiram Walker)*	62

anise-licorice liqueur:

anisette liqueur:

apricot liqueur:

blackberry liqueur:

brandy, flavored:

Liqueurs & Flavored Spirits, brandy, flavored, continued

ginger *(DuBouchett)*	75
ginger *(Garnier)*	74
ginger *(Hiram Walker)*	71
ginger *(Old Mr. Boston* Connoisseur 42 proof)	75
peach *(DuBouchett)*	88
(Brighton Punch)	89
butterscotch liqueur *(Hiram Walker)*	70

cherry liqueur:

(Bols)	96
(Cherry Heering)	80
(Dolfi)	87
(DuBouchett)	72
(Hiram Walker)	79
chocolate almond, Swiss *(Hiram Walker)*	91
chocolate cherry *(Hiram Walker* Cordial)	91
chocolate mint *(Hiram Walker)*	91
chocolate mint *(Vandermint)*	90

coffee liqueur:

(Coffee Southern)	85
(Kahlua)	106
(Kahlua Royale)	87
(Kahlua Stinger)	95
(Kahlua Untoasted Almond)	75
(Pusha Turkish)	100
(Tia Maria)	84
cranberry *(Hiram Walker* Cordial)	64

creme d'almond:

(Bols Creme de Noyaux)	115
(DuBouchett)	101
(Garnier Creme d'Amande)	111
(Hiram Walker Creme de Noyaux)	99
creme d'apricot *(Old Mr. Boston)*	66

creme de banana:

(Dolfi Creme de Banane)	100
(Garnier Creme de Banane)	96
(Hiram Walker)	96
(Old Mr. Boston)	66
creme de black cherry *(Old Mr. Boston)*	66
creme de blackberry *(Old Mr. Boston)*	66

Liqueurs & Flavored Spirits, continued

strawberry, wild, liqueur *(Dolfi* Fraise des Bois)	88
tangerine liqueur *(Dolfi)*	97
triple sec:	
(Bols)	113
(Dolfi)	107
(DuBouchett)	61
(Garnier)	83
(Hiram Walker)	90
(Leroux)	105
(Old Mr. Boston 60 proof)	105
(Old Mr. Boston Connoisseur 42 proof)	97
vodka, flavored:	
all varieties, except peppermint *(Old Mr. Boston)* . . .	100
peppermint *(Old Mr. Boston)*	90
yellow plum *(Dolfi* Mirabelle)	78
yellow plum *(Dolfi* Cordon d'Or Mirabelle)	83

BEER, ALE & MALT LIQUOR, 12 fluid ounces

	calories
ale *(McSorley's)*	166
ale *(Tiger Head)*	166
beer:	
(Anheuser Marzen)	168
(Beck's)	148
(Bud Light)	110
(Budweiser)	144
(Busch)	144
(Carlsberg)	149
(Carlsberg Light)	110
(Dribeck's)	94
(Knickerbocker)	140
(LA)	114
(Lite)	96
(Lite Genuine Draft)	98
(Lowenbrau Special/Special Dark)	158
(Meister Brau)	141
(Meister Brau Light)	98
(Michelob)	156

"HEALTHY WEIGHTS"
FOR MEN AND WOMEN*

Height (without shoes)	Weights in pounds (without clothing)	
	19 to 34 years	35 years and over
5'0"	97–128	108–138
5'1"	101–132	111–143
5'2"	104–137	115–148
5'3"	107–141	119–152
5'4"	111–146	122–157
5'5"	114–150	126–162
5'6"	118–155	130–167
5'7"	121–160	134–172
5'8"	125–164	138–178
5'9"	129–169	142–183
5'10"	132–174	146–188
5'11"	136–179	151–194
6'0"	140–184	155–200
6'1"	144–189	159–205
6'2"	148–195	164–210
6'3"	152–200	168–216
6'4"	156–205	173–222

*The lower weights generally apply to women, the higher to men.

Source: Report of the Dietary Guidelines Advisory Committee on the Dietary Guidelines for Americans, 1990.

HOW MANY CALORIES TO MAINTAIN YOUR DESIRABLE WEIGHT?

Desirable weight	18–35 years	35–55 years	55–75 years
WOMEN **DAILY MAINTENANCE CALORIES***			
99	1,700	1,500	1,300
110	1,850	1,650	1,400
121	2,000	1,750	1,550
128	2,100	1,900	1,600
132	2,150	1,950	1,650
143	2,300	2,050	1,800
154	2,400	2,150	1,850
165	2,550	2,300	1,950
MEN **DAILY MAINTENANCE CALORIES***			
110	2,200	1,950	1,650
121	2,400	2,150	1,850
132	2,550	2,300	1,950
143	2,700	2,400	2,050
154	2,900	2,600	2,200
165	3,100	2,800	2,400
176	3,250	2,950	2,500
187	3,300	3,100	2,600

*Based on moderate activity. If your life is very active, add calories; if you lead a sedentary life, subtract calories. Prepared by the Food and Nutrition Board of the National Academy of Sciences, National Research Council.

INDEX